W.B. SAUNDERS COMPANY
A Division of Elsevier Inc.

Elsevier, Inc., 1600 John F. Kennedy Blvd., Suite 1800, Philadelphia, PA 19103-2899

http://www.vetequine.theclinics.com

VETERINARY CLINICS OF NORTH AMERICA: Volume 22, Number 2
EQUINE PRACTICE ISSN 0749-0739
August 2006 ISBN 1-4160-3822-1
Editor: John Vassallo

Copyright © 2006 by Elsevier Inc. All rights reserved. No part of this publication may be reproduced or transmitted in any form or by any means, electronic or mechanical, including photocopy, recording, or any information retrieval system, without written permission from the Publisher.

Single photocopies of single articles may be made for personal use as allowed by national copyright laws. Permission of the publisher and payment of a fee is required for all other photocopying, including multiple or systematic copying, copying for advertising or promotional purposes, resale, and all forms of document delivery. Special rates are available for educational institutions that wish to make photocopies for non-profit educational classroom use. Permissions may be sought directly from Elsevier's Rights Department in Philadelphia, PA, USA: phone: (+1) 215 239 3804, fax: (+1) 215 239 3805, e-mail: healthpermissions@elsevier.com. Requests may also be completed on-line via the Elsevier homepage (http://www.elsevier.com/locate/permissions). In the USA, users may clear permissions and make payments through the Copyright Clearance Center, Inc., 222 Rosewood Drive, Danvers, MA 01923, USA; phone: (978) 750-8400, fax: (978) 750-4744, and in the UK through the Copyright Licensing Agency Rapid Clearance Service (CLARCS), 90 Tottenham Court Road, London WIP 0LP, UK; phone: (+44) 171 436 5931; fax: (+44) 171 436 3986. Other countries may have a local reprographic rights agency for payments.

The ideas and opinions expressed in *Veterinary Clinics of North America: Equine Practice* do not necessarily reflect those of the Publisher. The Publisher does not assume any responsibility for any injury and/or damage to persons or property arising out of or related to any use of the material contained in this periodical. The reader is advised to check the appropriate medical literature and the product information currently provided by the manufacturer of each drug to be administered to verify the dosage, the method and duration of administration, or contraindications. It is the responsibility of the treating physician or other health care professional, relying on independent experience and knowledge of the patient, to determine drug dosages and the best treatment for the patient. Mention of any product in this issue should not be construed as endorsement by the contributors, editors, or the Publisher of the product or manufacturers' claims.

Veterinary Clinics of North America: Equine Practice (ISSN 0749-0739) is published in April, August, and December by Elsevier Inc., 360 Park Avenue South, New York, NY 10010-1710. Business and Editorial Offices: 1600 John F. Kennedy Blvd., Suite 1800, Philadelphia, PA 19103-2899. Customer Service office: 6277 Sea Harbor Drive, Orlando, FL 32887-4800. Subscription prices are $150.00 per year for US individuals, $245.00 per year for US institutions, $75.00 per year for US students and residents, $175.00 per year for Canadian individuals, $300.00 per year for Canadian institutions, $190.00 per year for international individuals, $300.00 per year for international institutions and $95.00 per year for Canadian and foreign students/residents. To receive student/resident rate, orders must be accompanied by name of affiliated institution, date of term, and the *signature* of program/residency coordinator on institution letterhead. Orders will be billed at individual rate until proof of status is received. Foreign air speed delivery is included in all *Clinics* subscription prices. All prices are subject to change without notice. **POSTMASTER:** Send address changes to *Veterinary Clinics of North America: Equine Practice*, Elsevier Periodicals Customer Service, 6277 Sea Harbor Drive, Orlando, FL 32887-4800, USA; phone: 1-800-654-2452 [toll free number for US customers], or 1-407-345-4000 [customers outside US]; fax: 1-407-363-1354; e-mail: usjcs@elsevier.com

Reprints. For copies of 100 or more, of articles in this publication, please contact the Commercial Reprints Department, Elsevier Inc., 360 Park Avenue South, New York, New York 10010-1710. Tel. (212) 633-3813, fax: (212) 462-1935 email: reprints@elsevier.com.

Veterinary Clinics of North America: Equine Practice is covered in *Index Medicus*, *Excerpta Medica*, *Current Contents/Agriculture, Biology and Environmental Sciences*, and *ISI*.

Printed in the United States of America.

A. Simon Turner, BVSc, MS
CONSULTING EDITOR

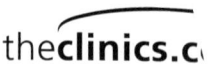

VETERINARY CLINICS OF NORTH AMERICA

Equine Practice

Advances in Diagnosis and Management of Infection

GUEST EDITOR
Louise L. Southwood, BVSc, PhD

August 2006 • Volume 22 • Number

SAUNDERS

An Imprint of Elsevier, Inc.
PHILADELPHIA LONDON TORONTO MONTREAL SYDNE

ADVANCES IN DIAGNOSIS AND MANAGEMENT OF INFECTION

CONSULTING EDITOR

A. SIMON TURNER, BVSc, MS, Diplomate, American College of Veterinary Surgeons; Professor, Department of Clinical Sciences, College of Veterinary Medicine and Biomedical Sciences, Colorado State University, Fort Collins, Colorado

GUEST EDITOR

LOUISE L. SOUTHWOOD, BVSc, PhD, Diplomate, American College of Veterinary Surgeons; Diplomate, American College of Veterinary Emergency and Critical Care; Assistant Professor, Large Animal Emergency and Critical Care, Department of Clinical Studies, New Bolton Center, University of Pennsylvania School of Veterinary Medicine, Kennett Square, Pennsylvania

CONTRIBUTORS

EMMA N. ADAM, BVetMed, Diplomate, American College of Veterinary Internal Medicine; Large Animal Surgery Resident, New Bolton Center, University of Pennsylvania School of Veterinary Medicine, Kennett Square, Pennsylvania

VALERIE A. BROWN, DVM, New Bolton Center, University of Pennsylvania School of Veterinary Medicine, Kennett Square, Pennsylvania

ANTONIO M. CRUZ, DVM, MVM, MSc, DrMedVet, Diplomate, European College of Veterinary Surgeons; Diplomate, American College of Veterinary Surgeons; Assistant Professor of Large Animal Surgery, Department of Clinical Studies, Ontario Veterinary College, University of Guelph, Guelph, Ontario, Canada

TRISHA DOWLING, DVM, MSc, PhD, Diplomate, American College of Veterinary Internal Medicine; Diplomate, American College of Veterinary Pharmacologists; Professor, Department of Veterinary Biomedical Sciences, Western College of Veterinary Medicine, University of Saskatchewan, Saskatoon, Saskatchewan, Canada

YVONNE A. ELCE, DVM, Diplomate, American College of Veterinary Surgeons; Assistant Professor of Surgery, College of Veterinary Medicine, North Carolina State University, Raleigh, North Carolina

DARIEN J. FEARY, BVSc, MS, Diplomate, American College of Veterinary Internal Medicine; Resident, Equine Emergency and Critical Care, Department of Medicine and Epidemiology, School of Veterinary Medicine, University of California-Davis, Davis, California

MELINDA A. FRYE, DVM, MS, PhD, Diplomate, American College of Veterinary Internal Medicine; Research Scholar, Department of Clinical Sciences, College of Veterinary Medicine and Biomedical Sciences, Colorado State University, Fort Collins, Colorado

EARL M. GAUGHAN, DVM, Diplomate, American College of Veterinary Surgeons; J.T. Vaughan Large Animal Hospital, Department of Clinical Sciences, College of Veterinary Medicine, Auburn University, Auburn, Alabama

MATHEW P. GERARD, BVSc, PhD, Diplomate, American College of Veterinary Surgeons; Clinical Assistant Professor, Equine Surgery, Department of Clinical Sciences, College of Veterinary Medicine, North Carolina State University, Raleigh, North Carolina

LAURIE R. GOODRICH, DVM, MS, PhD, Diplomate, American College of Veterinary Surgeons; Assistant Professor of Equine Surgery and Lameness, College of Veterinary Medicine and Biomedical Sciences, Colorado State University, Fort Collins, Colorado

DIANA M. HASSEL, DVM, PhD, Diplomate, American College of Veterinary Surgeons; Assistant Professor, Equine Emergency and Critical Care, Department of Clinical Sciences, College of Veterinary Medicine and Biological Sciences, Colorado State University, Fort Collins, Colorado

SOPHY A. JESTY, DVM, Cornell University Hospital for Animals, Ithaca, New York

ANDRÁS M. KOMÁROMY, Dr Med Vet, PhD, Diplomate, American College of Veterinary Ophthalmology; Diplomate, European College of Veterinary Ophthalmology; Assistant Professor of Ophthalmology, Department of Clinical Studies, School of Veterinary Medicine, University of Pennsylvania, Philadelphia, Pennsylvania

LEANDA C. LIVESEY, BVM&S, Cert VA, Cert EM (Int Med), MRCVS, Diplomate, American College of Veterinary Internal Medicine; Research Associate, J.T. Vaughan Teaching Hospital, College of Veterinary Medicine, Auburn University, Auburn, Alabama

KRISTINA G. LU, VMD, Hagyard Equine Medical Institute, Lexington, Kentucky

JOEL LUGO, DVM, MS, Diplomate, American College of Veterinary Surgeons; J.T. Vaughan Large Animal Hospital, Department of Clinical Sciences, College of Veterinary Medicine, Auburn University, Auburn, Alabama

PETER R. MORRESEY, BVSc, Rood and Riddle Equine Hospital, Lexington, Kentucky

ALESSANDRA PELLEGRINI-MASINI, DMV, PhD, Diplomate, American College of Veterinary Internal Medicine; Visiting Assistant Professor of Equine Medicine, Equine Section, Department of Clinical Sciences, College of Veterinary Medicine, Auburn University, Auburn, Alabama

VIRGINIA B. REEF, DVM, Diplomate, American College of Veterinary Internal Medicine; New Bolton Center, University of Pennsylvania School of Veterinary Medicine, Kennett Square, Pennsylvania

LUIS RUBIO-MARTINEZ, DVM, PhD, Resident in Large Animal Surgery, Department of Clinical Studies, Ontario Veterinary College, University of Guelph, Guelph, Ontario, Canada

ELIZABETH M. SANTSCHI, DVM, Diplomate, American College of Veterinary Surgeons; Clinical Associate Professor, Department of Surgical Sciences, School of Veterinary Medicine, University of Wisconsin, Madison, Wisconsin

LOUISE L. SOUTHWOOD, BVSc, PhD, Diplomate, American College of Veterinary Surgeons; Diplomate, American College of Veterinary Emergency and Critical Care; Assistant Professor, Large Animal Emergency and Critical Care, Department of Clinical Studies, New Bolton Center, University of Pennsylvania School of Veterinary Medicine, Kennett Square, Pennsylvania

PAMELA A. WILKINS, DVM, MS, PhD, Diplomate, American College of Veterinary Internal Medicine; Diplomate, American College of Veterinary Emergency and Critical Care; New Bolton Center, University of Pennsylvania School of Veterinary Medicine, Kennett Square, Pennsylvania

KATHRYN L. WOTMAN, DVM, Lecturer, Large Animal Internal Medicine, New Bolton Center, School of Veterinary Medicine, University of Pennsylvania School of Veterinary Medicine, Kennett Square, Pennsylvania

ADVANCES IN DIAGNOSIS AND MANAGEMENT OF INFECTION

CONTENTS

Preface xv
Louise L. Southwood

Principles of Antimicrobial Therapy: What Should We Be Using? 279
Louise L. Southwood

>Although the use of antimicrobials has had an insurmountable impact on preventing patient morbidity and mortality, problems with antimicrobial resistance and antimicrobial-induced diarrhea are becoming more apparent in human and veterinary medicine. The mortality associated with nosocomial infection with antimicrobial-resistant bacteria in human patients is alarming. Similarly, in veterinary medicine, the morbidity and high cost of treatment of patients with postoperative infection, for example, are concerns. Specifically in equine medicine, the high morbidity and mortality associated with antimicrobial-induced diarrhea have been devastating in many equine practices. Misuse of antimicrobials is extremely common in human and veterinary medicine. All clinicians have the responsibility to consider the appropriateness of their antimicrobial use carefully and, whenever possible, to minimize antimicrobial administration to patients.

New Antimicrobials, Systemic Distribution, and Local Methods of Antimicrobial Delivery in Horses 297
Antonio M. Cruz, Luis Rubio-Martinez, and Trisha Dowling

>The local delivery of antimicrobials is a valuable therapeutic tool with a low morbidity, is practical to use, and is well tolerated by horses. Clinically, its use has allowed equine practitioners to achieve better results when treating musculoskeletal infections, and it represents an extremely useful tool in the practitioner's armamentarium against these types of infections. The technique is indicated to combat orthopedic infections involving bones, joints, physes, tendon sheaths, and foot tissues. Optimal treatment must include other approaches, such as systemic antimicrobial therapy

and surgical debridement and lavage, and monitoring of the clinical progression of the patient can help to determine the ideal protocol for each patient.

Prevention of Postoperative Infections in Horses 323
Elizabeth M. Santschi

The best defense against postoperative infection is to use multiple strategies to minimize wound contamination, maintain wound tissue health, and provide rational antimicrobial strategies that do not promote the development of resistant bacteria and superinfections.

Surgical and Traumatic Wound Infections, Cellulitis, and Myositis in Horses 335
Emma N. Adam and Louise L. Southwood

Surgical site infections (SSIs) and traumatic wound management remain challenging clinical scenarios. The prevention of SSIs involves meticulous surgical technique and aftercare. Traumatic wounds require thorough evaluation to assess the involvement of synovial structures and radiographs to check for fractures. Chronic wounds can require a biopsy and histologic evaluation to obtain a diagnosis, because many underlying pathologic processes grossly appear similar but different treatment regimens are required. Early recognition and diagnosis of cellulitis and myositis enable the rapid aggressive intervention necessary for a positive outcome. Any delay in diagnosis and treatment increases the complication and mortality rates and makes these conditions difficult to treat successfully.

Septic Arthritis, Tenosynovitis, and Infections of Hoof Structures 363
Joel Lugo and Earl M. Gaughan

Infectious diseases of synovial and hoof structures in horses can be devastating to soundness and can result in life-threatening complications. Timely diagnosis and early aggressive treatment can result in successful outcomes and resumption of athletic careers; however, delays in recognition and therapy can be the most costly reasons for failure. Sterilization of affected compartments and tissues requires removal of microorganisms and compromised tissue. Debridement, lavage, and appropriate antimicrobial drug use are the most reliable avenues of treatment. Antimicrobial drugs can be administered by local, regional, and systemic routes. Lavage techniques and debridement typically require surgical manipulations.

Osteomyelitis in Horses 389
Laurie R. Goodrich

Much has been learned in the past decade about osteomyelitis. The inhibitory mechanisms of the "biofilm slime" layer that is formed by bacterial extracapsular exopolysaccharides and binds to bone, joints, and implants are now better understood than in the past. The surface colonization of bacteria that occurs within these biofilms is a biologic phenomenon that is somewhat unique to orthopedic infections. This survival strategy of bacteria is effective, and it is important for veterinarians who treat osteomyelitis to be aware of current diagnostic and therapeutic treatment modalities. The practitioner should be aware of the most common bacteria associated with osteomyelitis and the traditional treatments that are still used. Current therapeutic treatment modalities, such as antibiotic-impregnated polymethylmethacrylate, antibiotic-impregnated plaster of Paris, and regional perfusion, have become routine, however, and have been responsible for improving the prevention and outcome of osteomyelitis in the horse. It is the intent of this article to make equine veterinarians aware of current information as well as the future treatments of osteomyelitis.

Infections in the Equine Abdomen and Pelvis: Perirectal Abscesses, Umbilical Infections, and Peritonitis   419
Yvonne A. Elce

This article addresses the pathophysiology, diagnosis, management, and prognosis of several different infections within the equine abdomen and pelvic region. The latest advances in the diagnosis and treatment of perirectal abscesses, umbilical infections, and local and diffuse peritonitis are discussed. Emphasis is placed on recent advances in diagnostics and therapeutics with reference to human literature that may be useful in equine practice.

Enteritis and Colitis in Horses   437
Darien J. Feary and Diana M. Hassel

Enteritis and colitis remain challenging and life-threatening diseases despite many recent advances. Successful treatment is largely dependent on early recognition and directed therapy, which is facilitated by obtaining a complete history and physical examination. A number of new therapies and methods of monitoring critically ill patients have become integral components of treatment success. The critical monitoring of equine foals and adults continues to be an exciting and emerging field.

Septicemia and Cardiovascular Infections in Horses   481
Sophy A. Jesty and Virginia B. Reef

This article first reviews cardiovascular infections, including endocarditis, myocarditis, vasculitis, and pericarditis. It then addresses what is known at this stage about the effects of sepsis on the cardiovascular system. Some information is provided from current human literature to familiarize the reader with the diagnostics and therapeutics that may eventually be used in equine practice as well.

Pathophysiology, Diagnosis, and Management of Urinary Tract Infection in Horses 497
Melinda A. Frye

Equine urinary tract infection (UTI) most commonly occurs as a sequela to structural or functional inhibition of normal urine flow. Although it is an infrequent diagnosis in equids, the incidence of UTI in human beings is high and has inspired great investigative effort. The resultant findings with potentially broad application as well as current equine studies are reviewed here. Recent developments in the understanding of host-agent interactions and renal defense mechanisms, emerging antimicrobial resistance, and novel therapeutic alternatives to prophylactic antibiotic use are emphasized.

Reproductive Tract Infections in Horses 519
Kristina G. Lu and Peter R. Morresey

Diagnosis, treatment, and, ultimately, prevention of reproductive disease are vital components of equine veterinary medicine. A thorough understanding of anatomy and physiology is necessary to reconcile the pathologic findings of disease. Only then can a rational treatment plan be formulated. Many recent advances in knowledge about the reproductive system of multiple species have application to the mare and stallion.

Meningitis and Encephalomyelitis in Horses 553
Alessandra Pellegrini-Masini and Leanda C. Livesey

This article provides an overview of meningitis and encephalomyelitis in horses, including diagnostic tests, treatment developments, and preventative measures reported in the equine and human medical literature of the past few years.

Infections of the Head and Ocular Structures in the Horse 591
Mathew P. Gerard, Kathryn L. Wotman, and
András M. Komáromy

Infectious conditions of the equine head are commonly encountered in clinical practice. Pathogenic bacterial, viral, and fungal organisms may localize in the extensive nasal passages, paranasal sinuses, and guttural pouches, creating a range of clinical signs and conditions that can be severe enough to lead to unexpected fatality. Renewed interest in equine dentistry has led to a greater recognition of dental disease that is associated with infection. This article focuses on bacterial and fungal infections of the main anatomic regions of the equine head, where advances in diagnosis and management have been made or consolidated in recent years. It also addresses recent advances made in the area of infectious equine corneal disease, including bacterial, viral, and fungal etiologies. Recent developments in equine recurrent uveitis as it relates to infectious diseases and ocular manifestations of systemic disease are also discussed.

Advanced Techniques in the Diagnosis and Management of Infectious Pulmonary Diseases in Horses 633
Valerie A. Brown and Pamela A. Wilkins

Techniques for novel approaches to the diagnosis and management of equine pulmonary disease continue to be developed and used in clinical practice. Diagnostic techniques involving immunoassays and nucleic acid-based tests not only decrease the time in which results become available but increase the sensitivity and specificity of test results. These assays do not substitute for careful clinical evaluation but can shorten the time to a confirmed accurate diagnosis, and thus allow for early initiation of therapeutic strategies and prevention protocols. With further understanding of the molecular biology and immunology of equine pulmonary disease, diagnostic and management techniques should become further refined.

Index 653

GOAL STATEMENT

The goal of the *Veterinary Clinics of North America: Equine Practice* is to keep practicing veterinarians up to date with current clinical practice in equine medicine by providing timely articles reviewing the state of the art in equine care.

ACCREDITATION

The *Veterinary Clinics of North America: Equine Practice* offers continuing education credits, awarded by Cummings School of Veterinary Medicine at Tufts University, Office of Continuing Education.

Cummings School of Veterinary Medicine at Tufts University is a designated provider of continuing veterinary medical education. Veterinarians participating in this learning activity may earn up to 6 credits per issue up to a maximum of 18 credits per year. Credits awarded may not apply toward license renewal in all states. It is the responsibility of each participant to verify the requirements of their state licensing board.

Credit can be earned by reading the text material, taking the examination online at *http://www.theclinics.com/home/cme*, and completing the program evaluation. Following your completion of the test and program evaluation, and review of any and all incorrect answers, you may print your certificate.

TO ENROLL

To enroll in the *Veterinary Clinics of North America: Equine Practice* Continuing Veterinary Medical Education Program, call customer service at 1-800-654-2452 or sign up online at *http://www.theclinics.com/home/cme*. The CVME program is now available at a special introductory rate of $49.95 for a year's subscription.

FORTHCOMING ISSUES

December 2006
Reproduction
Elaine M. Carnevale, DVM, PhD, *Guest Editor*

April 2007
Trauma and Emergency Care
Eileen K. Sullivan, DVM, *Guest Editor*

August 2007
Evidence-Based Veterinary Medicine
David Ramey, DVM, *Guest Editor*

RECENT ISSUES

April 2006
Medical Case Management
Jennifer M. Macleay, DVM, PhD, *Guest Editor*

December 2005
Therapies for Joint Disease
Troy N. Trumble, DVM, PhD, *Guest Editor*

August 2005
Neonatal Medicine and Surgery
L. Chris Sanchez, DVM, PhD, *Guest Editor*

The Clinics are now available online!

Access your subscription at:
www.theclinics.com

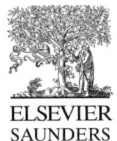

Preface

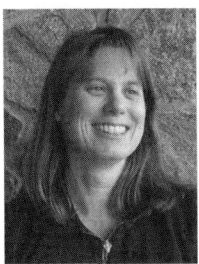

Louise L. Southwood, BVSc, PhD
Guest Editor

Infection is a common and often serious problem affecting human and veterinary patients. Despite the frequent occurrence of infection, diagnosis and treatment are a challenge in many cases. Infection can be diagnosed readily in patients with a fever, local redness, pain, heat, and swelling (color, dolor, rubor, and tumor), purulent drainage, and a positive culture. Many cases are not that straightforward, however. A recent case at our hospital exemplified the challenges with diagnosing an infection. A mature 500 kg gelding had sustained a puncture-wound kick injury to the proximal antebrachial area 7 to 10 days before presentation. The horse had been mildly lame since the injury and had become considerably lamer when the puncture wound had closed, which was the reason for referral. The horse showed signs of infection including a fever, lameness, pain on palpation, and hyperfibrinogenemia. After repeated physical examination by at least five veterinarians, hematological analysis, fibrinogen concentration monitoring, elbow joint arthrocentesis and synovial fluid analysis, numerous radiographs, and nuclear scintigraphy, it was still being debated whether the clinical signs and results of ancillary tests were associated with infection of the soft tissues of the antebrachium only and associated bone trauma as a result of the initial injury, or if the infection was in fact associated with the distal humerus and elbow joint. Similar challenges arise postoperatively in cases of suspected surgical site infection. In some cases, it is difficult to confirm the presence of osteomyelitis, peritonitis, and colitis, for example, as opposed to inflammation associated with the initial disease and surgery or an unrelated infection.

Early diagnosis and treatment are always critical for a favorable outcome. The incidence of infected synovial structures associated with a laceration, for example, has been reduced dramatically in some practices because of early recognition by referring veterinarians of synovial structure involvement, and this has led to rapid treatment and a very favorable outcome in most cases. The aim of this issue is to familiarize practitioners with the more basic and advanced diagnostic and treatment options for horses with infection so as to improve the prognosis for these patients.

Despite the emergence of new diagnostic techniques, such as scintigraphy, magnetic resonance imaging, and computerized tomography, history and physical examination are still critical for diagnosing infection. It is important that clinicians have a thorough understanding of the use and limitations of ancillary tests and interpret the results critically and in conjunction with other findings. Several articles in this issue address the use of ancillary diagnostic tests.

Morbidity and mortality associated with antimicrobial drug resistance and antimicrobial-induced diarrhea are major issues facing both medical and veterinary practitioners. Excessive antimicrobial use is common in both fields and is the major cause for antimicrobial drug resistance and antimicrobial-induced diarrhea. It should be the goal of every practitioner to critically evaluate antimicrobial-use practices and to minimize the use of antimicrobial drugs without compromising patient care. This issue provides the reader with some of the recent literature from the human and veterinary field on antimicrobial use and resistance prevention.

Last, but definitely not least, there are many people to acknowledge for their assistance and support with this issue. I would like to thank Dr. Simon Turner for the opportunity to edit this issue of *Veterinary Clinics of North America: Equine Practice*, and Mr. John Vassallo for his patience with article submission and my numerous questions. I appreciate all of the obvious effort that the authors put into writing the articles. Ms. Cindy Brockett worked tirelessly digitizing the editorial changes, communicating with the authors, proofreading the manuscripts, and checking the references for accuracy and completeness. Finally, I would like to thank my husband Eric Parente and sons Aiden and Kody for their ongoing love and support, particularly during the preparation of this issue.

Louise L. Southwood, BVSc, PhD
Department of Clinical Studies
New Bolton Center
University of Pennsylvania
382 West Street Road
Kennett Square, PA 19348, USA

E-mail address: southwoo@vet.upenn.edu

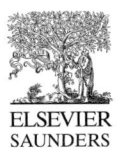

Principles of Antimicrobial Therapy: What Should We Be Using?

Louise L. Southwood, BVSc, PhD

*Department of Clinical Studies, New Bolton Center,
University of Pennsylvania, 382 West Street Road, Kennett Square, PA 19348, USA*

Antimicrobials have had an insurmountable positive impact on human and veterinary patient care. Prophylactic antimicrobial use in patients undergoing surgical procedures has reduced the incidence of postoperative infection and the associated morbidity, mortality, and high cost of treatment. Therapeutic use of antimicrobials has saved the lives of patients that would not have survived before the discovery of antimicrobials. Antimicrobials have relatively few side effects, are cost-effective to use, and are extremely effective at preventing and treating infection. Despite the undeniable benefits and convenience of antimicrobial use, there is considerable research, particularly in the human medical field, into the use and misuse of antimicrobial drugs.

Why should medical doctors and veterinarians be so concerned with antimicrobial use, and why are so much time, effort, and money being spent on investigating this particular area of medical practice? The major issue in human and veterinary medicine is the emergence of antimicrobial resistance and the serious morbidity and mortality occurring as a result of infection with a resistant microorganism. Additionally, the widespread occurrence of and high mortality associated with antimicrobial-induced diarrhea in equine patients have led equine veterinarians to reconsider antimicrobial use in this patient population.

Our goal as veterinarians should be to limit antimicrobial use without compromising our patient care. Although limiting antimicrobial use is important, an increase in surgical site infection (SSI) or distant site (respiratory or urinary tract) infection as a result of abstaining from prophylactic antimicrobial use, for example, ultimately requires more prolonged treatment with antimicrobial drugs. Guidelines for antimicrobial use in horses have

E-mail address: southwoo@vet.upenn.edu

been developed by the American Association of Equine Practitioners and endorsed by the American Veterinary Medical Association [1].

In reviewing the human literature on antimicrobial use, the focus of current clinical research is to slow the development of antimicrobial resistance by regulating and limiting antimicrobial use. Recommendations are made to accomplish these goals. Unfortunately, however, there is little experimental or clinical information in the veterinary literature from which guidelines regarding antimicrobial use can be drawn. The goal of this article is to introduce some of the current concepts on antimicrobial use in the human field and to provide points for discussion and future clinical studies on antimicrobial use in veterinary patients.

Antimicrobial prophylaxis

Postoperative infection increases patient morbidity and mortality, prolongs hospital stay, and substantially increases the cost of patient treatment. The discovery of antimicrobials and the subsequent implementation of prophylactic antimicrobial use were major milestones in the field of surgery, and "it has been suggested that antimicrobial prophylaxis has saved more lives than any other advance in surgery over the past 10 years" [2]. In human hospitals, surgical prophylaxis is one of the most frequent uses of antimicrobials and accounts for approximately half of the antimicrobials used [3]. Antimicrobial use should never replace aseptic and atraumatic surgical technique. Adherence to Halsted's principles of minimizing hemorrhage and trauma; using correct instrumentation, suture material, and implants; debriding devitalized tissue; and eradicating dead space are critical for preventing infection [4]. Although aseptic and atraumatic surgical technique is still the foundation for a successful outcome and infection prevention, the benefit of antimicrobials in preventing SSIs as well as infection at distant sites cannot be disputed. In more recent years, however, complications associated with perioperative antimicrobial use have been recognized and are becoming a major concern in human and veterinary surgery.

In 1961, Burke [5] was the first to demonstrate that antimicrobials should be administered before surgery to reduce the incidence of infection and that postoperative antimicrobial administration is ineffective. It is now common knowledge among human and veterinary surgeons that peak antimicrobial concentrations should be present during surgery to prevent infection [2]. Despite this knowledge, only 60% of human patients were administered antimicrobials before surgery (0–2 hours before the surgical incision was made) [6]. The SSI rate in patients administered preoperative antimicrobials was only 0.6%, which was significantly lower than that of patients receiving antimicrobials after surgery (more than 3 hours after the surgical incision was made: 3.3% SSI rate and 5.8 times increase in the relative risk of an SSI) or early (2–24 hours before the incision was made: 3.8% SSI rate and 6.7 times increase in the relative risk of an SSI) [6]. When preoperative orders were written or the antimicrobial was administered in the operating room, the patient was likely to receive an appropriate first prophylactic antimicrobial dose; however, when a patient had a β-lactam allergy or the surgery was performed on the day of admission, administration of an appropriate first prophylactic antimicrobial dose was less likely [7]. Antimicrobials should be administered immediately before induction of general anesthesia, and dosing should be repeated during prolonged surgical procedures to maintain adequate antimicrobial levels throughout the procedure. The challenge now is determining which patients require antimicrobials, the appropriate duration of antimicrobial use, and which antimicrobials to use.

Patients requiring prophylactic antimicrobials

Antimicrobial use should be restricted to surgical patients in which the incidence of infection exceeds 5% without prophylactic antimicrobial use [2], which generally includes patients undergoing clean-contaminated, contaminated, or dirty procedures (see article on surgical and traumatic wound infections, cellulitis, and myositis elsewhere in this issue). Antimicrobial prophylaxis can be used in patients undergoing clean procedures when the development of infection would be "devastating" and when implants are used. Prophylactic antimicrobial use is most controversial in patients undergoing clean-contaminated surgical procedures. The use of antimicrobials in patients undergoing dirty procedures becomes therapeutic rather than prophylactic, and an appropriate course of antimicrobials extending beyond the perioperative period should be prescribed. In these patients with dirty or infected wounds, antimicrobial "de-escalation" is recommended and involves initial treatment with appropriate empiric broad-spectrum antimicrobials for 24 to 48 hours only, followed immediately by narrow-spectrum antimicrobials based on culture and sensitivity test results from samples taken at surgery. This type of regimen improves individual patient care while minimizing the emergence of resistant organisms [8].

A review of patient- and surgery-related factors that predispose patients to SSIs is important in the decision as to which patients require prophylactic antimicrobials. Critically ill human patients are predisposed to developing SSIs as well as distant infections. Similarly, horses undergoing abdominal surgery on an emergency basis had a higher SSI rate (39%) compared with horses undergoing abdominal surgery on an elective basis (7%) [9]. Remote trauma and infection increased the incidence of SSI two- to threefold in human patients [10]. Geriatric human patients are predisposed to developing infection and have a threefold increase in mortality compared with younger patients with the same infection. Although the association between age and infection in veterinary patients is not as well established, older horses undergoing a celiotomy were also predisposed to developing infection compared with yearlings (43% versus 15%) [9]. Obesity is also associated with an increased risk of infection. Contamination of the wound with greater than 10^5 bacteria per gram of tissue is associated with infection, and it is important to remember that soil contains infection-potentiating factors [4]. Any foreign material decreases the inoculation dose of bacteria needed to cause infection by several fold [10]. Surgical factors that are associated with a reduction in infection rate include a decrease in the duration of surgery, patient and surgical preparation, and surgical technique [10]. Inexperienced surgeons may have an infection rate that is up to four times higher than that of more experienced surgeons [11]. In human pediatric patients, long duration of surgery, contamination at surgery, and an inexperienced surgeon as part of the surgical team predisposed patients to SSIs [12]. Interestingly, in this study, there was no association between SSIs and age, gender, American Society of Anesthesiologists preoperative assessment score, the presence of coexisting disease or remote site infection, or the use of perioperative antimicrobials [12].

Although the debate regarding the use of prophylactic antimicrobials has centered on surgical prophylaxis, there are numerous other indications. Whereas many of these indications are specific to the human field, such as partners of patients with sexually transmitted diseases and women prone to recurrent cystitis, the use of prophylactic antimicrobials in soft tissue trauma is particularly relevant to equine practice. Several studies have found no benefit to the use of prophylactic antimicrobials in human patients with simple soft tissue injuries (ie, not involving the underlying bone, joint, or body cavity) [13–15]. Meticulous surgical debridement was thought to be an important reason for the lack of difference between antimicrobial-treated and untreated groups [14]. The lack of difference in infection rates between patients treated with antimicrobial prophylaxis and those not treated may be because the duration of time after injury and wound contamination was greater than 3 hours [16]. It was proposed that soon after injury, the bacteria are enveloped in fibrin and inaccessible to antimicrobials. Therefore, antimicrobials should be administered immediately before surgical debridement [16]. The authors concluded that prolonged antimicrobial use beyond the surgical procedure is probably unnecessary [16]. Meticulous debridement is critical for a favorable outcome in patients with traumatic wounds so as to remove foreign material, nonviable tissue, and bacteria. Mizunaga and coworkers [17] showed that there was decreased bacteriocidal activity and postantibiotic effect of carbapenems and fluoroquinolones with a higher inoculum ($>10^8$ colony-forming units/mL) of *Staphylococcus aureus* and *Pseudomonas aeruginosa* compared with those with a lower inoculum.

Duration of perioperative antimicrobial use

Numerous studies have demonstrated that a single-dose prophylactic antimicrobial regimen is as effective as a multiple-dose prophylactic antimicrobial regimen [2]. Within 24 hours of a surgical procedure, the surgical site is believed to be sufficiently sealed and resistant to microorganism entry [18], and antimicrobial use beyond this time should be unnecessary. There was no difference in infection rates in human patients undergoing elective abdominal surgery (gastric, biliary, pancreatic, jejunal, ileal, or colorectal) who received a single versus triple dose of cefuroxime or cefuroxime plus metronidazole [19]. The wound infection rates were 1% (2 of 207) and 2% (5 of 221) and the deep SSI rates were 3% (6 of 207) and 4.5% (10 of 221) for patients receiving a single-dose versus triple-dose antimicrobial regimen, respectively [19]. Similarly, there was no difference in deep SSIs, length of hospital stay, duration of postoperative fever, or use of antimicrobials for postoperative infection in human patients receiving single-dose versus triple-dose antimicrobial prophylaxis with amoxicillin-clavulanic acid [20]. The infection rates were 10.7% (48 of 449) and 10.9% (49 of 451) in patients receiving a single-dose versus triple-dose antimicrobial regimen, respectively [20]. A single preoperative dose of an antimicrobial agent is recommended for obstetric and gynecologic surgical procedures as well as for major head and neck surgical procedures in human patients [21]. The use of a single dose of a long-acting antimicrobial is recommended because of the obvious longer duration of coverage after a single dose as well as the reduced drug costs and workload for personnel [2]. A single preoperative dose of ceftriaxone, a broad-spectrum cephalosporin administered every 24 hours, resulted in no difference in wound infection rate and postoperative intra-abdominal abscess formation and a lower incidence of urinary tract infections in patients undergoing abdominal surgery compared with patients administered three doses of cefazolin or cefotaxime (cephalosporin antimicrobials administered every 8 hours) [22]. Similarly, in a large meta-analysis comparing ceftriaxone with short-acting cephalosporins (cefamandole, cefazolin, cefotaxime, cefotiam, cefoxitin, or cefuroxime), there was 30% less risk of SSIs and 45% less risk of urinary tract infections in human patients administered ceftriaxone compared with the short-acting cephalosporins [23].

In a survey of American College of Veterinary Surgeons diplomates performing equine abdominal surgery, 72% to 78% of the respondents used antimicrobials for a duration of 1 to 5 days (most for 24 hours) after surgery if there was intestinal decompression only and no intestinal penetration [24]. All respondents used antimicrobials for 1 to 10 days if an enterotomy or enterectomy was performed, and 88% of respondents used antimicrobials for 1 to 10 days (most for 5 days) after surgery if there was intestinal ischemia [24]. In veterinary patients undergoing clean-contaminated or contaminated surgical procedures, such as gastrointestinal surgery, the optimal duration of antimicrobial use is unknown, particularly in critically ill patients or procedures performed on an emergency basis. It is likely, however, that prophylactic antimicrobial use beyond 24 hours is unnecessary in most patients.

Inappropriate prophylactic antimicrobial use is common in human (and veterinary) hospitals and was reported to range from 35% to 97% in various human hospitals [25–27]. There is increasing evidence that inappropriately timed or prolonged prophylactic antimicrobial use is not only ineffective but harmful to patients. In a recent study involving almost 3000 human hospitals in the United States, antimicrobials were administered within 1 hour before the surgical incision was made in only 55.7% of patients and were discontinued within 24 hours in only 40.7% of patients [25]. In another study evaluating surgical antimicrobial prophylaxis at a single human hospital, 65% of patients received inappropriate antimicrobial prophylaxis [26]. Appropriate antimicrobial prophylaxis was defined as the administration of a single dose before surgery and for up to 24 hours in high-risk patients; antimicrobials were not administered to patients undergoing clean procedures, and administration was limited to high-risk patients and patients with a prosthetic foreign body implant [26]. Prolonged duration of antimicrobial use was the most common reason for classification as "inappropriate use" and accounted for 24% of the cases classified as inappropriate antimicrobial use [26]. Inappropriate antimicrobial use was associated with a two to three times increase in the risk of nosocomial and SSI rates (11% versus 33%) [26]. Similar observations were made in canine and feline patients undergoing clean surgical procedures, where patients given antimicrobials in a manner other than the prescribed protocol had a higher infection rate compared with those patients not receiving antimicrobials (6.3% versus 4.4%) [27]. These studies emphasize the importance of appropriate antimicrobial use.

Local versus systemic antimicrobial delivery

The use of local versus systemic antimicrobials is reviewed in the article on new antimicrobials, systemic distribution, and local methods of antimicrobial delivery elsewhere in this issue. Systemic antimicrobial treatment combined with topical application of antimicrobials did not decrease the wound infection rate in human patients with peritonitis compared with patients treated with systemic antimicrobials alone. The incisional infection rate was 17% [28].

Antimicrobials to use

Perioperative antimicrobials should be selected based on the most likely organism(s) to cause an SSI. Pharmacokinetics, drug distribution, cost, and toxic side effects are all important considerations in antimicrobial selection. Bacteriocidal activity and antimicrobials with a long half-life are recommended [25]. In general, broad-spectrum antimicrobials are used prophylactically to prevent SSIs; however, the use of broad-spectrum antimicrobials increases the incidence of resistant bacteria [8]. The use of older antimicrobials is recommended, because the newer antimicrobials are used therapeutically and the routine use of these antimicrobial drugs is likely to increase the emergence of antimicrobial resistance. In human patients, vancomycin was reported to be used excessively for surgical prophylaxis [25]. In human hospitals, there are committees that make recommendations on the use or restriction of perioperative antimicrobials. The Netherlands, for example, has a restrictive antimicrobial policy; however, overall adherence to local hospital guidelines was achieved in only 28% of cases [29]. Inappropriate dosing interval and timing of the first dose of antimicrobials had the lowest adherence rates (43% and 50%, respectively) [29]. The poor rate of adherence was attributed to a lack of awareness because of ineffective distribution of the most recent version of the guidelines, lack of agreement by surgeons with the local hospital guidelines, and organizational constraints [29]. In equine surgery, antimicrobial selection is limited based on economic considerations and toxicity.

Critically ill surgical patients

Recommendations for antimicrobial use in critically ill surgical patients, particularly patients undergoing emergency abdominal surgery, are particularly challenging, and, unfortunately, there is a sparsity of information on antimicrobial use in these cases. When deciding on an antimicrobial regimen for these patients, considerations include the predisposition of these patients to antimicrobial-induced diarrhea and the high mortality rate associated with this complication. It is critical to ensure that we are treating these patients with an adequate dose of antimicrobials, particularly the aminoglycosides, in which 10 times the minimum inhibitory concentration (MIC) of common pathogens is recommended. Fluid therapy and endotoxemia have been shown to influence gentamicin pharmacokinetics [30]. In our hospital, a dose rate of 6.6 mg/kg often does not result in peak concentrations 10 times the MIC of common pathogens (3 µg/kg) (Pamela A. Wilkins, DVM, personal communication, 2005). Therefore, this area needs further investigation. Critically ill horses undergoing abdominal surgery are often showing signs of the systemic inflammatory response syndrome (SIRS), are leukopenic, or have ischemia-reperfusion injury to the intestine, and there is often gross contamination associated with an enterotomy during abdominal exploration. The effect of these factors on postoperative infection and the importance of perioperative antimicrobial drugs beyond 24 hours in preventing postoperative infection in these cases have not been investigated. Antiulcer medication has been shown to increase the risk of infection in human patients, because the low gastric pH is an important antibacterial defense mechanism [31]. Antiulcer medication could potentially increase the risk of nosocomial salmonellosis, for example, in equine patients. The significance of cardiovascular and nutritional support, in addition to meticulous surgical technique, is a critical component to any infection prevention regimen; it is likely underestimated and its importance is probably underappreciated in equine patients.

Antimicrobial therapy

When antimicrobials are used in patients with established infection or with contaminated or dirty surgical wounds, antimicrobial use is no longer prophylactic but therapeutic. The prognosis for patients with an infection is improved dramatically with early appropriate antimicrobial use. Early antimicrobial use necessitates treatment with broad-spectrum antimicrobial drugs on an empiric basis, which, unfortunately, increases the risk of antimicrobial drug resistance. Therefore, there is a balance between optimizing patient care with adequate empiric therapy and minimizing antimicrobial resistance by avoiding excessive antimicrobial use [8]. A delay in appropriate antimicrobial therapy was shown to be the strongest predictor of mortality in human patients with infection, and 30% of patients experienced a delay of 24 hours or more in initiation of treatment with appropriate antimicrobials [32].

Appropriate antimicrobial use in patients with infection depends on identification of the infecting pathogen and selecting an antimicrobial drug with adequate efficacy and minimal toxicity and cost [33]. While the results of culture and sensitivity testing are pending, antimicrobial drug selection is empiric and should be based on commonly infecting bacteria and sensitivity patterns specific for a particular hospital or geographic area [33].

The dose and timing of antimicrobial administration are critical for a favorable outcome as well as for reducing the emergence of antimicrobial resistance [34]. There are two general categories of antimicrobials: concentration-dependent and time-dependent. Examples of concentration-dependent antimicrobials commonly used in equine practice are aminoglycosides and fluoroquinolones. The efficacy of concentration-dependent antimicrobials is reliant on the ratio of the peak plasma concentration (PEAK) of the antimicrobial to the MIC (PEAK:MIC) and the area under the concentration-time curve (AUC) to the MIC (AUC:MIC) [34]. The optimal PEAK:MIC should be 10:1 to 12:1 for concentration-dependent antimicrobials [34]. A PEAK:MIC of 10:1 or greater for gentamicin prevented the emergency of antimicrobial resistance and resulted in an improved clinical response and the avoidance of toxicity [35]. In human patients, an AUC/MIC greater than 100 for fluoroquinolones has been associated with improved efficacy and low resistance [36]. When concentration-dependent antimicrobials are used, peak and trough concentrations should be monitored and antimicrobial therapy should be directed toward attaining a peak concentration that is at least 10 times the MIC of the target pathogen or of pathologic bacteria in the hospital. We routinely adjust the gentamicin dose in our hospital to attain an MIC of at least 30 μg/mL, because the MIC of commonly occurring pathologic bacteria in our hospital is 3 μg/mL. In most cases, the dose required to achieve these peak concentrations is in excess of the recommended 6.6 mg/kg and is often as high as 8 to 10 mg/kg. The trough concentration can be used to monitor renal clearance, and if a trough less than 2 μg/mL is not achieved within 20 hours, the dose interval may be increased [37].

β-Lactams (penicillins and cephalosporins) and macrolides (erythromycin and clarithromycin) are examples of time-dependent antimicrobials. Time-dependent antimicrobials have a saturable concentration-dependent increase in bacterial killing after drug concentrations reach two to four times the MIC, and bacterial killing is optimal when the drug concentration is greater than the MIC for a percentage of the dosing interval [34]. Continuous rate infusion of β-lactam antimicrobials has similar efficacy to intermittent dosing and is reported to be more cost-effective in human hospitals [34].

The duration of antimicrobial administration should be the shortest possible so as to minimize the emergence of resistance. Some authors recommend using higher doses for shorter periods than those currently recommended [33]. A recent study evaluated the efficacy of azithromycin administered as a single high dose or the same total dose divided into two or three doses and administered over 2 or 3 days, respectively, in mouse pneumonia, acute peritonitis, and neutropenic thigh infection models [38]. Azithromycin is a time-dependent antimicrobial, with concentration-dependent persistent effects [34]. A single dose resulted in higher survival rates and better bacterial clearance compared with the multidose regimens [38]. The AUC was similar for single- and multiple-dose regimens [38].

It is critical to select an antimicrobial that penetrates the infection site. The use of specific antimicrobial drugs for various infections is discussed in the articles addressing infections affecting individual organ systems elsewhere in this issue. Additionally, antimicrobial toxicities should be considered and have been addressed in other reviews [37].

Postoperative fever

Postoperative fever is one of the most challenging and frustrating complications after surgery. The problem is determining whether the fever is associated with a bacterial infection or not. Routinely treating patients with a postoperative fever with an empiric antimicrobial regimen is contraindicated. It is critical to determine whether or not an infection is present, identify the site of infection, and obtain fluid or tissue samples for antimicrobial culture and sensitivity testing. Common causes of postoperative fever in horses include SIRS, viral or bacterial respiratory tract infection, enterocolitis, intravenous catheter site infection, SSIs, and, less commonly, deep infection. The best approach to patients with a postoperative fever is to consider and rule out each potential site of infection sequentially.

In human patients undergoing abdominal surgery, 38% (163 of 434) developed a postoperative fever, but only 16% (24 of 163) of the febrile patients had a bacterial infection [39]. Bacterial infection was associated with (1) a leukocyte count less than 5000 or greater than 10,000 cells/μL, (2) blood urea nitrogen equal to or greater than 15 mg/dL, and (3) onset of fever after the second postoperative day [39]. When these index factors were used to assess the likelihood of a patient having a bacterial infection, there was an increase in the likelihood of bacterial infection, with an increase in the number of index factors identified (ie, zero, one, two, or three index factors were associated with a 2%, 14%, 45%, or 100% infection rate, respectively) [39]. In equine patients, leukopenia is most often associated with enterocolitis, and current recommendations are to discontinue antimicrobial drugs (except perhaps oral metronidazole) if enterocolitis is suspected. Blood urea nitrogen has not been evaluated in postoperative equine patients with fever. Anecdotally, the onset of fever after the second day may be a good indicator of bacterial infection in equine patients because they often have a mild intermittent fever for 24 to 48 hours after surgery that resolves spontaneously.

Antimicrobial drug resistance

Antimicrobial drug resistance is a serious issue facing human and veterinary medicine. The overall national costs of antimicrobial resistance were estimated to be $100 million to $30 billion annually in the human medical field [40]. In some cases of nosocomial infections with resistant organisms in human hospitals, there are no alternative antimicrobials available for treatment [41]. Methicillin-resistant *Staphylococcus aureus* (MRSA) has become the major *S aureus* phenotype in human hospitals (>60%) and is the predominant nosocomial gram-positive pathogen; it possesses a multidrug-resistant genotype, and infection with MRSA is associated with a high mortality rate [42].

Antimicrobial drug resistance is also a growing problem in veterinary medicine. In Germany, between 1992 and 1997, an increase in resistance to antimicrobial drugs was found in equine pathogens [43]. There was an increase in the resistance of *Escherichia coli* to tetracyclines (75% increase), ampicillin (80% increase), and sulfonamides (90% increase); a fourfold increase in gentamicin resistance; and a 50% to 60% increase in resistance to penicillin and amino-penicillins [43]. Outbreaks of infection with multidrug-resistant *Salmonella* spp have also been reported in equine hospitals in various countries [44,45]. Antimicrobial drug resistance, however, is not limited to hospital settings. Reservoirs of horses colonized with MRSA were identified on farms in Ontario and New York [46]. In this study, MRSA was isolated from 4.7% (46 of 972) horses and 13% (14 of 107) people, and the isolated MRSA was of one strain predominantly [46].

"Excessive and inappropriate use of antimicrobial agents remains one of the most important factors affecting antibiotic resistance patterns" [33]. The development of antimicrobial resistance is related to antimicrobial use, and administration of narrow-spectrum antimicrobials for a limited duration may reduce the emergency of resistant organisms [47]. Prevention of antimicrobial resistance is a balancing act between appropriate early empiric treatment and avoidance of unnecessary antimicrobial use [48]. In critically ill human patients, prolonged hospital stays, frequent exposure to invasive procedures, and the use of broad-spectrum antimicrobials have been associated with an increased risk of carrying resistant bacteria compared with the general hospital population [49]. In human ventilator patients receiving prophylactic antimicrobials for longer than 48 hours, pneumonia was diagnosed later and was more likely to be caused by resistant gram-negative bacteria compared with that in patients not receiving prolonged prophylactic antimicrobials [50].

Antimicrobial resistance delays the administration of adequate antimicrobial therapy and, as a consequence, increases the mortality rate of critically ill patients with infection [48]. The mortality rate of critically ill human patients treated with inappropriate antimicrobial therapy was 52.1% compared with 23.5% in patients treated with appropriate antimicrobial therapy [51]. Most of the patients who were treated with inappropriate antimicrobials were infected with antimicrobial-resistant bacteria [51]. The increase in mortality is not only associated with a delay in appropriate treatment but with an increase in virulence factors in resistant bacteria [51]. Unfortunately, mortality is not reduced after institution of appropriate antimicrobials based on culture and sensitivity testing after a period of inappropriate antimicrobial treatment [52]. In addition to the increase in mortality, the hospital stay is prolonged and the cost of treatment is increased, which are serious problems in veterinary and human patients.

Infection control strategies are critical in preventing the spread of resistant pathogens. Such strategies are as simple as hand washing, barrier nursing (ie, wearing gloves and gowns between high-risk patients), maintaining aseptic technique when placing intravenous catheters or other invasive devices, and reducing the duration of an intensive care unit or hospital stay [48].

Some of the strategies that have been developed in human hospitals to reduce antimicrobial resistance include hospital formulary restriction and antimicrobial heterogeneity. Hospital formulary restriction, as the name suggests, involves prohibiting the use of a particular antimicrobial. Hospital formulary restriction has been used for drugs with a broad spectrum of activity, rapid emergency or resistance, and toxicity [48]. This strategy has been effective in reducing the incidence of nosocomial infections associated with a particular pathogen that was resistant to the restricted antimicrobial (eg, restriction of clindamycin use during an outbreak of antimicrobial-induced diarrhea caused by clindamycin-resistant *Clostridium difficile*); however, invariably, resistance to nonrestricted antimicrobials increases [51]. Although some hospitals have reported a decrease in pharmacy expenses and adverse drug reactions with hospital formulary restriction [53], other hospitals have not experienced the same success and have reported an increase in expense [54]. Formulary restriction strategies are thought to be useful during outbreaks with antimicrobial-resistant pathogens; however, they should not be used in place of an overall policy of judicious antimicrobial use and infection control programs [51].

There are two types of antimicrobial heterogeneity strategies. The first type involves the development of antimicrobial practice guidelines and protocols with an automated system that uses patient-specific data, culture and sensitivity test results, and prior antimicrobial exposure to formulate an antimicrobial regimen for an individual patient based on bacterial culture and sensitivity testing and previous antimicrobial exposure. This system has been shown to maintain stable antimicrobial sensitivity patterns, most likely through promotion of heterogeneous antimicrobial use, prevention of unnecessary antimicrobial use, and minimizing ineffective antimicrobial therapy [55]. Antimicrobial practice guidelines reduced antimicrobial costs per patient ($123 to $52) and the number of antimicrobial doses for surgical prophylaxis per patient (19 versus 5.3 doses), decreased antimicrobial use by 23%, and increased the incidence of appropriately timed preoperative antimicrobial doses from 40% to 99% [55]. A sophisticated software package is necessary, however.

The second type involves antimicrobial cycling, which is when a scheduled change in the type of empiric and prophylactic antimicrobials used is instituted. Antimicrobials are cycled on a 3- to 6-month schedule. Antimicrobial cycling decreased the number of infections, the number of infectious deaths, and the percentage of infections caused by resistant bacteria [40], and it decreased the incidence of ventilator-associated pneumonia, the incidence of inadequate antimicrobial therapy, and hospital mortality in critically ill patients [51]. Compared with indiscriminate antimicrobial use, antimicrobial cycling on a quarterly basis resulted in a significant reduction in infection rate (42% versus 32%), infection caused by resistant bacteria (25% versus 18%), resistant gram-negative rods (13% versus 6%), and a 60% reduction in the mortality rate [56]. Kollef and coworkers [57] used ciprofloxacin and ceftazidime on a 6-month rotation schedule and reported an overall decrease in ventilator-associated pneumonia, primarily as a result of a decrease in antimicrobial-resistant gram-negative bacteria, compared with before the regimen was instituted. Antimicrobial cycling does not provide an immediate beneficial effect on resistance patterns [40]. Additionally, antimicrobial resistance has been reported to emerge to the antimicrobial that was in use [40,58–61]. For example, when aminoglycosides were replaced or rotated with cephalosporins to manage a problem with aminoglycoside-resistant *Acinetobacter* spp, there was an outbreak of cephalosporin-resistant *Klebsiella* spp, and when the *Klebsiella* spp were treated with imipenem, an imipenem-resistant strain of *Acinetobacter* spp emerged [60]. Mathematic models describing the effects of antimicrobial cycling on resistance patterns have shown that "cycling" is inferior to "mixing" of antimicrobials to reduce antimicrobial resistance [62] and that antimicrobial resistance drifted toward a level corresponding with maximal selection pressure and producing excess resistance ("ratchet effect") [63]. Antimicrobial heterogeneity may be effective in human hospitals; however, in veterinary, particularly large animal, patients, there is a limitation to the number of different types of antimicrobials that can be used. The major reason for this limitation is economics.

When treating patients with life-threatening infection empirically with antimicrobials, a de-escalating antimicrobial regimen should be used. De-escalation involves initial treatment with broad-spectrum empiric antimicrobials and then more narrow-spectrum antimicrobials once the results of culture and sensitivity testing are obtained [48]. The use of narrow-spectrum antimicrobials (eg, penicillin, gentamicin) has been successful in reducing the occurrence of *C difficile* infection in human patients [64] and is indicated in patients with infections that are community acquired and not life-threatening [48]. More recent clinical trials have found that reducing the duration of antimicrobial use in patients with infection decreases resistance without negatively affecting infection resolution [48]. Clinical trials have shown that treatment of nonbacteremic human patients with ventilator-associated pneumonia for 7 to 8 days [65], pyelonephritis for 7 days [66], and community-acquired pneumonia for 5 days [67] is as efficacious as treatment with the more traditional 14- to 21-day antimicrobial regimen.

In large veterinary hospitals, antimicrobial use, biosecurity, and infectious disease committees can be structured to monitor and make recommendations regarding hospital antimicrobial use as well as to monitor infection rates, common pathogens isolated, resistance patterns, and early signs of nosocomial disease outbreaks. Molecular techniques are also being used for earlier identification of resistant bacteria compared with traditional culture and sensitivity testing [68]. Additionally, hospital staff should be meticulous about hand washing between patients and gloves worn or barrier nursing practices used when treating or evaluating high-risk patients (most critically ill patients; Fig. 1).

Antimicrobial-induced diarrhea

Antimicrobial use has been associated with diarrhea caused by *Salmonella* species and *C difficile* in human and veterinary patients. In human patients undergoing colorectal surgery, preoperative administration of oral antimicrobials as part of the preoperative surgical preparation resulted in a higher rate of *C difficile* infection compared with patients not administered oral antimicrobials (7.4% versus 2.6%) [69]. In a study identifying risk factors for salmonellosis, horses treated with parenteral antimicrobials had a 6.4 times increased risk and horses treated with parenteral and enteral antimicrobials had a 40 times increased risk for salmonellosis compared with unaffected or nontreated horses [70]. Horses with gastrointestinal tract disease are particularly susceptible to salmonellosis; horses with colic had a 4.3 times increased risk for salmonellosis compared with unaffected horses [70]. *C difficile* has also been associated with antimicrobial-induced diarrhea, and this syndrome carries a high mortality rate of approximately 40% [71]. This mortality rate is similar with certain strains of *Salmonella* spp. Recommendations for antimicrobial use in veterinary patients undergoing gastrointestinal tract surgery are particularly difficult, because the procedure is often

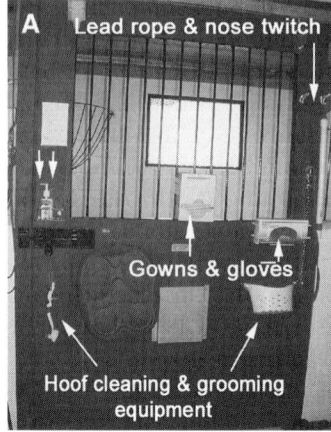
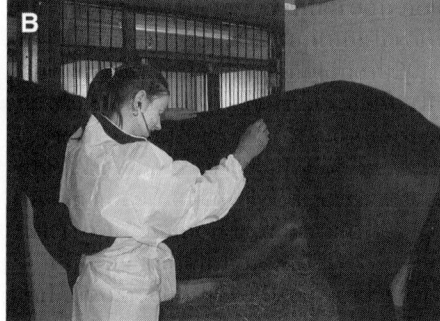
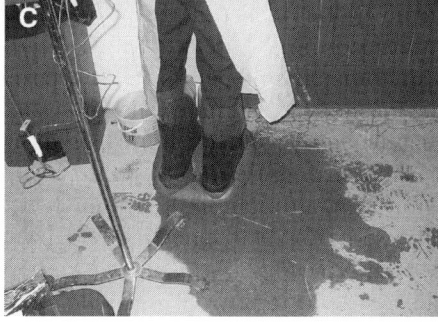

Fig. 1. Meticulous patient hygiene should always be practiced, and barrier nursing should be used for high-risk patients. Illustrated are some of the barrier nursing methods currently used at the New Bolton Center, University of Pennsylvania, for patients with gastrointestinal tract disease. (*A*) Each patient has its own hoof cleaning and grooming equipment (*arrow*) and lead rope and nose twitch (*arrow*), and there is hand disinfectant on each stall (*double arrow*) that can be used to clean the hands without the need for soap and water. (*B*) Gloves and gowns are worn by the nurse, student, or clinician when entering the stall. (*C*) There is a foot bath outside each stall to be used when entering or leaving the stall.

contaminated and the patient is systemically compromised. Because these patients are hospitalized in high-risk areas for nosocomial infections (ie, intensive care units), antimicrobial use increases their risks for antimicrobial-induced diarrhea and other nosocomial infections.

Summary

The use of perioperative antimicrobials should be limited for many reasons. Nevertheless, there are few to no studies on which recommendations can be based. Large, multicenter, prospective, randomized studies should be performed to evaluate the use of prophylactic antimicrobials in large- and small-animal patients. Studies should evaluate SSI and distant site infection rates. Complications associated with antimicrobial use, particularly diarrhea and the development of resistance, should also be included in any analysis.

References

[1] Traub-Dargatz JL, Dargatz DA, Morley PS. Antimicrobial resistance: what's the big deal? Importance of antimicrobial resistance to the equine practitioner. Proc Am Assoc Equine Pract 2002;48:138–44.
[2] Esposito S. Is single-dose antibiotic prophylaxis sufficient for any surgical procedure? J Chemother 1999;11:556–64.
[3] Bergquist EJ, Murphey SA. Prophylactic antibiotics for surgery. Med Clin North Am 1987; 71:357–68.
[4] Wong ES. Surgical site infections. In: Mayhall CG, editor. Hospital epidemiology and infection control. Baltimore (MD): Williams & Wilkins; 1996. p. 154–75.
[5] Burke JF. The effective period of preventive antibiotic action in experimental incisions and dermal lesions. Surgery 1961;50:161–8.
[6] Classen DC, Evans RS, Pestotnik SL, et al. The timing of prophylactic administration of antibiotics and the risk of surgical-wound infection. N Engl J Med 1992;326:281–6.
[7] Turnbull BR, Zoutman DE, Lam M. Evaluation of hospital and patient factors that influence the effective administration of surgical antimicrobial prophylaxis. Infect Control Hosp Epidemiol 2005;26:478–85.
[8] Imahara SD, Nathens AB. Antimicrobial strategies in surgical critical care. Curr Opin Crit Care 2003;9:286–91.
[9] Wilson DA, Baker GI, Boero MJ. Complications of celiotomy incisions in horses. Vet Surg 1995;24:506–14.
[10] Trostle SS, Hartmann FA. Surgical infection. In: Auer JA, Stick JA, editors. Equine surgery. 2nd edition. Philadelphia: WB Saunders; 1999. p. 47–54.
[11] Carlet J. General principles of choice of antibiotics for antibiotic prophylaxis in surgery. Ann Fr Anesth Reanim 1994;13(Suppl):10S–3S.
[12] Duque-Estrada EO, Duarte MR, Rodrigues DM, et al. Wound infections in pediatric surgery: a study of 575 patients in a university hospital. Pediatr Surg Int 2003;19:436–8.
[13] Haughey RE, Lammers RL, Wagner DK. Use of antibiotics in the initial management of soft tissue hand wounds. Ann Emerg Med 1981;10:187–92.
[14] Cassell OCS, Ion L. Are antibiotics necessary in the surgical management of upper limb lacerations? Br J Plast Surg 1997;50:523–9.
[15] Cummings P, Del Beccaro MA. Antibiotics to prevent infection of simple wounds: a meta-analysis of randomized studies. Am J Emerg Med 1995;13:396–400.
[16] Misra A, Iqbal M, Misra S. The use of antibiotics in simple soft-tissue trauma. Plast Reconstr Surg 2005;115:332–3.
[17] Mizunaga S, Kamiyama T, Fukuda Y, et al. Influence of inoculum size of Staphylococcus aureus and Pseudomonas aeruginosa on in vitro activities and in vivo efficacy of fluoroquinolones and carbapenems. J Antimicrob Chemother 2005;56:91–6.
[18] Altemeier WA, Culbertson WR, Hummel RP. Surgical considerations of endogenous infections—sources, types, methods of control. Surg Clin North Am 1968;48:227–40.
[19] Aberg C, Thore M. Single versus triple dose antimicrobial prophylaxis in elective abdominal surgery and the impact on bacterial ecology. J Hosp Infect 1991;18:149–54.
[20] Bates T, Roberts JV, Smith K, et al. A randomized trial of one versus three doses of Augmentin as wound prophylaxis in at-risk abdominal surgery. Postgrad Med J 1992;68:811–6.
[21] Van Scoy RE, Wilkowske CJ. Prophylactic use of antimicrobial agents in adult patients. Mayo Clin Proc 1992;67:288–92.
[22] Rotman N, Flamant Y, Hay JM, et al. Antibiotic prophylaxis in abdominal surgery. Prospective randomized study organized by the French Surgical Research Association. Presse Med 1991;20:1659–63.
[23] Bieser U, Dietrich ES, Frank U, et al. Meta-analysis of the perioperative prophylaxis of ceftriaxone versus other cephalosporins. Presented at the Fifth Annual Cochrane Colloquium. Amsterdam, The Netherlands. October 8–12, 1997.

[24] Traub-Dargatz JL, George JL, Dargatz DA, et al. Survey of complications and antimicrobial use in equine patients at veterinary teaching hospitals that underwent surgery because of colic. J Am Vet Med Assoc 2002;20:1359–65.
[25] Bratzler DW, Houck PM, Richards C, et al. Use of antimicrobial prophylaxis in major surgery. Arch Surg 2005;140:174–82.
[26] Fernández HA, Monge V, Garcinuño MA. Surgical antibiotic prophylaxis: effect in postoperative infections. Eur J Epidemiol 2001;17:369–74.
[27] Brown DC, Conzemius MG, Shofer F, et al. Injudicious antibiotic use may increase risk of postsurgical wound infection. J Am Vet Med Assoc 1997;210:1302–6.
[28] Moesgaard F, Nielson ML, Hjortrup A, et al. Intraincisional antibiotic in addition to systemic antibiotic treatment fails to reduce wound infection rates in contaminated abdominal surgery. A controlled clinical trial. Dis Colon Rectum 1989;32:36–8.
[29] van Kasteren MEE, Kullberg BJ, de Boer AS, et al. Adherence to local hospital guidelines for surgical antimicrobial prophylaxis: a multicenter audit in Dutch hospitals. J Antimicrob Chemother 2003;51:1389–96.
[30] van der Harst MR, Bull S, Laffont CM, et al. Influence of fluid therapy on gentamicin pharmacokinetics in colic horses. Vet Res Comm 2005;29:141–7.
[31] Merino PL. Gastrointestinal prophylaxis. In: The ICU book. 2nd edition. Philadelphia: Lippincott Williams & Wilkins; 1997. p. 94–105.
[32] Iregui M, Ward S, Sherman G, et al. Clinical importance of delays in the initiation of appropriate antibiotic treatment for ventilator-associated pneumonia. Chest 2002;122: 262–8.
[33] Niederman MS. Appropriate use of antimicrobial agents: challenges and strategies for improvement. Crit Care Med 2003;31:608–16.
[34] Goldberg J, Owens RC. Optimizing antimicrobial dosing in the critically ill patient. Curr Opin Crit Care 2002;8:435–40.
[35] Verpooten GA, Guiliano RA, Verbist L, et al. Once-daily dosing decreases renal accumulation of gentamicin and netilmicin. Clin Pharmacol Ther 1989;45:22–7.
[36] Schentag JJ, Gilliland KK, Paladino JA. What have we learned from pharmacokinetic and pharmacodynamic theories? Clin Infect Dis 2001;32(Suppl):S39–46.
[37] McKenzie MC III, Furr MO. Aminoglycoside antibiotics in neonatal foals. Compend Contin Educ Pract Vet 2003;25:457–69.
[38] Girard D, Finegan SM, Dunne MW, et al. Enhanced efficacy of single-dose versus multi-dose azithromycin regimens in preclinical infection models. J Antimicrob Chemother 2005;56:365–71.
[39] Mellors JW, Kelly JJ, Gusberg RJ, et al. A simple index to estimate the likelihood of bacterial infection in patients developing fever after abdominal surgery. Am Surg 1988;54: 558–64.
[40] Horner M. Judicious use of antimicrobials in the critical care setting. J Infus Nurs 2004;27: 79–84.
[41] Shlaes DM, Gerding DN, John JF Jr, et al. Society for Healthcare Epidemiology of America and Infectious Diseases Society of America Joint Committee on the Prevention of Antimicrobial Resistance: guidelines for the prevention of antimicrobial resistance in hospitals. Clin Infect Dis 1997;25:584–99.
[42] Barrett JF. MRSA: status and prospects for therapy? An evaluation of key papers on the topic of MRSA and antibiotic resistance. Expert Opin Ther Targets 2004;8:515–9.
[43] Trolldenier H, Kempf G. Resistance of equine pathogens—an overview of data recorded on the national level and recommendations for therapy. Prakt Tierarzt 2000;81:216–31.
[44] Dargatz DA, Traub-Dargatz JL. Multidrug-resistant Salmonella and nosocomial infections. Vet Clin North Am Equine Pract 2004;20:587–600.
[45] Amavisit P, Markham PF, Lightfoot D, et al. Molecular epidemiology of Salmonella Heidelberg in an equine hospital. Vet Microbiol 2001;80:85–98.

[46] Weese JS, Rousseau J, Traub-Dargatz JL, et al. Community-associated methicillin-resistant Staphylococcus aureus in horses and humans who work with horses. J Am Vet Med Assoc 2005;226:580–3.
[47] Franklin GA, Moore KB, Snyder JW, et al. Emergency of resistant microbes in critical care units is transient, despite and unrestricted formulary and multiple antibiotic trials. Surg Infect (Larchmt) 2002;3:135–44.
[48] Kollef MH, Micek ST. Strategies to prevent antimicrobial resistance in the intensive care unit. Crit Care Med 2005;33:1845–53.
[49] Archibald L, Phillips L, Monnet D, et al. Antimicrobial resistance in isolates from inpatients and outpatients in the Unites States: increasing importance of the intensive care unit. Clin Infect Dis 1997;24:211–5.
[50] Hoth JJ, Franklin GA, Stassen NA, et al. Prophylactic antibiotics adversely affect nosocomial pneumonia in trauma patients. J Trauma 2003;55:249–54.
[51] Kollef MH, Sherman G, Ward S, et al. Inadequate antimicrobial treatment of infections: a risk factor for hospital mortality among critically ill patients. Chest 1999;115:462–74.
[52] Luna CM, Vujacich P, Niederman MS, et al. Impact of BAL data on the therapy and outcome of ventilator-associated pneumonia. Chest 1997;111:676–85.
[53] McGowan JE Jr, Gerding DN. Does antibiotic restriction prevent resistance? New Horiz 1996;4:370–6.
[54] Rifenburg RP, Paladino JA, Hanson SC, et al. Benchmark analysis of strategies hospitals use to control antimicrobial expenditures. Am J Health Syst Pharm 1996;53:2054–62.
[55] Pestotnik SL, Classen DC, Evans RS, et al. Implementing antibiotic practice guidelines through computer-assisted decision support: clinical and financial outcomes. Ann Intern Med 1996;124:884–90.
[56] Raymond DP, Pelletier SJ, Crabtree TD, et al. Impact of rotating empiric antibiotic schedule on infectious mortality in an intensive care unit. Crit Care Med 2001;29:1101–8.
[57] Kollef MH, Vlasnik J, Sharpless L, et al. Scheduled rotation of antibiotic classes: a strategy to decrease the incidence of ventilator-associated pneumonia due to antibiotic resistant gram-negative bacteria. Am J Respir Crit Care Med 1997;156:1040–8.
[58] Gruson D, Hibert G, Vargas F, et al. Rotation and restricted use of antibiotics in a medical intensive care unit: impact on the incidence of ventilator-associated pneumonia caused by antibiotic-resistant gram-negative bacteria. Am J Respir Crit Care Med 2000;162:837–43.
[59] Kollef MH, Ward S, Sherman G, et al. Inadequate treatment of nosocomial infections is associated with certain empiric antibiotic choices. Crit Care Med 2000;28:3456–64.
[60] Meyer KS, Urban C, Eagan JA, et al. Nosocomial outbreak of *Klebsiella* infection resistant to late-generation cephalosporins. Ann Intern Med 1993;119:353–8.
[61] Rahal JJ, Urban C, Horn D, et al. Class restriction of cephalosporin use to control total cephalosporin resistance in nosocomial Klebsiella. JAMA 1998;280(14):1233–7.
[62] Bergstrom CT, Lo M, Lipsitch M. Ecological theory suggests that antimicrobial cycling will not reduce antimicrobial resistance in hospitals. Proc Natl Acad Sci USA 2004;101: 13285–90.
[63] Magee JT. The resistance ratchet: theoretical implications of cyclic selection pressure. J Antimicrob Chemother 2005;56:257–8.
[64] McNulty C, Logan M, Donald IP, et al. Successful control of Clostridium difficile infection in an elderly care unit through use of a restrictive antibiotic policy. J Antimicrob Chemother 1997;40:707–11.
[65] Micke ST, Ward S, Fraser VJ, et al. A randomized controlled trial of an antibiotic discontinuation policy for clinically suspected ventilator-associated pneumonia. Chest 2004;125: 1791–9.
[66] Talan DA, Stamm WE, Hooton TM, et al. Comparison of ciprofloxacin (7 days) and trimethoprim-sulfamethoxazole (14 days) for acute uncomplicated pyelonephritis in women: a randomized trial. JAMA 2000;283:1583–90.

[67] Dunbar LM, Wunderink RG, Habib MP, et al. High-dose, short-course levofloxacin for community-acquired pneumonia: a new treatment paradigm. Clin Infect Dis 2003;37: 752–60.
[68] Woodford N, Sundsfjord A. Molecular detection of antibiotic resistance: when and where? J Antimicrob Chemother 2005;56:259–61.
[69] Wren SM, Ahmed N, Jamal A, et al. Preoperative oral antibiotics in colorectal surgery increase the rate of Clostridium difficile colitis. Arch Surg 2005;140:752–6.
[70] Hird DW, Casebolt DB, Carter JD, et al. Risk factors for salmonellosis in hospitalized horses. J Am Vet Med Assoc 1986;188:173–7.
[71] Båverud V, Gustaffson A, Franklin A, et al. Clostridium difficile associated with acute colitis in mature horses treated with antibiotics. Equine Vet J 1997;29:279–84.

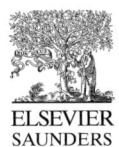

New Antimicrobials, Systemic Distribution, and Local Methods of Antimicrobial Delivery in Horses

Antonio M. Cruz, DVM, MVM, MSc, DrMedVet[a],*, Luis Rubio-Martinez, DVM, PhD[a], Trisha Dowling, DVM, MSc, PhD[b]

[a]*Department of Clinical Studies, Ontario Veterinary College, University of Guelph, Guelph, Ontario, Canada N1G 2W1*
[b]*Department of Veterinary Biomedical Sciences, Western College of Veterinary Medicine, University of Saskatchewan, Saskatoon, Saskatchewan, Canada*

Infection is a common occurrence in equine practice. Prompt and effective treatment must be instituted to maximize the chances of a successful outcome. A synovial cavity, bone, or implant, for example, once colonized by bacteria, constitutes problematic environments with which to deal. Although other aspects of treatment, such as surgical debridement of necrotic debris, control of inflammation, and appropriate rehabilitation, are important, prompt elimination of the invading bacterial population is paramount for a favorable outcome.

Antimicrobial selection

Because of the variety of pathogens involved in musculoskeletal infections, appropriate samples must be submitted for microbiologic culture and susceptibility testing. While awaiting culture results, initial antimicrobial selection can be chosen based on the clinical case characteristics and retrospective studies. In septic neonates, infections with gram-negative pathogens, such as *Escherichia coli*, *Klebsiella* spp, *Salmonella* spp, and *Actinobacillus* spp, predominate [1,2]. Traumatic wounds are often contaminated and infected with *Streptococcus zooepidemicus*, *E coli*, *Enterobacter*

---

* Corresponding author.
E-mail address: acruz@uoguelph.ca (A.M. Cruz).

spp, and other gram-negative opportunists [2,3]. Iatrogenic infections from joint injections or incisional contamination commonly yield *Staphylococcus aureus*, and methicillin-resistant *Staphylococcus aureus* (MRSA) is of increasing concern in equine infections [3–5].

Penicillin, ampicillin, and ceftiofur are all highly efficacious against *S zooepidemicus* and most other gram-positive bacteria involved in equine infections, but increasing resistance to trimethoprim-sulfonamides has been documented [3,6]. Ceftiofur is the only cephalosporin antimicrobial approved for horses, and it is only labeled for *S zooepidemicus* respiratory infections. When administered, ceftiofur is rapidly metabolized to the active metabolite desfuroylceftiofur [7]. Desfuroylceftiofur is less active than ceftiofur against *S aureus* and *Proteus* spp. Because of the instability of desfurolyceftiofur, only ceftiofur is used in susceptibility testing; thus, results for staphylococci and *Proteus* spp isolates should be interpreted with caution [7]. It can be used for regional perfusion and intra-articular injection in horses [8]. Other cephalosporins approved for human use have been investigated for their use in horses and foals. Most are administered parenterally and could be used in local drug delivery systems. Some are suitable for oral administration. Clinical use is often limited by the expense of these drugs. Cefpodoxime proxetil is a third-generation cephalosporin that can be administered orally to horses, but expense limits its use to foals [9]. Cefotaxime is an injectable third-generation cephalosporin that reaches therapeutic concentrations in the synovial fluid of adult horses [10]. Cefepime is a fourth-generation cephalosporin with strong gram-negative activity, at the expense of gram-positive and anaerobic activity. It seems to be suitable for intravenous administration in septic foals [11] but is associated with adverse gastrointestinal effects in adult horses [12].

The new extended-spectrum macrolides are being investigated for use in horses. Their spectrum of activity includes gram-positive bacteria, gram-negative respiratory bacteria, anaerobes, and mycoplasma. They are characterized by high distribution and good oral absorption in foals. Parenteral products are irritating and would not be recommended for local drug delivery. Azithromycin and clarithromycin are used in the treatment of *Rhodococcus equi* pneumonia in foals but have the potential to be effective against streptococcal and staphylococcal musculoskeletal infections [13]. Tilmicosin and tulathromycin are new macrolides developed for use in cattle and swine, but they also have potential for use in horses. Pharmacokinetic and safety studies of tilmicosin are in progress.

Resistance in gram-negative bacteria has led to a reduction in the use of gentamicin, but it remains efficacious against most staphylococci and streptococci [3]. Although it is more effective than gentamicin against gram-negative bacteria and staphylococci, amikacin has poor activity against streptococci and should not be used as a single agent for traumatic wounds [3]. The aminoglycosides are well tolerated when administered by local drug delivery methods, which reduces costs and avoids systemic toxicity [14].

Fluoroquinolones, such as enrofloxacin, typically have excellent activity against staphylococci and gram-negative bacteria, including *Pseudomonas* spp, but activity against streptococci and enterococci is variable. The pharmacokinetics of enrofloxacin, ciprofloxacin, marbofloxacin, and orbifloxacin have been described in horses. Because of the potential for fluoroquinolones to cause cartilage erosion [15], their use is not recommended in young growing horses, but they have been used successfully [16]. Intravenous use of cattle injectable formulations is safe in adult horses [17].

Antimicrobials that are used to treat resistant infections in human patients, such as imipenem and vancomycin, should be reserved for cases with no alternative treatment options [18]. The carbapenems, imipenem, and meropenem have the broadest antimicrobial spectrum of activity of any antimicrobial group. Their broad spectrum of activity is attributable to their capacity to penetrate the bacteria, their stability toward β-lactamases, and their affinity for specific penicillin-binding proteins that cause the lysis of the bacteria [19]. They are the most potent of the newer agents against gram-positive cocci and anaerobes, and more than 90% of gram-negative organisms are susceptible, including those resistant to other β-lactam antimicrobials and the aminoglycosides. The carbapenems are highly resistant to most β-lactamases, with meropenem being the most active against *Pseudomonas* spp and Enterobacteriaceae [19]. Imipenem is extensively metabolized by the renal tubules to a potentially nephrotoxic compound [20]. Therefore, imipenem is combined with the drug cilastatin, which inhibits renal tubular enzymes [20]. The combined product avoids renal toxicity and achieves high urine concentrations of the active antimicrobial [20]. In dogs, meropenem, another carbapenem not yet studied in horses, causes fewer gastrointestinal side effects and is not nephrotoxic or neurotoxic [19,20]. Meropenem has fewer adverse effects and can be administered intravenously in a more concentrated solution than imipenem, so it may be useful for regional limb perfusion (RLP) in horses. The pharmacokinetic parameters of systemically administered imipenem have been described in horses [20]. After a 10-minute intravenous infusion of an imipenem solution (100 mg/mL) at doses of 10 and 20 mg/kg, a three-compartment model can describe the kinetics of imipenem in plasma and synovial fluid [20]. Maximum concentrations (C_{max}s) of synovial fluid of 4.78 ± 1.52 and 10.12 ± 2.95 μg/mL for systemic intravenous doses of 10 and 20 mg/kg, respectively, are obtained [20]. Plasma concentrations decrease to less than 1 μg/kg by 3 hours after infusion [20]. The times to C_{max}s in synovial fluid are 30 and 60 minutes for the 10- and 20-mg/kg doses, respectively [20]. A dose of 10 to 20 mg/kg administered by slow intravenous infusion every 6 hours is well tolerated in adult horses and maintains concentrations above the minimum inhibitory concentration (MIC) for most bacteria [20].

Antimicrobial pharmacokinetics and pharmacodynamics

The pharmacokinetic-pharmacodynamic (PK-PD) relation between an antimicrobial and a pathogen determines the dosage regimen. Antimicrobials are broadly classified as concentration dependent or time dependent for their antibacterial activity. For antimicrobials whose efficacy is concentration dependent, a high C_{max} of plasma relative to the MIC of the pathogen (C_{max}/MIC) and an area under the plasma concentration-time curve (AUC_t) that is greater than the bacterial MIC during the dosage interval (area under the inhibitory curve [AUIC] = AUC/MIC) are the major determinants of clinical efficacy (Fig. 1A) [21]. The aminoglycosides and fluoroquinolones are concentration-dependent antimicrobials [21]. These drugs also have long postantibiotic effects (PAEs), where bacterial growth remains suppressed for a period after drug concentration has decreased below the MIC, thereby allowing long dosing intervals with maximum clinical efficacy. The PAE is defined as the time required for an organism to demonstrate viable regrowth after the removal of an antimicrobial. The higher the aminoglycoside dosage, the greater is the PAE up to a certain maximal response.

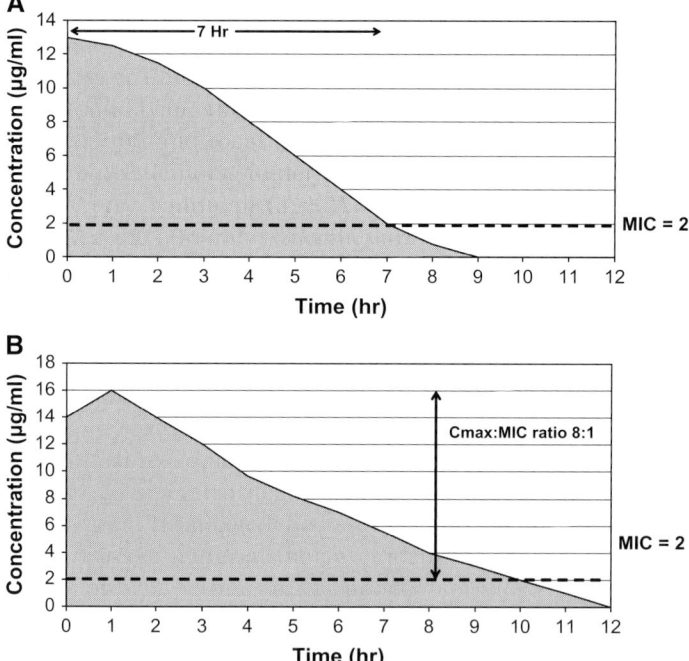

Fig. 1. (*A*) The efficacy of a concentration-dependent antimicrobial, such as a fluoroquinolone or aminoglycoside, depends on achieving a C_{max}/MIC ratio of 8 to 10. (*B*) The efficacy of a time-dependent antimicrobial, such as a penicillin or cephalosporin, depends on keeping the antimicrobial concentration above the bacterial MIC for at least 50% of the dosing interval.

In vivo, the PAE for aminoglycosides is prolonged by the synergistic effect of host leukocyte activity. It is believed that leukocytes have enhanced phagocytosis and killing activity after exposure to aminoglycosides [22].

For time-dependent antimicrobials, the time during which the antimicrobial concentration exceeds the MIC of the pathogen determines the clinical efficacy (see Fig. 1B) [21]. The time greater than the MIC should be at least 50% for most patients and should be closer to 100% for bacteriostatic drugs and for patients that are immunosuppressed [21]. All the penicillin, cephalosporins, carbapenems, tetracyclines, macrolides, and trimethoprim-sulfonamide combinations are considered time-dependent antimicrobials [21,23]. For these drugs, bactericidal activity does not increase with increasing plasma concentrations; once the MIC of the bacteria is exceeded, only increasing the dosage frequency increases efficacy.

Glycopeptide antimicrobials, such as vancomycin, showed concentration-dependent and time-dependent killing in mouse models of peritonitis [24]. Because of its importance in human medicine, vancomycin should only be used in equine patients with serious infections from pathogens, such as MSRA, when no other treatment options exist. The concentration of systemically administered antimicrobials in a target region depends on many factors affecting local vascular supply, which is commonly altered in infected sites. Inflammation, vascular thrombosis, pannus formation, accumulation of necrotic debris, and acidosis associated with infected sites reduce the penetration and activity of systemically administered antimicrobials. Obtaining appropriate antimicrobial concentrations by systemic administration at infected sites has remained a limiting factor in the successful treatment of musculoskeletal infections, particularly those affecting synovial cavities. To overcome the limitations of systemic antimicrobial delivery, local delivery systems have been developed and applied successfully.

Local methods of antimicrobial delivery

Local delivery of antimicrobials to the infected site offers major advantages over traditional systemic therapy. A high local drug concentration at the site of infection can be achieved with a local drug delivery system while maintaining low systemic drug levels, thereby avoiding possible side effects. The modes of local antimicrobial administration involve biodegradable and nonbiodegradable implants, constant rate infusion (CRI) or indwelling systems, and RLP by intravenous or intraosseous routes.

Nonbiodegradable antimicrobial-impregnated implants

Polymethylmethacrylate

Polymethylmethacrylate (PMMA) is a synthetic polymer product marketed in a powder form. It is also marketed in combination with gentamicin in the form of premade beads (Septopal; Biomet Canada, Oakville, Ontario, Canada) (Fig. 2A); however, the clinician could manufacture antimicrobial-impregnated PMMA beads at the time of implantation (see Fig. 2B). The combination of the liquid monomer and the powder polymer to produce the characteristic PMMA hard bead produces an exothermic reaction that could produce soft tissue burns and destabilize certain antimicrobials, such as ampicillin. Therefore, it is important to place the beads in the tissue when they are cold. The antimicrobial used to impregnate the beads must be thermostable and have adequate elution characteristics to produce sustained and appropriate release from the bead [25]. The elution of the antimicrobial from the PMMA bead depends on the pore size, permeability, size and shape of the implant, type of antimicrobial, and amount of antimicrobial present in the bead. The amount and rate of wound exudate alter the elution kinetics of an antimicrobial from the bead [26,27]. In general, the larger the PMMA bead, the less elution of antimicrobial there is, because the surface-to-volume ratio is also smaller. In horses, gentamicin, amikacin, cefazolin, tobramycin, vancomycin, ceftiofur, and enrofloxacin have been used successfully [18,25,28–34]. Release of the antimicrobial from PMMA is bimodal [29]. There is rapid release during the first 24 hours after implantation, followed by continuous sustained release that can last from weeks to years [29]. Typically, antimicrobial at a dose of 1 to 2 g is mixed with cement powder (40 g) [25]. A larger amount of antimicrobial could potentially prevent hardening of the PMMA [29] or affect its mechanical strength [35] in cases in which the cement is used to increase the stability of other implants. Ideally, it is best if the powder form of the antimicrobial is added, because use of the liquid form may also compromise the strength of the implant [26]. The authors have added gentamicin in the liquid (100 mg/mL) form, and although the exothermic reaction takes longer to complete, no problems have been encountered. The use of gentamicin-impregnated PMMA beads for treatment of equine osteomyelitis is widespread. Bactericidal concentrations of gentamicin are achieved for at least 30 days [31]. When compared with amikacin and ceftiofur, it was found that liquid and powder forms of

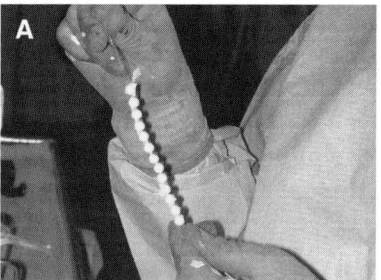
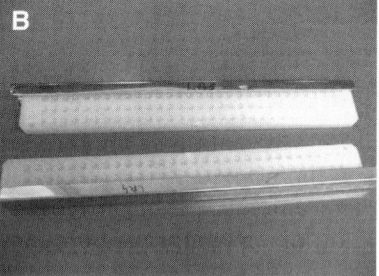

Fig. 2. Commercially available gentamicin-impregnated PMMA beads (*A*) and mold used to prepare gentamicin-impregnated PMMA beads (*B*).

gentamicin behaved similarly [31]. The powder form of amikacin had better elution characteristics than the liquid form, however [31]. The aminoglycosides eluted better than ceftiofur, which did not produce sustained long-term release [31]. In addition, the liquid form of amikacin at a dose of 250 mg in PMMA powder (2 g) was superior to the liquid form of amikacin at a dose of 125 mg [20]. Other cephalosporins have been used successfully in human patients, with sustained elution for up to 26 weeks in vitro [36]. Although the release of cephalosporins seems to be more rapid than the release of aminoglycosides, cephalosporins also seem to be effective in controlling infection [26]. Combination of antimicrobials in the same bead could affect the elution characteristic of either antimicrobial [35]. In addition, some antimicrobial groups are antagonistic, and their use in combination is not recommended [37]. Such is the case with the aminoglycosides and β-lactams [37]. At the present time, it is recommended to use one antimicrobial per PMMA bead preparation, although we have used beads impregnated with two different antimicrobials within the same infected region.

Antimicrobial-impregnated PMMA caused synovial irritation, cartilage erosion, and lameness when placed intra-articularly; therefore, its use is not recommended in joints [33]. Antimicrobial-impregnated PMMA has been used frequently in cases of bone and soft tissue infections [25]. Perhaps the most negative aspect of its use is that it is nonbiodegradable. Although most tissues seem to have a minimal inflammatory reaction to the presence of the beads, tissue irritation is also possible. In these cases, implant removal is recommended. Alternatively, PMMA beads can be left in place if no tissue reactivity is apparent.

Biodegradable antimicrobial-impregnated implants

Biodegradable implants offer the advantages of not needing a second operation for removal and potentially being more biocompatible than nonbiodegradable implants. Biodegradable implants should produce sustained release of high concentrations of antimicrobial, avoid tissue irritation, and not change their biologic properties in the presence of an antimicrobial. Ideally, they should not be cost-prohibitive, and they should be user-friendly.

Collagen

Commercially available gentamicin-impregnated collagen sponges (Collatamp; Syntacoll AG, Herisau, Switzerland) (Fig. 3) are readily available in Europe but not in Canada or the United States. Clinical use of Collatamp has been reported in cattle [38], dogs [39], and horses [40]. Because the product is not available or approved for use in Canada, its use in our practice requires that a special drug release form be filed with our pharmacy to import the product. We have used Collatamp successfully in horses and cattle

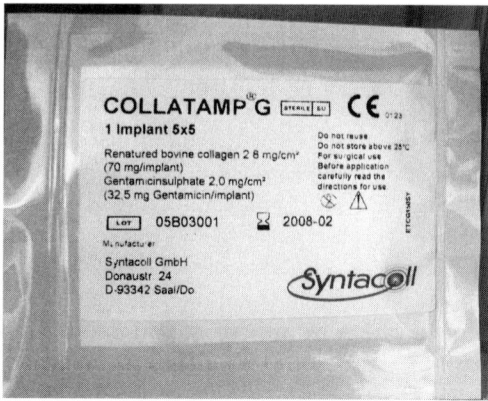

Fig. 3. Commercially available gentamicin-impregnated collagen sponges.

in cases of open fractures, infected arthrodesis, and soft tissue infections in more than a dozen cases with no identified side effects. The contribution of the collagen-impregnated sponges to the successful outcome of the case was difficult to ascertain. There is conflicting information pertaining to their clinical applicability. Although in vitro studies have reported excessively rapid antimicrobial release, which prevents sustained release over time [41], in vivo studies support this therapeutic modality in combination with systemic antimicrobials and surgical debridement [38,39]. Gentamicin-impregnated collagen sponges are easy to implant; prevent subinhibitory antimicrobial concentration, which could occur with PMMA beads; and obviate the need for implant removal [39]. Complete elution occurs over a period of 2 weeks, with high elution rates during the first week [42]. Gentamicin-impregnated collagen (3 mg/kg) was implanted into the femoral medullary canal of 45 adult white rabbits, and the average bone gentamicin concentration was greater than 600 µg/mL during the initial 48 hours [42]. Collagen impregnated with gentamicin proved to be an effective biodegradable carrier of gentamicin in the healthy rabbit; it provided local bone concentrations greater than the MIC of gentamicin and serum concentrations lower than levels associated with systemic toxicity for as long as 28 days after implantation [42].

Perhaps the main disadvantage of gentamicin-impregnated collagen is its cost, approximately CAN $135 per square (5 in × 5 in). Collagen used in the manufacturing of these implants is extracted from bovine (Collatamp G; Syntacoll AG) or equine (Collatamp EG; Syntacoll AG) species. The collagen extraction process is in accordance with strict European regulations, and the source of bovine collagen is compliant with the regulations of the European Directorate for the Quality of Medicines, ensuring the absence of microorganisms and prions. In human patients, there is a 3% incidence of hypersensitivity to collagen, but because of the purification process during manufacturing, the immune reactivity is greatly reduced. Collatamp G has been used in more than 1.5 million human patients to date without any report of a serious adverse event (David Prior, PhD, Vice-president, Innocoll Corporation, personal communication, 2006).

Hydroxyapatite

Hydroxyapatite cement (HAC) implanted within bone and subcutaneous tissue is reabsorbed, and it has osteoconductive properties in bone [43]. HAC is fabricated with water, which can be replaced with the antimicrobial drug in liquid form, eliminating the concern of implanting liquid rather than powder onto the cement. In an in vitro study, gentamicin, amikacin, or ceftiofur eluted at a greater concentration from the HAC than from PMMA, creating concerns about possible toxic side effects [31]. Although HAC seems to have optimal qualities for a biodegradable delivery system in vivo, studies are necessary to determine its overall safety and efficacy.

Plaster of Paris

Plaster of Paris (POP) is an inexpensive and readily available material that has been investigated for use as an antimicrobial delivery system. POP gentamicin-impregnated beads are inexpensive, biocompatible, biodegradable, osteoconductive, and easily manufactured using a liquid antimicrobial and a bead mold [44]. Its use in vivo has been documented in equine odontology [45], and an in vitro study has documented the release of gentamicin from POP for at least 14 days [44]. Eighty percent of the gentamicin was released within the first 48 hours, and *E coli* growth was inhibited for the duration of the study [44]. In addition, POP gentamicin-impregnated beads released bactericidal concentrations of drug after ethylene oxide sterilization and 5 months of storage at room temperature [44]. The gentamicin concentrations obtained after 48 hours were not high (~ 4 μg/mL), however, and may be insufficient to kill the bacteria responsible for biomaterial-centered orthopedic infections. This relatively short duration of a high gentamicin concentration may suggest that POP beads may be ideal for antimicrobial prophylaxis in high-risk cases, such as fracture repair [44].

Polyanhydrides

Septacin (Abbott Laboratories, Abbott Park, Illinois) is a polyanhydride implant containing gentamicin for local antimicrobial delivery. In vitro and in vivo studies, including a horse model of tarsocrural joint septic arthritis, have demonstrated clinical efficacy and high local gentamicin concentrations [46]. In horses, an experimental model of septic arthritis involving inoculation of the tarsocrural joint with *S aureus* was used to evaluate Septacin [46]. Twenty-four hours after injection, Septacin was placed into the dorsal and plantar joint pouches [46]. Infection was eliminated in two of six joints within 3 days and in four of six joints within 13 days [46]. A mild to moderate synovitis was elicited by the presence of Septacin beads, but there was no detectable lameness or joint pain [34]. The elution of gentamicin from Septacin occurs over a period of 4 weeks, after an initial burst (40% elution) within the first week [46]. A clinical trial in human patients has confirmed its applicability for synovial infection and lack of toxic effects; however, its clinical use has not been reported in horses.

Hyaluronan

Hyaluronan has been investigated as an antimicrobial carrier for synovial cavity infections [47]. Because it is bioabsorbable and innocuous to the joint environment, hyaluronan could potentially constitute an optimal antimicrobial carrier for synovial infections [47]. Rapid release of amikacin occurred from a ferric hyaluronan implant with sustained concentrations greater than the MIC for a period of approximately 24 hours [47]. Although infection was eliminated within 24 hours of implantation in this in vivo study, the rapid release of amikacin makes it impractical for a long-term antimicrobial delivery system. Modifications to this system are required to ensure a high in vivo elution of amikacin for a longer period to make it practical in a clinical situation.

Polylactide-polyglycolide

An in vitro study using equine synovial explants and comparing poly (DL)-lactide and poly(DL)-lactide-co-glycolide showed equivalent controlled release of gentamicin at high concentrations for 10 days and elimination of infection with no adverse effects on synovial viability or synovial hyaluronan production [48]. The release of gentamicin was biphasic. There was a slow induction period and then a period of rapid release. The period of rapid release consisted of a high-burst release of gentamicin in the first 24 hours and then sustained release for 10 days, after which the gentamicin concentration was less than 10 µg/mL until 14 days [48]. To the authors' knowledge, no clinical reports exist on the use of this delivery system in horses.

Constant rate infusion or indwelling systems

Constant delivery of antimicrobials is best suited for synovial cavities, such as joints or tendon sheaths. The use of commercially available CRI pumps (MILA International, Florence, Kentucky) (Fig. 4A) has been reported with amikacin or gentamicin [49]. Alternatively, the use of an in-house–manufactured delivery system has also been reported [50] by using an intravenous fluid bag and fenestrated catheter placed inside the joint or affected area (see Fig. 4B). In this report [50], 32 cases of synovial sepsis

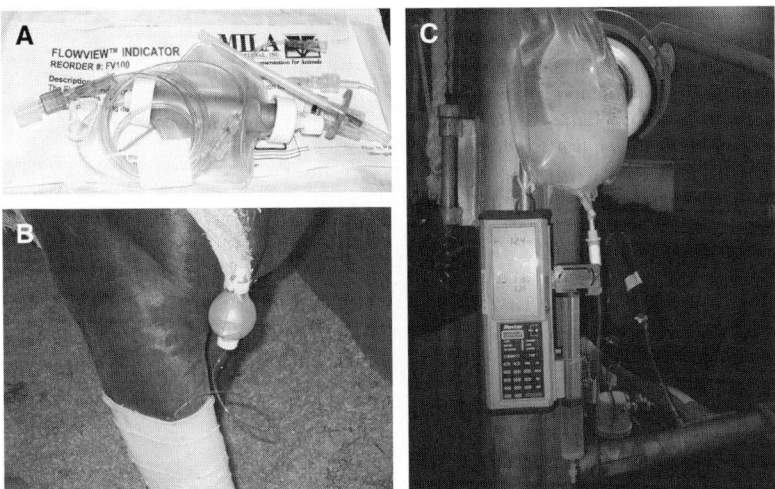

Fig. 4. (*A*) Commercial CRI pump for antimicrobial delivery. (*B*) Commercial CRI in a case with infectious tenosynovitis. Please note the balloon containing the antimicrobial solution and the line going into the bandage and connecting to the catheter part of the infusion system and in-house manufactured system. (*C*) Electronic syringe to infuse at a predetermined and constant rate using the in-house manufactured infusion system.

were resolved. Infected synovial structures treated with this system included the distal interphalangeal, metacarpophalangeal/tarsophalangeal, intercarpal, radiocarpal, scapulohumeral, tarsocrural, and medial femoropatellar joints; the carpal canal; and the digital, tarsal, and extensor carpi radialis tendon sheaths. Horses tolerate the tubing well with no apparent discomfort and with mild soft tissue swelling as the only reported complication [50].

Advantages of a CRI delivery system manufactured in-house include the ability to provide high concentrations of the appropriate antimicrobial to the site frequently and conveniently, ease of application, the possibility of lavaging the joint (if needed) using the same system, and comfort to the horse. In the authors' experience with the commercially available CRI system, intrasynovial catheter problems, such as blockage and breakage, are not uncommon. The advantage of the commercially available system is the small size of the intrasynovial catheter, which may minimize inflammation, and the constant drug release, which may be more relevant for time-dependent antimicrobials than for concentration-dependent antimicrobials. Previous studies investigating the CRI of gentamicin into a synovial cavity in horses have shown that there were no significant effects on histologic scores of articular cartilage damage or synovial membrane inflammation [51]. At a gentamicin dose rate of 0.17 ± 0.02 mg/kg/h, intra-articular CRI resulted in synovial fluid gentamicin concentrations greater than 100 times the MIC reported for common equine pathogens [51]. Aminoglycosides exert an important PAE as described previously.

Direct intra-articular injection

Antimicrobials, such as gentamicin, amikacin, and ceftiofur, can also be administered in a joint by direct daily injection [52]. This technique results in high concentrations of intrasynovial antimicrobials; however, it requires daily preparation of the joint for injection and involves repeated trauma to the synovial capsule and membrane. It is unknown whether daily injection is preferable over the placement of an infusion system. In our practice, the prophylactic use of direct intra-articular antimicrobials during joint surgery is replacing their systemic use in an effort to avoid gastrointestinal tract side effects associated with systemic antimicrobial use.

Regional perfusion

Antimicrobial concentrations several times higher than the MIC of common equine pathogens in a region of interest of the distal extremity can be achieved by the administration of a drug solution into the vasculature of a selected portion of the extremity that has been previously isolated from the systemic circulation by the controlled application of a tourniquet. This is termed *regional limb perfusion*, and, in our opinion, it has greatly contributed to the successful treatment of musculoskeletal infections. Adequate vascular isolation is essential to perform this procedure successfully [53].

Penetration of the perfusate into tissues of a selected area has been demonstrated by venography [54]. During RLP, high concentration and pressure gradients between the intravascular and extravascular compartments are obtained, allowing diffusion of the antimicrobial into the surrounding tissues, including the poorly vascularized tissues where bacteria are protected from systemically circulating antimicrobials [54].

RLP techniques are limited to the distal extremity because it is impossible to isolate regions of the proximal extremity. Therefore, areas above the midradius and midtibia in the forelimb and hind limb, respectively, are not good candidates for this therapeutic modality. In these regions, the local use of alternative delivery systems, such as CRI devices or placement of PMMA beads or antimicrobial-impregnated collagen in the infected area, is better indicated.

There are two modalities for performing RLP: intravenous and intraosseous. During intravenous regional limb perfusion (IVRLP), the veins selected include the cephalic, saphenous, and palmar or plantar metacarpal or metatarsal veins. Any visible and accessible vein can be used safely to administer antimicrobials, however. The arterial route is discouraged because it has been associated with severe side effects, such as endothelial damage [55]. The antimicrobial solution can also be administered via an intraosseous route using a specially designed screw with a luer connection attached to a previously cannulated cortical screw. The specially designed screw is placed into the medullary cavity of the metacarpal or metatarsal bone, tibia, or radius.

To perform RLP in standing horses, adequate chemical restraint by conventional means is recommended. Ideally, the area to be perfused should be exsanguinated by using an Esmarch bandage (Fig. 5A). When the intravenous route is to be used, superficial vein catheterization before the exsanguination is recommended, because the vein collapses after exsanguination and catheterization can be difficult. RLP can be performed without previous exsanguination [53,56,57].

A tourniquet is applied proximal to the proposed injection site. Although tourniquets should ideally fulfill certain requirements of pressure and width, clinically, it seems that the use of manual systems, such a rubber band 10 to 15 cm in width, is adequate (see Fig. 5B). For intravenous administration, after the placement of a tourniquet, an 18- or 20-gauge, 1-in (adults) or 22-gauge, 1-in (foals) butterfly needle or an intravenous over-the-needle catheter can be used to access the selected vein. Smaller diameter needles can also be used and cause less damage to the blood endothelium, which is important if repeated perfusions are to be performed [58]. When using smaller needles, however, rapid injection of the perfusate should be avoided. The selection of an intraosseous route is mostly based on the clinician's preference and whether or not a vein can be identified. In cases with extensive posttraumatic cellulitis, the identification of a vascular portal may be difficult and the use of the intraosseous route would be preferable. When using the intraosseous route, a cannulated screw can be placed in the standing horse under sedation and using local anesthesia. The procedure should be performed aseptically in a clean and well-lit area (Fig. 6). The placement of a cannulated screw or even the end of an intravenous administration system requires the creation of a hole in the medullary cavity of the selected bone [59]. Under standing sedation and local anesthesia or general anesthesia, hole creation is performed by making small skin and periosteum incisions and drilling the bone. The portal should ideally be located far from

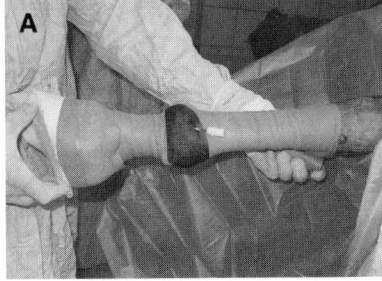 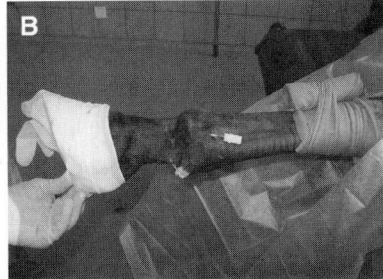

Fig. 5. Esmarch bandage (*A*) and tourniquet (*B*).

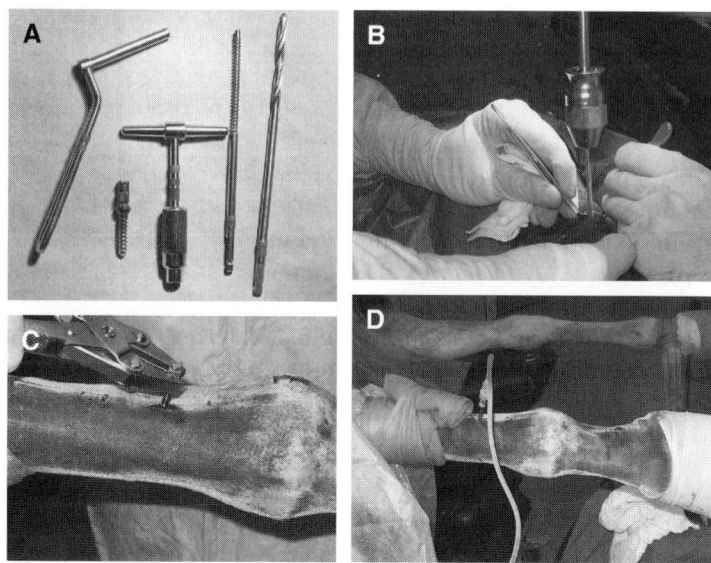

Fig. 6. Technique for RLP using the intraosseous technique. (*A*) Equipment needed to place a cannulated intraosseous screw system (drill not shown). From left to right, a 4.5-mm guide, an in-house manufactured cannulated 4.5-mm cortical screw 26 mm in length with a luer attachment welded to the screw head, a T-shaped handle to tap the screw hole, a 4.5 tap, and a 3.2 drill bit. (*B*) Tapping of the hole after drilling. (*C*) Placing the screw in the hole. (*D*) Intravenous infusion set attached to the screw head to perform perfusion. Please note the tourniquet in place proximad to the perfusion point.

any major vessel, nerve, synovial structure, or tendon [60]. During intraosseous perfusion, high medullary pressures are created, which can cause leakage of perfusate at the interface between the bone and the intraosseous needle or intravenous tube [59]. Leakage of perfusate can be reduced by sealing the interface with cyanoacrylate ester glue [60] or by using a well-fitted cannulated screw [59,61,62].

During IVRLP, maximal infusion pressures are usually less than 15 psi, and during intraosseous regional limb perfusion (IORLP), pressures of 450 psi have been reached [60]. This high pressure may be painful [63,64], because lower values of intramedullary pressure have been found to cause lameness in a horse [65]. Clinically, horses seem to tolerate IORLP. A small percentage of horses may react to the injection process. In these horses, a small volume (2 to 3 mL) of local anesthetic could be perfused ahead of time into the medullary cavity to minimize the painful response in the awake horse. Nonetheless, after IORLP, horses do not usually show evidence of lameness, possibly because the defect left open in the bone allows the intramedullary pressure to equilibrate with the outside pressure [60]. The cannulated screw is usually left in place for the duration of the treatment, and the screw head must be protected by a bandage, because screw head breakage may occur and result in the permanent implantation of a screw in the medullary cavity (see Fig. 6).

The antimicrobial solution can be administered as a bolus, commonly by hand [59], or as a slow controlled infusion, usually at a rate of 2 mL/min [60,62,66], by hand or using an electronic injection pump (see Fig. 6). For the IORLP technique, high intramedullary pressures offer more resistance to injection. Therefore, small-volume syringes (2–5 mL) are needed for IORLP by hand [61,63], whereas slow-controlled IORLP requires high-pressure pumps, such as angiographic injectors (see Fig. 6) [60]. In cases in which vancomycin is administered via IVRLP, the infusion rate should be limited to 2 mL/min and at a C_{max} of 5 mg/mL because of its irritating nature and the possibility of thrombophlebitis [67]. Once the injection is complete, no special care is required at the injection site.

Antimicrobial selection for regional perfusion

The antimicrobial to be perfused must be hydrosoluble and soluble in a balanced polyionic solution (0.9% sodium chloride or Ringer's lactate). Antimicrobial selection should be based on culture and sensitivity results from infected tissue samples taken before the initiation of antimicrobial therapy. Initial antimicrobial selection can be made according to the most common pathogens and the clinical case characteristics [1,2,4,68,69]. In studies on the susceptibility of equine isolates, amikacin has demonstrated the greatest efficacy against pathogens seen in horses with orthopedic problems, including gram-positive and gram-negative bacteria [69,70]. The use of gentamicin has been reduced because of the emergence of resistance [3]. Third-generation cephalosporins, such as ceftiofur, also show high activity [70] and have been experimentally administered using RLP in cattle [71]. In cases of iatrogenic infections caused by multiresistant bacteria, such as MRSA, local administration of highly effective narrow-spectrum antimicrobial drugs has been necessary [18], but their use in clinical cases by RLP has not been described.

RLP maintains high antimicrobial concentrations for a period approximating or exceeding 24 hours in some cases [14,60]. The PK-PD properties of the antimicrobial dictate dosage and schedule regimens of the drug. Time-dependent antimicrobials, such as penicillins, cephalosporins, carbapenems, and macrolides, require maintenance of a concentration greater than the MIC for antibacterial activity [72,73], and increases in the C_{max} do not augment the killing rate [74–76]. Conversely, maximal efficacy of concentration-dependent antimicrobials, such as aminoglycosides or fluoroquinolones, is determined by a high C_{max}, because these drugs exert prolonged persistent postadministration effects [72,73].

These characteristics allow aminoglycosides to be administered once daily, whereas β-lactams require maintenance of a minimum concentration during a high proportion of the dosing interval for adequate antibacterial activity [74]. In clinical practice, RLP is usually performed once daily or once every 2 to 3 days. According to this schedule, concentration-dependent antimicrobials are more suitable for proper antibacterial activity. The use of time-dependent antimicrobials for RLP can be justified, however, because this technique is likely to result in therapeutic concentrations of the antimicrobial in infected ischemic tissues for a longer time than is possible with systemic administration [21]. In addition, once the tourniquet is released, the high antimicrobial concentrations achieved in the surrounding tissues serve as an antimicrobial depot as the drug slowly elutes [54]. Concentrations of aminoglycosides in the target region have remained above the desired level for periods equal to or longer than 24 hours in healthy horses [14,60]. We have investigated the use of RLP-delivered vancomycin, a time-dependent glycopeptide, in horses. Synovial fluid concentrations in the metacarpophalangeal joint remained above the MIC value for approximately 20 hours, whereas plasma concentrations associated with toxic side effects were avoided [67,77]. Further studies on the regional pharmacokinetics of time-dependent antimicrobials administered by RLP would be important, however, so as to avoid possible misuse of these antimicrobials in clinical cases.

The pharmacodynamic particularities of each drug must be considered. For instance, because of the strong affinity of ceftiofur for proteins (a time-dependent cephalosporin antimicrobial) and its active metabolite desfuroylceftiofur, the higher the concentrations that can be achieved with RLP, the longer the drug remains above therapeutic concentrations. This prolongs the dosing interval and makes RLP a more practical therapy than systemic administration. Regional plasma and synovial fluid concentrations of ceftiofur were much higher than MIC values even for resistant organisms after its regional administration in cattle [56] and horses [78].

Many commonly used antimicrobials in equine medicine can be delivered using RLP. Several studies have investigated the clinical efficacy, safety, distribution, and pharmacokinetics of the most frequently used antimicrobials for orthopedic infections in horses [59,60,62,66,79]. The use of antimicrobials causing vascular toxicity, such as enrofloxacin, has been questioned [58], and excessive doses of antimicrobials commonly administered by RLP can also be harmful to the vessels [80,81]. Nevertheless, in a recent study, it was documented that the experimental use of enrofloxacin (1.5 mg/kg) delivered via IVRLP achieved sustained concentrations greater than the MIC in subcutaneous tissues, radiocarpal joint synovial fluid, and bone marrow of the third metacarpal bone without documented side effects [82].

The medullary cavities of bones are composed of large numbers of venous sinusoids surrounded by bone marrow cells and provide ready access to the systemic circulation [83]. Therefore, although no studies have been performed to evaluate the effect of antimicrobial delivery using RLP on the medullary sinusoids, similar reactions to those occurring in the vascular endothelium could be expected.

Clinical use

Synovial antimicrobial concentrations after RLP are not as high as those achieved after direct intra-articular injection [84], but concentrations as high as 100 times greater than the MIC for periods of up to 36 hours have been reported [14,57,59,60,62,79]. Compared with systemic antimicrobial delivery, RLP produces higher regional antimicrobial concentrations and C_{max}/MIC ratios 3 to 30 times higher than the target ratios of systemic therapy [59,60,62].

Intravenous and intraosseous techniques have been used for perfusion of digital structures of horses [14,57,59,79]. Infusion into the first phalanx is an alternative, but antimicrobial concentrations in the metacarpophalangeal joint were lower compared with IORLP in the distal metacarpus or IVRLP via the cephalic vein [57]. Higher C_{max}s and areas under the curve (AUCs) were observed in the distal interphalangeal joint after intravenous infusion compared with the intraosseous route, but no differences were observed in the fetlock joint [59]. For tarsal joint perfusion, intravenous infusion into the saphenous vein is preferred to intraosseous delivery into the distal tibia or proximal metacarpus, because higher concentrations are achieved in synovial fluid and the procedure is easier to perform [62]. Both intraosseous routes delivered adequate concentrations of the antimicrobial to the tibiotarsal joint, however [62].

Fewer studies have been performed to investigate the antimicrobial concentrations in osseous tissues [14,79]. Bones located in the region subjected to RLP are also perfused [67,77,79], which has been questioned after intra-articular administration of antimicrobials [85]. Intra-articular administration and RLP produced bone concentrations of gentamicin that were not significantly different, however [52]. Standing intraosseous distal limb perfusion resulted in local gentamicin concentrations in the digital bones that exceeded the reported MIC of pathogens commonly implicated in equine orthopedic infections [14]. Comparison of perfusate distribution to the different tissues and structures has not been thoroughly studied. The times to reach C_{max} and maximal elimination half-life in each digital synovial structure were similar using both delivery routes [59,67]. Antimicrobial concentrations achieved in the digital tendon sheath were similar [59] or lower [57] than those observed in joints. After IVRLP with amikacin at a dose of 125 mg, similar amikacin concentrations in synovium were found in the metacarpophalangeal and distal interphalangeal joints [79]. We found significantly higher concentrations of vancomycin after IVRLP in the distal interphalangeal joint compared with the metacarpophalangeal joint, however [67]. Surrogate parameters (slope of the elimination phase of the concentration-time curve [β (min^{-1})], elimination half-life [$t_{1/2}$ β (min)], AUC_t

[μg · min/mL], and mean residence time of vancomycin [MRT_t (μg · min/mL)]) were different after IVRLP between metacarpophalangeal and distal interphalangeal joints (see Fig. 1) [67].

All these studies on regional pharmacokinetics of antimicrobials have been conducted in healthy animals. It is important to note that vascularity can change in septic conditions, thus altering antimicrobial concentrations and pharmacokinetics. Because antimicrobial activity at infected sites can be reduced compared with noninfected sites, pharmacokinetic investigations under septic conditions and more case studies are necessary.

RLP has been more effective than systemic antimicrobial administration for the treatment of experimentally induced joint infections [60] and has resulted in the elimination of infection in clinical cases of septic arthritis and osteomyelitis [66,81]. In experimental chronic infections in rabbits, antimicrobial RLP produced negative bone cultures in 70% of the animals, whereas in those rabbits treated with systemic antimicrobials, only 35% of the animals yielded negative cultures [85]. The efficacy of the RLP technique was evaluated in the horse using experimentally induced septic arthritis [66]. In this study, four horses were treated with IVRLP of gentamicin after an experimental infection of the antebrachiocarpal joint with *S aureus*. Three horses were successfully perfused, and two (66%) of those three horses had culture-negative synovial fluid and membrane within 24 hours after bacterial inoculation [66]. The synovial fluid white blood cell count was also significantly decreased [66]. The efficacy of RLP is difficult to assess in clinical cases, however, because it is usually used as an adjunct to conventional therapy (systemic antimicrobials, lavage, debridement, anti-inflammatory drugs, and rest). Treatment and management strategies vary between cases, which precludes direct comparison between cases and valid conclusions unless an extremely large case study is undertaken to control for the effect of different treatments. It is our impression that the favorable clinical response of cases in which antimicrobial RLP has been performed supports the clinical application of the RLP technique [82,85,86]. Survival rates are high (>80%), with many horses returning to riding soundness [82,85,86].

Antimicrobial dose for regional perfusion

The optimal antimicrobial dose for RLP is not known. Doses of amikacin as low as 125 mg produced extremely high concentrations (235 ± 82 μg/mL) in synovial fluid [79], and doses of amikacin from 125 to 250 mg or of gentamicin from 100 to 300 mg have been used successfully in adult horses [82]. Higher doses of aminoglycosides, between 500 mg [35,47,57,59,72,82] and 1 g [60,62,66,86], are commonly used clinically, however. β-Lactams have been used less commonly, but RLP with sodium or potassium penicillin (dose of 1×10^6 IU) [60,86,87], ticarcillin–clavulanic acid (1 g) [88], and sodium ampicillin (9 g) [60] has produced satisfactory clinical outcomes. For young foals, lower doses of amikacin, such as 50 mg, are recommended [81], but doses as high as 500 mg have also been used with a satisfactory outcome [61]. High interindividual variability of tissue concentrations has been observed in experimental studies [59,60,62]. Dosing according to the limb volume or weight has been indicated as the most accurate method [60,79]; however, this is not practical. Some authors recommend the administration of one third of the daily systemic antimicrobial dose as the RLP dose [35,54]. This would mean gentamicin or amikacin at a dose of approximately 1 g for RLP of a 450- to 500-kg horse, which has been frequently used clinically [86]. In our practice, we administer gentamicin or amikacin at a dose of 500 mg for each RLP in an adult horse.

Occasionally, two different antimicrobials (eg, a β-lactam and an aminoglycoside) have been combined in the same RLP [61,86]. Some drugs show synergistic effects when administered concurrently [85]; however, other combinations can inactivate each other. Aminoglycosides and β-lactams are synergistic against some pathogens; the cell wall disruption caused by the β-lactam allows for increased intracellular accumulation of the aminoglycoside for a synergistic effect. Care must be taken in the administration of such a combination, however, because aminoglycosides can be inactivated in vitro by some β-lactams [37]. After their combined administration using separate syringes in a clinical case, successful results were observed [61], but it is generally recommended that RLP be performed with a single antimicrobial, with antimicrobial selection based on culture and sensitivity test results [81].

When antimicrobials with known systemic toxic effects, such as aminoglycosides, are used for RLP, concurrent systemic administration of the antimicrobial should be avoided or plasma drug concentrations should be monitored for toxicity, because plasma concentrations may rise considerably after releasing the tourniquet [60,61]. Although this is unlikely to cause complications in adult horses, it may be important in systemically compromised foals.

Volume of perfusate solution for regional perfusion

The optimal volume of perfusate is not known. As a general rule, the higher the volume perfused, the higher is the intravascular pressure that is achieved, and thus the higher is the drug diffusion rate into the surrounding tissues [54,89].

Antimicrobial perfusion distal to the antebrachium of adult equine limbs has been commonly performed using perfusate solution at a volume of 60 mL [59,60,66,79,81], whereas 20 mL [86], and 40 mL [57] have also been used clinically, and the results were satisfactory in 18 of 24 horses surviving in one study [86]. Similar volumes have been used for perfusion of other anatomic locations, such as the carpus and tarsus [60,62,66]. In foals, smaller volumes from 10 to 35 mL are recommended for IORLP or IVRLP [61,81].

After carpal perfusion with a perfusate volume of 60 mL, an even distribution of contrast media and India ink through the pericarpal tissues, synovial membranes, and carpal bones was evident [60]. Contrast was observed radiographically within the carpal joints [60]. Similarly, after distal limb perfusion with radiopaque dye at a volume of 40 mL, radiography showed complete distribution of the contrast through the digital tissues [86]. Using radiographic contrast at a rate of 50 to 60 mL for horses undergoing digital venography, we have observed complete digital perfusion. We routinely use a volume of 60 mL for antimicrobial RLP in the adult horse. In a recent study, the perfusate volume was determined according to the horse's weight (0.1 mL/kg), which could be more proportional to the animal size and weight [14]. When perfusate volumes of 30 mL and 60 mL were compared for tarsal perfusion, higher antimicrobial concentrations in synovial fluid were reached after administration of the higher volume [62].

Distribution of perfusate after regional perfusion

Because the perfusate is injected intravenously, the first investigators recommended that the antimicrobial should be infused from a point located distal to the infection site [54,60]. In more recent studies, however, RLP with radiopaque dye injected into the lateral digital vein at the level of the proximal sesamoid bone confirmed complete perfusion of the digit within seconds after intravenous injection [86]. Therefore, an injection portal distal to the infection site is no longer considered necessary. In the case of infections involving the hoof, a superficial proximally located vein should be catheterized with the catheter directed distad toward the foot [60].

Perfusions with radiopaque dye and India ink have shown that with the intravenous or intraosseous route, the perfusate distributes following the venous system [60,62,86]. When the tourniquet is applied around the diaphysis, the perfusate may enter the medullary cavity and reach the systemic circulation through the proximal diaphyseal and epiphyseal vessels [66]. In a radiographic study comparing both techniques, greater density of contrast material was observed in the tarsal venous system after intravenous perfusion compared with intraosseous perfusion [62]. Perfusion with 99m-technetium pertechnetate resulted in the same radionuclide activity in the distal equine limb after intravenous and intraosseous techniques, however [53].

Antimicrobial concentrations achieved in structures located distal to the infusion site may reach 25 to 100 times the MIC [57,59,62,79]; recently, we obtained significantly higher synovial antimicrobial concentrations in the distal interphalangeal joint compared with the metacarpophalangeal joint after intravenous perfusion of the distal limb of horses at the level of the proximal sesamoid region [67].

Number of perfusions and selection of regional perfusion procedure

There is no one general treatment protocol (ie, the number and frequency of RLP or dose) to achieve the resolution of orthopedic infections. One to nine procedures have been used for different clinical cases, and they are usually performed once daily or every 2 or 3 days. In human patients with long-standing infections, the antimicrobials were regionally infused twice daily for 5 to 7 days [54], which might be indicated in equine patients when using time-dependent antimicrobials. Other equine patients have responded after a single perfusion. Factors determining the efficacy of the RLP procedure include the characteristics of the infectious process being treated, the duration of the septic process before treatment, the ability to debride the infected and necrotic tissue, the susceptibility pattern of the organism, the dose and action mechanism of the antimicrobial, the chronicity and extent of the infection, and the technique used for RLP [61]. In practice, the number of perfusions is usually determined on the basis of clinical evidence of improvement. In foals undergoing IVRLP, systemic administration of antimicrobials before the procedure has been recommended to prevent septicemia [81], although in most cases, foals are already undergoing systemic antimicrobial treatment.

Comparative studies have not been conducted to determine the optimum duration of each perfusion. The time that the tourniquet should be maintained could be dependent on the physicochemical, pharmacologic, and pharmacodynamic characteristics of the antimicrobial; microbiologic factors; and individual attributes of the patient and the clinical case. In those cases in which the antimicrobial solution is slowly infused, tourniquet maintenance for a longer period than the infusion time is preferred so as to allow the antimicrobial to distribute completely into the tissues [67].

The prophylactic use of antimicrobial RLP before long surgical procedures seems interesting, and its efficacy has been reported in human patients before implantation of knee prostheses [90]. In a prospective study including 160 patients and 205 prostheses, only one superficial infection was detected and no deep infections involving the prosthesis were identified during a 2-year follow-up period. This has not been described in horses; however, prophylactic RLP could be of benefit for long surgical procedures (eg, complex fractures, difficult arthrodesis) that are associated with a higher risk of infection [91].

Summary

Overall, the local delivery of antimicrobials is a valuable therapeutic tool with a low morbidity, is practical to use, and is well tolerated by horses. Clinically, its use has allowed equine practitioners to achieve better results when treating musculoskeletal infections, and it represents an extremely useful tool in the practitioner's armamentarium against these types of infections.

The technique is indicated to combat orthopedic infections involving bones, joints, physes, tendon sheaths, and foot tissues. Optimal treatment must include other approaches, such as systemic antimicrobial therapy and surgical debridement and lavage, and monitoring of the clinical progression of the patient can help to determine the ideal protocol for each patient.

References

[1] Steel CM, Hunt AR, Adams PL, et al. Factors associated with prognosis for survival and athletic use in foals with septic arthritis: 93 cases (1987–1994). J Am Vet Med Assoc 1999; 215:973–7.
[2] Meijer MC, van Weeren PR, Rijkenhuizen AB. Clinical experiences of treating septic arthritis in the equine by repeated joint lavage: a series of 39 cases. J Vet Med A Physiol Pathol Clin Med 2000;47:351–65.
[3] Clark C, Greenwood S, Dowling PM, et al. A review of bacterial isolates of equine origin (1998–2003) and implications for antimicrobial therapy. J Vet Pharmacol Ther 2004;27: 385–7.
[4] Schneider RK, Bramlage LR, Moore RM, et al. A retrospective study of 192 horses affected with septic arthritis/tenosynovitis. Equine Vet J 1992;24:436–42.
[5] Weese JS, Archambault M, Willey BM, et al. Methicillin-resistant Staphylococcus aureus in horses and horse personnel, 2000–2002. Emerg Infect Dis 2005;11:430–5.
[6] Albihn A, Baverud V, Magnusson U. Uterine microbiology and antimicrobial susceptibility in isolated bacteria from mares with fertility problems. Acta Vet Scand 2003;44:121–9.
[7] Salmon SA, Watts JL, Yancey RJ Jr. In vitro activity of ceftiofur and its primary metabolite, desfuroylceftiofur, against organisms of veterinary importance. J Vet Diagn Invest 1996;8: 332–6.
[8] Mills ML, Rush BR, St. Jean G, et al. Determination of synovial fluid and serum concentrations, and morphologic effects of intraarticular ceftiofur sodium in horses. Vet Surg 2000;29: 398–406.
[9] Carrillo NA, Giguere S, Gronwall RR, et al. Disposition of orally administered cefpodoxime proxetil in foals and adult horses and minimum inhibitory concentration of the drug against common bacterial pathogens of horses. Am J Vet Res 2005;66:30–5.
[10] Orsini JA, Moate PJ, Engiles J, et al. Cefotaxime kinetics in plasma and synovial fluid following intravenous administration in horses. J Vet Pharmacol Ther 2004;27:293–8.
[11] Gardner SY, Papich MG. Comparison of cefepime pharmacokinetics in neonatal foals and adult dogs. J Vet Pharmacol Ther 2001;24:187–92.
[12] Guglick MA, MacAllister CG, Clarke CR, et al. Pharmacokinetics of cefepime and comparison with those of ceftiofur in horses. Am J Vet Res 1998;59:458–63.
[13] Jacks SS, Giguere S, Nguyen A. In vitro susceptibilities of Rhodococcus equi and other common equine pathogens to azithromycin, clarithromycin, and 20 other antimicrobials. Antimicrob Agents Chemother 2003;47:1742–5.
[14] Mattson SE, Bouré LP, Pearce SG, et al. Intraosseous gentamicin perfusion of the distal metacarpus in standing horses. Vet Surg 2004;33:180–6.
[15] Vivrette SL, Bostian A, Bermigham E, et al. Quinolone-induced arthropathy in neonatal foals. Proc Am Assoc Equine Pract 2001;47:376–7.
[16] Rodger LD, Carlson GP, Moran ME, et al. Resolution of a left ureteral stone using electrohydraulic lithotripsy in a Thoroughbred colt. J Vet Intern Med 1995;9:280–2.
[17] Bertone AL, Tremaine WH, Macoris DG, et al. Effect of long-term administration of an injectable enrofloxacin solution on physical and musculoskeletal variables in adult horses. J Am Vet Med Assoc 2000;217:1514–21.

[18] Trostle SS, Peavey CL, King DS, et al. Treatment of methicillin-resistant Staphylococcus epidermidis infection following repair of an ulnar fracture and humeroradial joint luxation in a horse. J Am Vet Med Assoc 2001;218:554–9.
[19] Bidgood T, Papich MG. Plasma pharmacokinetics and tissue fluid concentrations of meropenem after intravenous and subcutaneous administration in dogs. Am J Vet Res 2002;63: 1622–8.
[20] Orsini JA, Moate PJ, Boston RC, et al. Pharmacokinetics of imipenem-cilastatin following intravenous administration in healthy adult horses. J Vet Pharmacol Ther 2005;28:355–61.
[21] McKellar QA, Sanchez Bruni SF, Jones DG. Pharmacokinetic/pharmacodynamic relationships of antimicrobial drugs used in veterinary medicine. J Vet Pharmacol Ther 2004;27: 503–14.
[22] Craig WA, Gundmundson S. Postantibiotic effect. In: Lorian V, editor. Antibiotics in laboratory medicine. 3rd edition. Baltimore (MD): Williams & Wilkins; 1991. p. 403–31.
[23] Ariano RE, Nyhlen A, Donnelly JP, et al. Pharmacokinetics and pharmacodynamics of meropenem in febrile neutropenic patients with bacteremia. Ann Pharmacother 2005;39: 32–8.
[24] Knudsen JD, Fuursted K, Raber S, et al. Pharmacodynamics of glycopeptides in the mouse peritonitis model of Streptococcus pneumoniae or Staphylococcus aureus infection. Antimicrob Agents Chemother 2000;44:1247–54.
[25] Holcombe SJ, Schneider RK, Bramlage LR, et al. Use of antibiotic-impregnated polymethyl methacrylate in horses with open or infected fractures or joints: 19 cases (1987–1995). J Am Vet Med Assoc 1997;211:889–93.
[26] Streppa HK, Singer MJ, Budsberg SC. Applications of local antimicrobial delivery systems in veterinary medicine. J Am Vet Med Assoc 2001;219:40–8.
[27] Baxter GM. Instrumentation and techniques for treating orthopaedic infections in horses. Vet Clin North Am Equine Pract 1996;12:303–35.
[28] Schneider RK, Andrea R, Barnes HG. Use of antibiotic-impregnated polymethyl methacrylate for treatment of an open radial fracture in a horse. J Am Vet Med Assoc 1995;207: 1454–7.
[29] Tobias KM, Schneider RK, Besser TE. Use of antimicrobial-impregnated polymethyl methacrylate. J Am Vet Med Assoc 1996;208:841–5.
[30] Butson RJ, Schramme MC, Garlick MH, et al. Treatment of intrasynovial infection with gentamicin-impregnated polymethylmethacrylate beads. Vet Rec 1996;138:460–4.
[31] Ethell MT, Bennett RA, Brown MP, et al. In vitro elution of gentamicin, amikacin, and ceftiofur from polymethylmethacrylate and hydroxyapatite cement. Vet Surg 2000;29:375–82.
[32] Booth TM, Butson RJ, Clegg PD, et al. Treatment of sepsis in the small tarsal joints of 11 horses with gentamicin-impregnated polymethylmethacrylate beads. Vet Rec 2001;148: 376–80.
[33] Farnsworth KD, White NA II, Robertson J. The effect of implanting gentamicin-impregnated polymethylmethacrylate beads in the tarsocrural joint of the horse. Vet Surg 2001; 30:126–31.
[34] Richardson DW. Local antibiotic delivery in equine orthopaedics. In: Proceedings of the 13th Annual American College of Veterinary Surgeons Veterinary Symposium. Washington (DC); 2003.
[35] Murray WR. Use of antibiotic-containing bone cement. Clin Orthop 1984;190:89–95.
[36] Hughes S, Field CA, Kennedy MR, et al. Cephalosporins in bone cement: studies in vitro and in vivo. J Bone Joint Surg Br 1979;61:96–100.
[37] Wallace SM, Chan LY. In vitro interaction of aminoglycosides with beta-lactam penicillins. Antimicrob Agents Chemother 1985;28:274–81.
[38] Steiner A, Hirsbrunner G, Rytz U, et al. The treatment of articular and bone infections in large animals with gentamicin-impregnated collagen sponges. Schweiz Arch Tierheilkd 2000;142:292–8.

[39] Owen MR, Moores AP, Coe RJ. Management of MRSA septic arthritis in a dog using a gentamicin-impregnated collagen sponge. J Small Anim Pract 2004;45:609–12.
[40] Summerhays G. Treatment of traumatically induced synovial sepsis in horses with gentamicin-impregnated collagen sponges. Vet Rec 2000;147:184–8.
[41] Sorenson TS, Sorenson AI, Merser S. Rapid release of gentamicin from collagen sponge: in vitro comparison with plastic beads. Acta Orthop Scand 1990;61:353–6.
[42] Humphrey SJ, Mehta S, Seaber AV, et al. Pharmacokinetics of a degradable drug delivery system in bone. Clin Orthop 1998;349:218–24.
[43] Costantino PD, Friedman CD, Jones K, et al. Hydroxyapatite cement. I. Basic chemistry and histologic properties. Arch Otolaryngol Head Neck Surg 1991;117:379–84.
[44] Santschi EM, McGarvey L. In vitro elution of gentamicin from plaster of Paris beads. Vet Surg 2003;32:128–33.
[45] Trostle SS, Juzwiak JS, Santschi EM. How to use antibiotic impregnated plaster of Paris for alveolar packing after tooth removal. In: Proceedings of the 45th Meeting of the American Association of Equine Practitioners. San Antonio (TX); 2000. p. 180–1.
[46] Li LC, Deng J, Stephens D. Polyanhydride implant for antibiotic delivery—from the bench to the clinic. Adv Drug Deliv Rev 2002;54:963–86.
[47] Cribb NC, Boure LP, Weese JS, et al. Development of amikacin-impregnated hyaluronan implants for the treatment of septic arthritis in horses. Vet Surg 2005;34:E5.
[48] Cook VL, Bertone AL, Kowalski JJ, et al. Biodegradable drug delivery systems for gentamicin release and treatment of synovial membrane infection. Vet Surg 1999;28:233–41.
[49] Adams SB, Lescun TB. How to treat septic joints with constant intra-articular infusion of gentamicin or amikacin. In: Proceedings of the 45th Meeting of the American Association of Equine Practitioners, San Antonio, TX. 2000;45:188–92.
[50] Hogan PM. How to treat synovial sepsis using a modified indwelling extension set tubing. In: Proceedings of the 49th Meeting of the American Association of Equine Practitioners, Denver, CO. 2004;49:224–6.
[51] Lescun TB, Adams SB, Wu CC, et al. Continuous infusion of gentamicin into the tarsocrural joint of horses. Am J Vet Res 2000;61:407–12.
[52] Werner LA, Hardy J, Bertone AL. Bone gentamicin concentration after intra-articular injection or regional intravenous perfusion in the horse. Vet Surg 2003;32:559–65.
[53] Mattson SE, Bouré LP, Pearce SG, et al. Comparison of standing intraosseous and intravenous 99m technetium pertechnate infusion of the distal limb in horses using scintigraphic imaging. In: Proceedings of the 12th Annual Meeting of the American College of Veterinary Surgeons, San Diego, CA. 2002:16.
[54] Finsterbusch A, Weinberg H. Venous perfusion of the limb with antibiotics for osteomyelitis and other chronic infections. J Bone Joint Surg Am 1972;54:1227–34.
[55] Gottlob R. Endothelschäden nach intravasalen Injektionen und Infusionen. Verh Dtsch Ges Pathol 1972;56:563–5.
[56] Navarre CB, Zhang L, Sunkara G, et al. Ceftiofur distribution in plasma and joint fluid following regional limb injection in cattle. J Vet Pharmacol Ther 1999;22:13–9.
[57] Harriss FK, Galupo LD, Van Hoomgmoed LM, et al. Antibiotic delivery to the forelimb digital flexor tendon sheath and metacarpophalangeal joint of horses by three regional limb perfusion techniques. In: Proceedings of the 29th Annual Conference of the Veterinary Orthopedic Society. 2002:63.
[58] Richardson DW. Local antimicrobial delivery in equine orthopedics. In: Proceedings of the 13th Annual Symposium of the American College of Veterinary Surgeons, Washington, DC. 2003:479.
[59] Butt TD, Bailey JV, Dowling PM, et al. Comparison of 2 techniques for regional antibiotic delivery to the equine forelimb: intraosseous perfusion vs. intravenous perfusion. Can Vet J 2001;42:617–22.
[60] Whitehair KJ, Blevins WE, Fessler JF, et al. Regional perfusion of the equine carpus for antibiotic delivery. Vet Surg 1992;21:279–85.

[61] Kettner NU, Parker JE, Watrous BJ. Intraosseous regional perfusion for treatment of septic physitis in a two-week-old foal. J Am Vet Med Assoc 2003;222:346–50.
[62] Scheuch BC, Van Hoogmoed LM, Wilson WD, et al. Comparison of intraosseous or intravenous infusion for delivery of amikacin sulfate to the tibiotarsal joint of horses. Am J Vet Res 2002;63:374–80.
[63] Whitehair KL. Regional limb perfusion with antibiotics. In: Proceedings of the Fifth Annual Symposium of the American College of Veterinary Surgeons, Chicago. 1995:59–61.
[64] Welch RD, Waldron MJ, Hulse DA, et al. Intraosseous infusion using the osteoport implant in the caprine tibia. J Orthop Res 1992;10:789–99.
[65] Morisset S, Hawkins JF, Kooreman K. High intraosseous pressure as a cause if lameness in a horse with a degloving injury of the metatarsus. J Am Vet Med Assoc 1999;10:1478–80.
[66] Whitehair KJ, Bowersock TL, Blevins WE, et al. Regional perfusion for antibiotic treatment of experimentally induced septic arthritis. Vet Surg 1992;21:367–73.
[67] Rubio-Martínez L, López-Sanromán J, Cruz AM, et al. Intravenous distal limb perfusion with vancomycin in the horse. Am J Vet Res 2005;66:2107–13.
[68] Lapointe JM, Laverty S, Lavoie JP. Septic arthritis in 15 Standardbred racehorses after intra-articular injection. Equine Vet J 1992;24:430–4.
[69] Moore RM, Schneider RK, Kowalski J, et al. Antimicrobial susceptibility of bacterial isolates from 233 horses with musculoskeletal infection during 1979–1989. Equine Vet J 1992;24:450–6.
[70] Adamson PJ, Wilson WD, Hirsh DC, et al. Susceptibility of equine bacterial isolates to antimicrobial agents. Am J Vet Res 1985;46:447–50.
[71] Gagnon H, Ferguson JG, Papich MG, et al. Single-dose pharmacokinetics of cefazolin in bovine synovial fluid after intravenous regional injection. J Vet Pharmacol Ther 1994;17:31–7.
[72] Craig WA. Pharmacokinetic/pharmacodynamic parameters: rationale for antibacterial dosing of mice and men. Clin Infect Dis 1998;26:1–10.
[73] Zhanel GG. Influence of pharmacokinetic and pharmacodynamic principles on antibiotic selection. Curr Infect Dis Rep 2001;3:29–34.
[74] Silley P, Brewster G. Kill kinetics of the cephalosporin antibiotics cephalexin and cefuroxime against bacteria of veterinary importance. Vet Rec 1988;123:343–5.
[75] Burgess DS. Pharmacodynamic principles of antimicrobial therapy in the prevention of resistance. Chest 1999;115(Suppl):19S–23S.
[76] Woodnutt G. Pharmacodynamics to combat antibiotic resistance. J Antimicrob Chemother 2000;46:25–31.
[77] Rubio-Martínez L, López-Sanromán J, Cruz AM, et al. Intraosseous distal limb perfusion with vancomycin in the horse. In: Proceedings of the 12th Congress of European Society of Veterinary Orthopaedics and Traumatology. 2004:249.
[78] Pille F, DeBaere S, Ceelen L, et al. Synovial fluid and plasma concentrations of ceftiofur after regional intravenous perfusion in the horse. Vet Surg 2005;34:610–7.
[79] Murphey ED, Santschi EM, Papich MG. Regional intravenous perfusion of the distal limb of horses with amikacin sulfate. J Vet Pharmacol Ther 1999;22:68–71.
[80] Steiner A, Ossent P, Mathis GA. Die intravenöse Stauungsanästhesie/-antibiose beim Rind—Indikationen, Technik, Komplikationen. Schweiz Arch Tierheilkd 1990;132:227–37.
[81] Santschi EM, Adams SB, Murphey ED. How to perform equine intravenous digital perfusion. In: Proceedings of the 44th Annual Convention of the American Association of Equine Practitioners, Baltimore, MD. 1998:198–201.
[82] Parra A, Lugo J, Boothe D, et al. Pharmacokinetics of enrofloxacin and amikacin after intravenous regional perfusion of the distal limb in standing horses. Vet Surg 2005;34:E20.
[83] Nickel R, Schurmman A, Wille KH, et al. Osteology. In: Nickel R, Schummer A, Seiferle E, editors. The anatomy of the domestic animals, vol. 1. The locomotor system of domestic mammals. 5th edition. Berlin-Hamburg: Verlag Paul Parey; 1986. p. 9–168.
[84] Tate LP, Berry CR, King C. Comparison of peripheral-to-central circulation delivery times between intravenous and intraosseous infusion in foals. Equine Vet Educ 2003;15:201–6.

[85] Bertone AL. Infectious arthritis. In: Ross MW, Dyson SJ, editors. Diagnosis and management of lameness in the horse. 1st edition. Philadelphia: WB Saunders; 2003. p. 598–605.
[86] Lloyd KC, Stover SM, Pascoe JR, et al. Synovial fluid pH, cytologic characteristics and gentamicin concentration after intra-articular administration of the drug in an experimental model of infectious arthritis in horses. Am J Vet Res 1990;51:1363–9.
[87] Finsterbusch A, Argaman M, Sacks T. Bone joint perfusion with antibiotics in the treatment of experimental Staphylococcal infection in rabbits. J Bone Joint Surg Am 1970;52:1424–32.
[88] Palmer SE, Hogan PM. How to perform regional limb perfusion in the standing horse. In: Proceedings of the 45th Annual Convention of the American Association of Equine Practitioners, Albuquerque, NM. 1999:124–7.
[89] Cimetti LJ, Merriam J, D'Oench SN. How to perform intravenous regional limb perfusion using amikacin and DMSO. In: Proceedings of the 50th Annual Convention of the American Association of Equine Practitioners, Denver, CO. 2004:1429.
[90] Dietz O, Kehnscherper G. Intravenöse Stauungsantibiose bei pyogenen Infektionen der distalen Gliedmassenabschnitte des Pferdes. Prakt Tierarzt 1990;71(8):30–3.
[91] Hershberger E, Aeschlimann JR, Moldovan T, et al. Evaluation of bactericidal activities of LY333328, vancomycin, teicoplanin, ampicillin-sulbactam, trovafloxacin, and RP59500 alone or in combination with rifampin or gentamicin against different strains of vancomycin-intermediate Staphylococcus aureus by time-kill curve methods. Antimicrob Agents Chemother 1999;43:717–21.

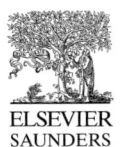

Prevention of Postoperative Infections in Horses

Elizabeth M. Santschi, DVM

Department of Surgical Sciences, School of Veterinary Medicine, University of Wisconsin, 2015 Linden Drive Madison, Wisconsin 53706, USA

Postoperative infection (POI) is a common problem in equine surgery and can result in significant patient morbidity and even mortality. The seriousness of the consequences of POI is generally related to the depth of the infection. The incidence of POI is, in large part, determined by the type, number, and virulence of infecting bacteria, but it is also dependent on the surgical procedure performed. Infection is more common in emergency versus elective procedures and in orthopedic surgery as compared with soft tissue surgery [1]. Although it is impossible to reduce infection rates to none, every surgeon should aim to reduce the incidence of POI. Most wound infections are established during surgery [2,3]. All surgical wounds have bacterial contamination; however, few contaminated surgical wounds become infected. The breakpoint for POI risk is 10^5 microorganisms per gram of tissue [4], but this dose is reduced logarithmically when foreign material is present [5,6]. The goal of the surgeon is to minimize wound contamination and maximize the ability of the wound to resist the establishment of infection. The paradox in the prevention of POI is that in creating the wound, the surgeon is the proximate cause of the contamination; however, wound access also allows the surgeon to take the steps necessary to prevent POI. Because the decisive period in the establishment of infection is within 2 hours of contamination [3], the best opportunity to interdict infection is during surgery.

The four major areas that should be addressed in the control of POI are the patient, the wound environment, systemic antimicrobials, and surgical procedures. Many strategies that are used to reduce POI target more than one of these areas, and the overlapping tactics strengthen the defense against POI.

E-mail address: santsche@svm.vetmed.wisc.edu

Patient

Immune system

The efficacy of the postoperative host defense determines, in large part, whether a surgical wound becomes infected [3]. The immune system of the horse has only been investigated in a preliminary way, but it is known that many of the major components of immunity described in other species do exist in the horse. Immunity to bacteria can be roughly divided into two related categories: the nonspecific innate system and the specific adaptive system [7]. Innate immunity is the first defense against bacteria and is probably the major component of the immune response engaged in POI prevention. The first defense is the physical barrier of the skin and mucosal surface, which are supplemented by surface factors (eg, mucus) and resident microflora. Of course, at surgery, this defense layer is compromised by skin preparation and the scalpel blade. The second layer of the innate defense recognizes broad characteristics of bacteria (eg, cell wall components, including lipopolysaccharide) rather than specific epitopes as in adaptive immunity. Some constituents of the humoral innate system include acute-phase proteins, antimicrobial peptides and enzymes, complement, lectins, and integrins [7]. The major sites of expression of these factors are in plasma [7]. The final layer of innate immunity is membrane-bound factors, such as lectins, scavenger receptors, surface proteins and integrins, which are found on macrophages and natural killer cells [7]. After the surgeon must compromise the innate immune response by breaching its first barrier, the second and final layers of the innate immune response should be maximized. One potential method to improve the innate response is the addition of plasma to the surgical wound, which is discussed in the section on surgical procedures in this article.

The adaptive immune response is the immune mechanism that is specific to a pathogen. The process requires immunoglobulins secreted by plasma cells, which are specific for a particular extracellular bacteria or toxin. The immunoglobulins bind to the bacteria or toxin and initiate neutralization or lysis, opsonization, and phagocytosis by neutrophils and macrophages. Oxidative killing of bacteria by neutrophils is a major part of the defense against bacteria [8]. Unfortunately, the adaptive response requires previous priming of the immune response; however, if present, it can have a powerful role in the prevention of POI.

Immunocompromise is a relatively infrequent concern of the equine surgeon; however, it can be an issue in neonates. The neonatal immune response is naive; despite having all the constituent parts of the adult response, it is simply not as effective as the adult immune response to infection (D.P. Lunn, BVSc, PhD, MRCVS, personal communication, 2005). The easiest constituent to measure and, to a certain extent, to correct is failure of passive transfer. All neonates undergoing surgery should have a serum IgG concentration greater than 800 mg/dL. If colostral antibody absorption is not sufficient, a plasma transfusion should be performed.

Other patient factors

Other patient factors that may play a role in supporting the wound's ability to resist infection are wound temperature and tissue oxygenation [3]. Neither of these patient factors has been investigated in the horse. The impact of hypothermia on wound infection has been debated in the field of human surgery [9], and there is evidence that lowered temperatures increase wound infection [2,10]. Lower body temperatures are not a significant concern in adult horses but can be an issue in foals, particularly if the skin and hair coat become wet. Mild hypothermia before induction of peritonitis reduced survival in a rat model, and impairment of granulocyte recruitment and changes in cytokine expression indicated that the mechanism was immunosuppression [11]. The frequency of sepsis in neonates and the difficulty in treatment of sepsis suggest that avoidance of hypothermia in these patients is important. Local wound temperature may be an issue in adult horses when limbs are suspended in dorsal recumbency or are isolated for long periods by a tourniquet; for this reason, the author limits the use of both techniques when the risk of POI is high (Table 1).

The supply of oxygen to the wound tissues is believed to be important for the prevention of POI [3,12,13], although, as always, there is some disagreement [14]. The mechanism by which oxygen may help to prevent POI is by providing a critical substrate for the killing of bacteria by neutrophils [8]. Wound infection rates decrease as tissue oxygen tensions increase to 100 mm Hg [13]. In the equine surgical patient, efforts should be made to ensure the best perfusion and oxygenation to the surgical wound that is practical and possible. In the author's hands, this means that tourniquet use is uncommon unless already dealing with an infection or in a situation in which hemorrhage makes visibility of the surgical field difficult.

Wound environment

The pathogens causing POI in the horse are described only for orthopedic infection but are probably also those often responsible for soft tissue infections. The major agents include Enterobacteriaceae, *Streptococcus* spp, *Staphylococcus* spp, *Pseudomonas* spp, and anaerobes [15,16]. These bacteria enter the wound during surgery and originate from the skin, mucous membranes, and intestinal flora of the patient as well as from the operating room personnel, materials (including instruments) entering the operative field, and operating room [17]. To reduce the incidence of POI, the number of bacteria coming from these sources should be reduced.

Table 1
Guidelines for antimicrobial prophylaxis in the horse based on the relative risk of postoperative surgical infection

POI risk	Likely pathogens	Systemic drug guidelines	Administration	Alternative drugs
Low	Staph, Strep	IV penicillin (crystalline) or IM (procaine G), 22,000 IU/kg	Before surgery only (IV within 1hour before incision, IM within 3 hours)	Other β-lactams
Moderate	Staph, Strep and gram-negative	IV penicillin (22,000 IU/kg) and gentamicin (6.6 mg/kg)	IV only, start within 1hour before incision, end by 24 hours after surgery	Other β-lactams
High	Staph, Strep, gram-negative, and nosocomial (if applicable)	IV penicillin (22,000 IU/kg) and gentamicin (6.6 mg/kg)	IV only, start within 1hour before incision, end by 72 hours after surgery	Dependent on nosocomial resistance patterns

Low postoperative infection (POI) risk, for all elective procedures without implants (eg, arthroscopy, upper airway surgery, superficial urogenital procedures); moderate POI risk, for nonarthroscopic elective orthopedic procedures, urogenital procedures involving the peritoneum, procedures with minor implants (laryngoplasty, <3 lag screws), and emergency procedures without gross contamination or traumatic tissue damage; high risk, for all procedures requiring substantial implant materials (eg, dynamic compression plate, mesh), procedures with gross contamination with infectious materials, procedures with persisting compromised tissue, and immunocompromised patients (neonates).

Abbreviations: IM, intramuscular; IV, intravenous; Staph, *Staphylococcus* spp; Strep, *Streptococcus* spp.

Patient

The cornerstone of patient bacterial reduction is preparation of the wound site, which includes removal of gross foreign material, clipping of hair, shaving the wound site (in some cases), and disinfecting the skin surface. Methods for local presurgical preparation are well covered in general surgery textbooks. This author prefers to wait until the horse is under general anesthesia to prepare all skin sites. If the operation involves the hoof or an adjacent area, however, the hoof should soak in antiseptic overnight before surgery. Some surgeons prefer to perform at least an initial preparation of the surgical site before anesthesia to save time under general anesthesia. This is perfectly acceptable, except when it involves shaving surgical sites. If done, shaving increases POI rates when performed hours before surgery and should be performed only immediately before surgery to reduce the possibility of bacterial contamination of small dermal abrasions [18,19].

Other general strategies to reduce bacterial contamination from the patients are cleaning the coat of loose hair, dandruff, and debris; picking their feet; and covering all limbs and the tail with clean plastic covers (usually rectal sleeves). Patients with concomitant infections, such as pneumonia or superficial wounds, should have their operation delayed if possible until that infection is resolved.

Sterile surgical drapes are used to create a barrier between the patient and the surgical field. There are few data to indicate that draping reduces POI, but a barrier between the surgical field and nonsterile areas should reduce wound contamination with bacteria. Disposable drapes have been shown to be superior to cotton drapes in the prevention of wound infection [20], and the drapes should be impervious to liquids [21].

Operating room personnel

Bacteria entering the surgical field can be brought in by operating room personnel, who should be limited to those individuals necessary to perform the procedure. Although there are few supporting data, barrier use on personnel would seem to be prudent. Strategies recommended by the Centers for Disease Control Hospital Infection Control Practices Advisory Committee for general operating room personnel include not wearing jewelry; wearing scrub suits, which should be changed when soiled; and wearing a surgical mask and cap or hood to cover hair on head and face fully [17]. Additionally, for personnel who enter the operative field, the fingernails should be kept short, a preoperative scrub should be performed with an appropriate antiseptic for 2 to 5 minutes, barrier-type surgical gowns should be worn, and an appropriate aseptic technique should be used [17]. Sterile gloves should be worn by all scrubbed personnel; for orthopedic procedures, double gloving can reduce the incidence of glove punctures that expose hand skin.

Materials

All materials entering the surgical field should be sterilized according to approved methods (eg, steam under pressure, dry heat, ethylene oxide, gas plasma). It is important to monitor the quality of sterilization routinely. Detailed recommendations are published elsewhere [22,23].

Operating room

The greatest concern in the operating room is the presence of airborne bacteria and debris. In collaboration with the United States Department of Health and Human Services, the American Institute of Architects has published guidelines for human hospitals, which recommend positive pressure in the operating room, air filtration greater than 90%, 15 air exchanges per hour, and air introduction at the ceiling and exhausting at the floor [24]. These benchmarks can be difficult to achieve in an equine operating room because of cost and room size but should serve as guidelines. It is known that ultraclean air does reduce the incidence of POI [25]; thus, it follows that the cleaner the air, the greater is the effect on the reduction of POI. Another facet of the effect of the operating room on POI is the overall room cleanliness. Rooms should be uncluttered and have minimal horizontal surfaces, and dust should be controlled. Routine cleaning of surfaces should be performed, but disinfecting between procedures in the absence of contamination or soiling is unnecessary [17]. If soiling is present, use of an approved hospital disinfectant is appropriate [17].

Systemic antimicrobials

Systemic antimicrobial prophylaxis to reduce the occurrence of POI is a widely accepted surgical practice [26]. Responsible use of antimicrobials is directed toward achieving therapeutic concentrations in tissues during surgery. The antimicrobials should have activity against likely pathogens. At the same time, it is important to minimize the emergence of bacterial resistance and the occurrence of superinfections. In human surgery, the most common failures in prophylactic antimicrobial use are inappropriate timing (the antimicrobial drug should be administered within 1 hour of making the incision, and this was reported to occur in only 56% of patients), drug selection inconsistent with published guidelines (not a common problem, occurring in only 7% of patients), and excess duration of antimicrobial administration (common, occurring in 59% of patients) [26]. There are probably similar occurrences of inappropriate antimicrobial prophylaxis in equine patients. With regard to the antimicrobial drug used for prophylaxis, front-line broad-spectrum agents should not be used systemically. Antimicrobial drugs chosen for prophylaxis of POI in equine surgery should be based on a clinical estimation of the risk of POI; guidelines are suggested by risk level in Table 1.

Route of systemic administration of antimicrobials

Oral administration of prophylactic antimicrobials is not recommended because of variations in absorption, which could result in less than minimal inhibitory concentration (MIC) levels at surgery. Drugs should be given parenterally, preferably intravenously, within 1 hour of making the incision. When a specific resistant nosocomial infection is feared, the author reserves the use of more powerful antimicrobials for local use and administers routine agents systemically. One exception to this rule is the substitution of amikacin sulfate for gentamicin sulfate in neonates because it is less nephrotoxic. Additional doses of antimicrobials should be administered during surgery if the duration of the surgical procedure exceeds one to two times the half-life of the drug [27]. As a practical matter, for horses, this necessitates redosing of β-lactam antimicrobials during operations lasting more than 2 hours.

Duration

This is the most difficult topic for the equine surgeon. The overwhelming seriousness of POI, especially in orthopedic patients, results in routine durations of antimicrobial prophylaxis of a week or more. We have little good information to guide us. In human surgery, there is little evidence that continuing antimicrobials after 24 hours, even when drains are present, decreases the incidence of infection [27]. One could argue for prolonged use of antimicrobials by pointing to the environment in which our patients live (contaminated with hay, straw, and large amounts of feces and urine). The frequency of resistant nosocomial infections in human hospitals does not suggest (from an outcome perspective) that environment is better than barns and stalls, however. There is an alarming increase in the occurrence of superinfections in some equine hospitals with high population densities. The most common problem is multiple drug-resistant *Salmonella* spp, which often results in fatal colitis. In human patients, it is known that prolonged use of antimicrobials does not reduce the incidence of POI, alters the skin and gut flora, and encourages the development of antimicrobial resistance [28–32]. Equine surgeons should take a hard look at reducing the duration of prophylactic antimicrobial use in their patients and consider the following: "The selection and duration of antimicrobial prophylaxis should have the smallest impact possible on the normal bacterial flora of the patient and the microbiologic ecology of the hospital" [27]. For further discussion on prophylactic antimicrobial use, the reader is referred to the article by Southwood elsewhere in this issue.

Surgical procedure

Factors at surgery that can have an impact on POI include duration, operative technique, the use of tourniquets and drains, and wound irrigation.

Prolonged surgical duration has frequently been associated with an increase in POI [33–36]. A confounding factor is that more complicated procedures take longer to perform; thus, statements that equine orthopedic procedures taking longer than 90 minutes are 3.6 times more likely to develop POI than procedures taking less than 90 minutes [34] are of little practical benefit. For example, most long bone fractures requiring a dynamic compression plate (DCP) cannot be repaired in less than 90 minutes, and they do have a higher incidence of infection compared with fractures that can be repaired using lag screws alone. Other factors (eg, quality of skin barrier, stability of repair, soft tissue damage, extent of dissection) are probably much more important to the risk of POI than an operative time longer than 90 minutes. The goal is not to have all operations complete in less than 90 minutes but to get the best fixation possible without infection. A short operative time is only a part of the defense against POI.

Excellent surgical technique, such as gentle tissue handling, effective hemostasis, removal of devitalized tissues, eradication of dead space, and appropriate use of drains and suture material, is widely believed to reduce the incidence of POI [17]; however, for some of these strategies, there are few data to support these conclusions. It is intuitive that gentle tissue handling, removal of dead tissue, and eradicating dead space support uncomplicated wound healing. Hemostasis is indicated for hemorrhage that obscures the surgical field or has the potential to result in significant blood loss. Because bleeding is the first defense against infection, however, the extreme use of ligation and electrocautery to achieve a dry wound may potentiate POI. Although this has not been directly investigated, it is known that coagulation current increases the likelihood of infection in experimental laparotomies as compared with scalpel incision [37].

Allowing healthy wound bleeding is different from leaving blood clots and serum that have exhausted its beneficial plasma components in a wound. Excessive fluid accumulation should not persist in a wound because it promotes dead space. Some surgeons use drains to remove fluid that collects in a surgical wound, but such drains can act as portals for bacteria to enter a surgical wound. Drains have been shown not to be helpful in reducing infection in orthopedic trauma surgery that is clean and not urgent [38] and should be used sparingly in orthopedic and soft tissue surgery. For orthopedic procedures, this author prefers to rely on bandages to reduce dead space and edema as well as to support venous and lymphatic return rather than using drains.

Tourniquets are used for the isolation of a portion of a limb from the systemic vasculature and are most commonly employed to reduce hemorrhage and improve visibility of the surgical field. Because tourniquets have the potential to reduce oxygenation, lower the tissue temperature, and impede the innate immune system, their use should be limited to procedures that cannot be completed if hemorrhage is present.

Wound irrigation is used to remove contaminants physically, deliver drugs (eg, antiseptics, antimicrobials), cool the tissues and instruments, and remove blood to enhance visibility [39–48]. The ideal irrigation solution should decontaminate the tissues in a reasonable time frame and not damage healthy tissues [48]. Additionally, because of the cost and difficulty in the treatment of infection caused by resistant bacteria, strategies (eg, lavage) that do not promote antimicrobial resistance are desirable. There are probably as many ways to lavage a wound as there are surgeons because of individual hospital factors and a lack of data about the superiority of any lavage solution. Factors to consider include the base fluid, the volume of fluid, any additives and their concentrations, and the pressure of the fluid delivered and whether it is delivered as a pulse or continuously. There are insufficient data to make firm recommendations in horses, but the following guidelines may be useful as recommendations:

1. All fluids should be sterile and isotonic.
2. Fluid volume is dependent on the wound surface area and the degree of contamination. A rough guideline is that a moderately contaminated wound with a 20-cm^3 defect should be lavaged with fluid (at least 1 L). For elective wounds, this volume can be reduced by 50%; however, the wound tissues should not be allowed to dry.
3. Antimicrobials in lavage are useful as a prophylaxis against infection but are insufficient to control infection in heavily contaminated or infected wounds.
4. Pulsed delivery is superior to continuous lavage for cleaning traumatic contaminated wounds. The pressure generated from a bulb syringe is sufficient for elective wounds.
5. High-pressure lavage should only be used for heavily contaminated and infected wounds because of its capability of causing tissue damage.

The base component of any irrigation fluid should be isotonic and sterile [50]. Saline, lactated Ringer's solution, or proprietary fluids (eg, Plasmalyte; Baxter Health Care Corporation, Deerfield, Illinois) are all suitable. Additions to the fluid include antiseptics, antimicrobials, soaps, and plasma or immunoglobulins alone. Concerns about tissue damage limit the use of antiseptics. Antimicrobials have been widely used and proven effective in reducing contamination or infection as additives to lavage solutions [39,41,44–47]. There are many agents used and at many differing concentrations. In the horse, the use of local agents that cannot be given systemically (eg, neomycin) has been advocated, and it is in this local application where front-line antimicrobials, such as vancomycin, should be sparingly used for prophylaxis if necessary. Consideration should be given to the local effects of some antimicrobials, such as the fluoroquinolones and aminoglycosides. These drugs can be quite irritating and toxic to cells [51], and they should only be used in a diluted form.

Soap has been shown to be more effective than antimicrobial solutions in removing some bacteria as well as in improving wound healing in open fractures [40,49]. Soap is not recommended for prophylactic use to prevent infection but may be useful in the horse for irrigation of contaminated wounds.

The local addition of plasma or immunoglobulins has been suggested to be a complementary therapy to the prevention of bacterial adhesion and infection [52,53] and has been shown to reduce bacterial adhesion to bone in an experimental equine model [54]. Plasma has the potential to deliver many components of the first-line innate immune response, and immunoglobulins added to an experimental site of sepsis have been shown to enhance bacterial opsonization and phagocytosis [55]. This author uses hyperimmune plasma (Polymune plasma; Veterinary Dynamics, Templeton, California) for POI prophylaxis in operations that require major implants, such as DCPs and mesh. The plasma is diluted 50% with saline, and amikacin sulfate is added to a final concentration of lavage solution of 500 mg/L. Although a limited number of operations have been performed using this lavage, it has been effective in the prevention of POI in the horse.

Summary

The best defense against POI is to use multiple strategies to minimize wound contamination, maintain wound tissue health, and provide rational antimicrobial strategies that do not promote the development of resistant bacteria and superinfections.

References

[1] Santschi EM. Diagnosis and management of surgical site infection and antimicrobial prophylaxis. In: Auer JA, Stick JA, editors. Equine surgery. 2nd edition. Philadelphia: WB Saunders; 1999. p. 54–60.
[2] Kurz A, Sessler DI, Lenhardt R. Perioperative normothermia to reduce the incidence of surgical-wound infection and shorten hospitalization. Study of Wound Infection and Temperature Group. N Engl J Med 1996;334:1209–15.
[3] Sessler DI, Akca O. Nonpharmacological prevention of surgical wound infections. Clin Infect Dis 2002;35:1397–404.
[4] Raahave D, Friis-Moller A, Bjerre-Jepsen K, et al. The infective dose of aerobic and anaerobic bacteria in postoperative wound sepsis. Arch Surg 1986;121:924–9.
[5] Brote L. Wound infections in clean and potentially contaminated surgery. Importance of bacterial and non-bacterial factors. Acta Chir Scand 1976;142:191–200.
[6] Merritt K, Hitchins VM, Neale AR. Tissue colonization from implantable biomaterials with low numbers of bacteria. J Biomed Mater Res 2000;44:261–5.
[7] Giguère S, Prescott JF. Equine immunity to bacteria. Vet Clin North Am Equine Pract 2000; 16:29–47.
[8] Babior BM. Oxygen-dependent microbial killing by phagocytes (first of two parts). N Engl J Med 1978;298:659–68.
[9] Barone JE, Tucker JB, Cecere J, et al. Hypothermia does not result in more complications after colon surgery. Am Surg 1999;65:356–9.
[10] Sessler DI. Perioperative heat balance. Anesthesiology 2000;92:578–96.
[11] Torossian A, Ruehlmann S, Middeke M, et al. Mild preseptic hypothermia is detrimental in rats. Crit Care Med 2004;32:1899–903.

[12] Greif R, Akca O, Horn EP, et al. Supplemental perioperative oxygen to reduce the incidence of surgical-wound infection. N Engl J Med 2000;342:161–7.
[13] Hopf HW, Hunt TK, West JM, et al. Wound tissue oxygen tension predicts the risk of wound infection in surgical patients. Arch Surg 1997;132:997–1004.
[14] Pryor KO, Fahey TJ III, Lien CA, et al. Surgical site infection and the routine use of perioperative hyperoxia in a general surgical population: a randomized controlled trial. JAMA 2004;291:79–87.
[15] Moore RM, Schneider RK, Kowalski J, et al. Antimicrobial susceptibility of bacterial isolates from 233 horses with musculoskeletal infection during 1979–1989. Equine Vet J 1992;24:450–6.
[16] Snyder JR, Pascoe JR, Hirsh DC. Antimicrobial susceptibility of microorganisms isolated from equine orthopedic patients. Vet Surg 1987;16:197–201.
[17] Mangram AJ, Horan TC, Pearson ML, et al. Guideline for prevention of surgical site infection, 1999. Hospital Infection Control Practices Advisory Committee. Infect Control Hosp Epidemiol 1999;20:250–78.
[18] Cruse PJ, Foord R. The epidemiology of wound infection: a 10-year prospective study of 62,939 wounds. Surg Clin North Am 1980;60:27–40.
[19] Mishriki SF, Law DJ, Jeffery PJ. Factors affecting the incidence of postoperative wound infection. J Hosp Infect 1990;16:223–30.
[20] Moylan JA, Fitzpatrick KT, Davenport KE. Reducing wound infections. Improved gown and drape barrier performance. Arch Surg 1987;122:152–7.
[21] Blom A, Estela C, Bowker K, et al. The passage of bacteria through surgical drapes. Ann R Coll Surg Engl 2000;82(6):405–7.
[22] Association of Operating Room Nurses. Standards, recommended practices, guidelines. Denver (CO): Association of Operating Room Nurses; 1999.
[23] Favero MS, Bond W. Sterilization, disinfection, and antisepsis in the hospital. In: Balows A, Hausler WJ Jr, Herrmann KL, et al, editors. Manual of clinical microbiology. 5th edition. Washington (DC): American Society of Microbiology; 1991. p. 183–200.
[24] American Institute of Architects. Guidelines for design and construction of hospital and health care facilities. Washington (DC): American Institute of Architects Press; 1996.
[25] Friberg B. Ultraclean laminar airflow ORs. AORN J 1998;67:841–2.
[26] Bratzler DW, Houck PM, Richards C, et al. Use of antimicrobial prophylaxis for major surgery: baseline results from the National Surgical Infection Prevention Project. Arch Surg 2005;140:174–82.
[27] Bratzler DW, Houck PM. Surgical Infection Prevention Guideline Writers Workgroup. Antimicrobial prophylaxis for surgery: an advisory statement from the National Surgical Infection Prevention Project. Am J Surg 2005;189:395–404.
[28] Harbarth S, Samore MH, Lichtenberg D, et al. Prolonged antibiotic prophylaxis after cardiovascular surgery and its effect on surgical site infections and antimicrobial resistance. Circulation 2000;101:2916–21.
[29] Hecker MT, Aron DC, Patel NP, et al. Unnecessary use of antimicrobials in hospitalized patients: current patterns of misuse with an emphasis on the antianaerobic spectrum of activity. Arch Intern Med 2003;163:972–8.
[30] Hoth JJ, Franklin GA, Stassen NA, et al. Prophylactic antibiotics adversely affect nosocomial pneumonia in trauma patients. J Trauma 2003;55:249–54.
[31] Takesue Y, Yokoyama T, Akagi S, et al. Changes in the intestinal flora after the administration of prophylactic antibiotics to patients undergoing a gastrectomy. Surg Today 2002;32: 581–6.
[32] Archer GL. Alteration of cutaneous staphylococcal flora as a consequence of antimicrobial prophylaxis. Rev Infect Dis 1991;18(Suppl 10):S805–9.
[33] Killian CA, Graffunder EM, Vinciguerra TJ, et al. Risk factors for surgical-site infections following cesarean section. Infect Control Hosp Epidemiol 2001;22:613–7.

[34] MacDonald DG, Morley PS, Bailey JV, et al. An examination of the occurrence of surgical wound infection following equine orthopedic surgery. Equine Vet J 1994;26:323–6.
[35] Nicholson M, Beal M, Shofer F, et al. Epidemiologic evaluation of postoperative wound infection in clean-contaminated wounds: a retrospective study of 239 dogs and cats. Vet Surg 2002;31:577–81.
[36] Wilson DA, Baker GJ, Boero MJ. Complications of celiotomy incisions in horses. Vet Surg 1995;24:506–14.
[37] Soballe PW, Nimbkar NV, Hayward I, et al. Electric cautery lowers the contamination threshold for infection of laparotomies. Am J Surg 1998;175:263–6.
[38] Lang GJ, Richardson M, Bosse MJ, et al. Efficacy of surgical wound drainage in orthopedic trauma patients; a randomized prospective trial. J Orthop Trauma 1998;12:348–50.
[39] Acar O, Mutlu B, Cimen N, et al. The role of intraoperative antibiotic irrigation and postoperative antibiotic therapy for contaminated implantable prosthesis: in a rat model in vivo. Int J Impot Res 2000;12:285–8.
[40] Anglen JO. Comparison of soap and antibiotic solutions for irrigation of lower-limb open fracture wounds. A prospective, randomized study. J Bone Joint Surg Am 2005;87:1415–22.
[41] Bingham R, Fleenor WH, Church S. The local use of antibiotics to prevent wound infection. Clin Orthop 1974;99:194–200.
[42] Leslie LF, Faulkner BC, Woods JA, et al. Wound cleansing by irrigation for implant surgery. Journal of Long-Term Effects of Medical Implants 1995;5:111–28.
[43] Badia JM, Torres JM, Tur C, et al. Saline wound irrigation reduces the postoperative infection rate in guinea pigs. J Surg Res 1996;63:457–9.
[44] Martin C, Viviand X, Potie F. Local antibiotic prophylaxis in surgery. Infect Control Hosp Epidemiol 1996;17:539–44.
[45] Maurice-Williams RS, Pollock J. Topical antibiotics in neurosurgery: a re-evaluation of the Malis technique. Br J Neurosurg 1999;13:312–5.
[46] Rosenstein BD, Wilson FC, Funderburk CH. The use of bacitracin irrigation to prevent infection in postoperative skeletal wounds. J Bone Joint Surg Am 1989;71:427–30.
[47] Simons JP, Johnson JT, Yu VL, et al. The role of topical antibiotic prophylaxis in patients undergoing contaminated head and neck surgery with flap reconstruction. Laryngoscope 2001;111:329–35.
[48] Anglen J, Apostoles PS, Christensen G, et al. Removal of surface bacteria by irrigation. J Orthop Res 1996;14:251–4.
[49] Conroy BP, Anglen JO, Simpson WA, et al. Comparison of Castile soap, benzalkonium chloride, and bacitracin as irrigation solutions for complex contaminated orthopaedic wounds. J Orthop Trauma 1999;13:332–7.
[50] Buffa EA, Lubbe AM, Verstraete FJ, et al. The effects of wound lavage solutions on canine fibroblasts: an in vitro study. Vet Surg 1997;26:460–6.
[51] Miclau T, Edin ML, Lester GE, et al. Bone toxicity of locally applied aminoglycosides. J Orthop Trauma 1995;9:401–6.
[52] Poelstra KA, Barekzi NA, Rediske AM, et al. Prophylactic treatment of gram-positive and gram-negative abdominal implant infections using locally delivered polyclonal antibodies. J Biomed Mater Res 2002;60:206–15.
[53] Poelstra KA, van der Mei HC, Gottenbos B, et al. Pooled human immunoglobulins reduce adhesion of Pseudomonas aeruginosa in a parallel plate flow chamber. J Biomed Mater Res 2000;51:224–32.
[54] Bauer SM, Santschi EM, Fialkowski J, et al. Quantification of *Staphylococcus aureus* adhesion to equine bone surfaces passivated with Plasmalyte™ and hyperimmune plasma. Vet Surg 2004;33:376–81.
[55] Barekzi NA, Felts AG, Poelstra KA, et al. Locally delivered polyclonal antibodies potentiate intravenous antibiotic efficacy against gram-negative infections. Pharmacol Res 2002;19: 1801–7.

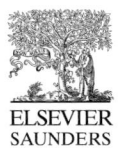

Surgical and Traumatic Wound Infections, Cellulitis, and Myositis in Horses

Emma N. Adam, BVetMed[a],*,
Louise L. Southwood, BVSc, PhD[b]

[a]New Bolton Center, University of Pennsylvania, 382 West Street Road,
Kennett Square, PA 19348–1692, USA
[b]Department of Clinical Studies, New Bolton Center,
University of Pennsylvania, 382 West Street Road, Kennett Square, PA 19348–1692, USA

Wound infection

Wound infection and healing are subjects of intense research but clinically remain sources of considerable morbidity and mortality in human and veterinary patients. Whether a wound was created surgically or through trauma, fundamental principles need to be considered for successful management. Key considerations include tissue integrity, perfusion, bacterial challenge and host responses, and tissue repair processes.

Surgical wound infection

In 1992, the Centers for Disease Control [1] proposed guidelines for the surveillance and epidemiologic study of surgical site infections (SSIs). Distant site surgery-related infections are not considered SSIs; for example, postanesthetic pneumonia is considered a surgical complication and not an SSI. Superficial incisional infections are those defined as occurring within 30 days of surgery and involving only the skin or subcutaneous tissues [1]. Deep incisional infections are regarded as occurring within 30 days of surgery if no implant was left in place and within 1 year if an implant was placed at surgery [1]. These infections are considered to be related to the surgical procedure and involve muscle or fascial layers. Organ or space SSIs

* Corresponding author.
E-mail address: eadam@vet.upenn.edu (E.N. Adam).

involve any part of the anatomy other than the incision that was opened or manipulated at surgery. Again, the timeline is within 30 days of surgery if no implant was left in place and within 1 year if an implant was placed at surgery [1].

The National Research Council Operative Wound Classification is based on intrinsic microbial contamination (Table 1). It must be placed in context with other risk factors that have been identified in human and veterinary studies.

Pathophysiology

The development of infection at any site involves the attachment and multiplication of microbes. For this to occur, bacteria and host factors define a balance that falls in favor of microbial colonization. The most significant microbe-related factor is the bacterial inoculation dose [2]. An inoculum size of 10^5 organisms per gram of tissue is a bacterial challenge below which soft tissue wounds may heal without infection [2]. This value was determined using experimental models and is likely to be lower when considering a patient with an impaired immune response, poor tissue perfusion, or the presence of a foreign body. Other considerations include the virulence of the organism, its ability to evade the host immune system, adhesion mechanisms, the presence of a capsule, and the organism's ability to secrete exotoxins that impair tissue viability or host defenses. The placement of an implant markedly reduces the inoculum size necessary to produce an infection [3]. Doses of 10^2 *Staphylococcus pyogenes* organisms per gram of tissue produced infection in the presence of foreign material, such as suture in human beings [4], and a dose of 10^2 *Staphylococcus aureus* organisms per gram of tissue was able to produce a 60% implant-related infection rate in a rabbit femoral screw model [3]. The development of device-related infections is a growing problem in human surgery, where the use of prostheses is increasing in soft tissue and orthopedic operations [5]. The formation of a biofilm on prostheses is a well-recognized phenomenon in human and veterinary

Table 1
National Research Council Operative Wound Classification

Wound category	Characteristics of the wound
Clean	Nontraumatic, primary closure, elective wound without drain; no break in aseptic technique; not infected or inflamed
Clean-contaminated	Respiratory, gastrointestinal, or urogenital tract entered under conditions; break in aseptic technique minor
Contaminated	Fresh, open traumatic wound; gross gastrointestinal tract contamination, spillage from biliary or urinary tract; incisions in inflamed sites; major break in aseptic technique
Infected or dirty	Traumatic wound with organic debris, foreign body, and devitalized tissue; viscus perforation; purulent debris encountered

surgery [5,6]. Many bacteria are capable of causing implant-associated infections, but those that are capable of producing exopolysaccharide (glycocalyx) are more virulent [7]. *S aureus* is the most common musculoskeletal pathogen of human beings and animals [8], and it has been reported to be responsible for 19% of equine orthopedic infections [9]. Virulence factors include the ability to adhere to bone sialoprotein, collagen, and fibronectin [10]. Bacterial adhesion molecules are referred to as microbial surface components recognizing adhesive matrix molecules (MSCRAMMs) [10]. Two fibronectin-binding genes, *fnbA* and *fnbB*, were detected in 98% and 99% of *S aureus* recovered from 191 human orthopedic infections, respectively [7]. Coagulase-negative staphylococci (CNS) have traditionally been considered to have low pathogenic potential [11,12]. *Staphylococcus epidermidis*, the most common CNS, is an opportunistic pathogen and a habitual inhabitant of human skin [11]. It is frequently associated with postsurgical infections, especially those involving a prosthesis [12]. Thirty-six percent of *S epidermidis* isolated from 342 orthopedic implant infections was found to produce exopolysaccharide based on the presence of *icaA* and *icaB* genes [12]. Products of the *ica* locus, polysaccharide intercellular adhesion (PIA), are essential components of biofilm [12]. These strains were also more likely to have multiple antimicrobial resistance patterns. Eighty percent of all isolates were β-lactam resistant, 31% were aminoglycoside resistant, and 37% were methicillin/oxacillin resistant [12]. Methicillin-resistant *S epidermidis* has been reported as an orthopedic implant-related infection in the horse [13].

Bacterial adherence to foreign material in tissue makes their elimination difficult. Bacteria in a biofilm exhibit greater resistance to antimicrobials [14]. Proposed mechanisms include low diffusion or failure of antimicrobial penetration, slow bacterial growth within mature biofilms because of lack of nutrients and biofilm thickness heterogeneity, slower growth as a stress response to biofilm formation, and induction of a biofilm phenotype characterized by activated multidrug efflux pumps and altered membrane-protein composition [14]. The clinical relevance of this information is that any foreign material represents a potential source of infection and that speciation of and antibiograms for all staphylococcal organisms are important.

SSIs are not strictly proportional to the degree of contamination at surgery [15,16]. For example, horses undergoing exploratory laparotomy were more likely to develop an SSI when an enterotomy was performed versus a resection and anastomosis, which are clean-contaminated procedures [15,16]. In equine orthopedic surgery, however, wound classification and SSIs are strongly associated. Clean-contaminated wounds are 24 times more likely to develop SSIs than clean wounds [16].

Patient-related SSI risk factors in human general surgery include increasing age [17], diabetes, and obesity [18]. With respect to equine celiotomy surgery, horses less than 1 year of age but older than 1 month of age had an SSI rate of 15% compared with a 43% SSI rate in horses older than 1 year of age [19]. The role of concurrent endocrinopathy in the equine patient is hard to establish. The roles of old age and endocrine diseases, such as pituitary pars intermedia dysfunction, have yet to be defined in the equine patient. Horses weighing more than 300 kg and undergoing a ventral midline celiotomy were twice as likely to develop incisional complications [19]. This may be a function of anesthesia-related hypotension and tissue perfusion [19]. Hypovolemia and perioperative blood loss are consistently identified as risk factors for incisional infection and tissue dehiscence in human patients [20]. It has been suggested that the immunomodulatory effects of an allogenic blood transfusion given to compensate for perioperative hemorrhage may have been a confounding factor, however [21]. Patients undergoing emergency gastrointestinal operations are at increased risk of wound complications, such as infection and dehiscence, compared with similar procedures performed electively in human patients [22]. The reported incidence of wound complications varies, but in a recent publication, it was reported that the incidences of wound complications were 6% and 16% in elective and emergency gastrointestinal surgeries, respectively [22]. In this study, wound complications were defined as superficial or deep wound infection, wound or intra-abdominal abscess, or disruption of sutured tissue (wound, fascia, or anastomosis). Interestingly, in the study by Sorensen and colleagues [22], an elective procedure was twice as likely to be performed by a specialist surgeon as an emergency procedure. Celiotomies performed in horses for acute abdominal disease (gastrointestinal and nongastrointestinal) had a 39% incidence of incisional complications; elective celiotomies had a 7% incidence [19]. The role of the surgeon's experience versus the elective or emergency nature of the procedure needs to be differentiated.

Cardiovascular compromise and severe metabolic derangements are important risk factors for the development of SSIs [18]. They represent and encompass all the negative aspects of the sick patient, such as poor immune function, circulating volume/perfusion mismatch, coagulopathies, and endotoxemia, to name a few. Remote infections pose a two- to threefold increase in SSI development in human patients [18]. This is not well investigated in the veterinary literature but is a worthy consideration for elective procedures. Other risk factors found in the human literature include smoking cigarettes, cardiovascular disease, lung disease, and male gender. Most of these risk factors are not issues in veterinary patients, except for gender. The major difference is that we tend to deal with intact female animals and castrated male animals, and the association between gender and SSIs is not well investigated in the veterinary literature.

The presence of foreign material and organic debris acts as a nidus for infection and biofilm formation. Soil contamination merits mention, because certain soil particles can interfere with leukocyte function and render them ineffective phagocytes [23]. Montmorillonite clay (hydrated sodium calcium aluminum magnesium silicate hydroxide), a common component of clay soils in the United States, is a highly charged particle that is one of the most potent soil infection potentiators [23]. In vitro, it causes neutrophil lysis and impairs complement activity. These effects were offset by pretreatment of clay with 0.1% albumin [23].

Length of surgery time is a huge risk factor for SSIs in human and veterinary patients. It is probably a composite of the operation being a more complicated procedure, the effects of prolonged anesthesia affecting tissue perfusion, drying of tissues at the surgery site, contamination of the surgery site, and increased tissue trauma from extensive manipulation. Incisional complications were twice as likely to occur after ventral midline celiotomies taking longer than 2 hours [19], and equine patients undergoing orthopedic procedures were 3.6 times more likely to develop an SSI when the surgery time was greater than 90 minutes [16].

Other surgery-related factors include the amount of tissue trauma during surgery and at the clipping and preparing stage, inadequate hemostasis, inappropriate instrumentation, suture and suture pattern used, insufficient debridement of devitalized tissues, the creation of dead space, and the experience of the surgeon [24]. Fortunately, many of these factors can be overcome with a skilled and experienced surgical team.

Diagnosis and treatment

Obtaining culture samples from infected surgical sites should be the mainstay of directed therapy wherever possible. Samples should be taken on a sterile swab from deep within the infected site or tract after cleansing of the wound with dilute povidone-iodine or chlorhexidine scrub, followed by thorough lavage with sterile isotonic fluid or by harvesting fresh exudate on a sterile swab. Every effort should be made to reduce the likelihood of culturing surface contaminants, which may be misleading. Various commercially available products are intended for use in maintaining the viability of aerobic and anaerobic microorganisms during transport from the patient to the laboratory, for example, Septi-Chek (Becton-Dickinson, Franklin Lakes, New Jersey) and Port-A-Cul (BBL Microbiology, Becton-Dickinson, Franklin Lakes, New Jersey). Although there is no replacement for a representative culture and antibiogram, it is helpful to have an idea of the organisms to expect when faced with the need for therapy in the absence of this information. After arthroscopic surgery in horses, the bacterial isolates obtained from SSIs were commonly coagulase-positive and -negative *Staphylococcus* spp, in addition to Enterobacteriaceae, *Streptococcus* spp, *Pseudomonas* spp, and anaerobes [25,26]. Enterobacteriaceae and *Streptococcus* spp were the most common bacterial isolates obtained from orthopedic procedures or fracture repair and were often mixed infections [9,16]. In these studies, not all sites were cultured for anaerobes [9,16]. Antimicrobial susceptibility of *Pseudomonas* spp can be unpredictable, and therapy should be based on antibiograms [27]. *Staphylococcus* spp were isolated from 31% of postoperative synovial structure infections [26]. Amikacin or cephalothin was a good treatment choice [9,28]. Aminoglycosides have a concentration-dependent bactericidal action and a good concentration-dependent "postantibiotic effect" [29]. The postantibiotic effect is that bactericidal concentrations remain for several hours after the dose is administered and bacteria continue to take up the drug through a combination of passive and oxygen-dependent facilitated processes [29]. Amikacin or gentamicin is currently the drug of choice for the treatment of orthopedic SSIs [28]. Their concentration-dependent bactericidal effect lends itself to their use as a regional perfusate. Their elution from polymethylmethacrylate (PMMA) and bioabsorbable compounds, such as collagen sponges, is supported by in vitro and clinical findings [26,30]. This is discussed in more detail in the article on new antimicrobials, systemic distribution, and local methods of antimicrobial delivery elsewhere in this issue.

Mixed bacterial infections were isolated from SSIs after gastrointestinal, urogenital, and respiratory tract operations [24]. Bacterial isolates were of patient origin in equine patients with celiotomy infections [31]. Studies using human albumin tracer particles on patient skin distant to the surgical site showed that these particles could be recovered from the incision, indicating that bacteria on the skin from a distant site can migrate to the surgery site [32]. Infection of soft tissue surgery sites has been reported with *Actinobacillus* spp [33]. Although *Actinobacillus* spp are often susceptible to penicillin and potentiated sulfonamides [28], one report of 10 cases had different antibiograms, which included penicillin resistance [33]. Monitoring of SSI isolates is crucial in the recognition of surgery-related and nosocomial SSIs, however.

Traumatic wound infection

The principles relating to SSIs are valuable as a basis for considering traumatic wound infection, tissue viability, and the wound's response to surgical debridement. The National Research Council Operative Wound Classification provides guidance; however, in addition to frank bacterial contamination, emphasis should be placed on tissue viability, edema, hemorrhage, loss of tissue architecture and function, lymphatic drainage, wound location, and patient age. Horses are presented to the practitioner with a challenging array of lesions that must be thought through and evaluated carefully to bring about a satisfactory outcome.

A complete physical examination is essential when evaluating any patient. The cardiovascular status of the horse should be investigated, paying particular attention to heart rate, oral mucous membrane color and texture, and peripheral pulse quality. Any hemorrhage should be controlled as a priority. There may have been sufficient hemorrhage to warrant volume resuscitation with fluid therapy before further diagnostics and treatment are performed, particularly if general anesthesia is necessary [34]. The physical and physiologic state of the horse should be assessed before chemical restraint for examination whenever possible.

Wound healing

Wound healing merits a brief review, particularly with respect to the differences between trunk and limb wounds and between horses and ponies. Wound healing is broadly divided macroscopically into four sequential but overlapping phases: inflammation, granulation, wound contraction, and epithelialization [35]. The severity of trauma determines the magnitude of the resulting cellular and vascular response (ie, the inflammatory response). After the initial vasoconstriction of blood vessels, vasodilation occurs, promoting the passage of cells, platelets, fluid, and protein into the wound space. Products of the coagulation cascade and platelet aggregation form a clot, providing hemostasis and a scaffold for cellular infiltration. Neutrophils phagocytose bacteria and, with platelets, release chemoattractants to recruit monocytes. Once in the tissue, monocytes become macrophages and play a central role in debridement, microbe killing, and the orchestration of wound repair [35].

Transforming growth factor-β (TGFβ) is released by platelets, neutrophils, and macrophages and is a potent chemoattractant for these cells [36]. The recruitment of leukocytes in wounds in ponies is faster and more numerous compared with that in horses, and pony leukocytes produce more reactive oxygen species, which are necessary for microbial killing [37]. It is not surprising then that ponies are capable of producing a healthy granulation bed more rapidly than horses, leading to the elimination of wound infection more rapidly. Ponies also produce higher levels of other inflammatory mediators that play a key role in the efficacy of the inflammatory response, production of granulation tissue, and wound contraction [36]. The positive feedback loop that is created is likely the reason why ponies have a stronger inflammatory response and better prevention of wound infection compared with horses [37]. The weak inflammatory response seen in wounds in horses results in chronic inflammation, leading to prolonged release of degradative enzymes and TGFβ, which overstimulates fibroblasts, causing excessive fibroplasia and exuberant granulation tissue (EGT) and inhibiting wound contraction [36,37]. In terms of wound management, this emphasizes the care that needs to be taken in meticulous wound debridement and cleansing so that the process may start off with minimal bacterial infection, thus helping to avoid a chronic inflammatory response, which is more likely to lead to EGT formation [37].

The proliferative phase of wound healing involves endothelial, fibroblast, and epithelial proliferation. Macrophages stimulate angiogenesis and fibroplasia [35] by secreting growth factors, stimulating other cells to secrete growth factors, and degrading connective tissue matrix to facilitate endothelial cell migration [38]. Fibroblast migration precedes endothelial cell migration but follows macrophage matrix degradation [38].

Initially, a loose provisional matrix is deposited, consisting of a fibronectin framework. The framework is critical to wound repair. Porcine small intestine and bladder submucosa products are available commercially, and it has been suggested that they may provide this meshwork, along with various growth factors and inhibitors, to enhance wound repair [38]. In a study comparing split-thickness allogeneic skin, allogeneic peritoneum, and xenogenic porcine small intestinal submucosa with conventional nonbiologic dressings, however, no difference was found in terms of wound healing, infection, or inflammatory response [39]. Validation of the use of these products in equine wound repair is eagerly anticipated.

A variety of mediators stimulate fibroblasts to deposit extracellular matrix (ECM), mainly via upregulation of fibroblast growth factor (FGF) [40]. FGF inhibits ECM degradation by upregulating tissue inhibitors of metalloproteases (TIMPs) [40]. It is thought that the chronic inflammatory response seen in wounds on the distal limbs of horses is the reason why their granulation tissue is irregular, chaotic, and exuberant, with delayed epithelialization as compared with ponies [37].

Matrix remodeling in the later stages (7–21 days) of wound repair involves removal of the provisional matrix and replacement with organized components that increase the resilience and tensile strength of the ECM [38]. For example, type III collagen is replaced by type I collagen. Fibroblasts undergo apoptosis or differentiate into myofibroblasts that bring about wound contraction [38]. Although myofibroblast contractility in ponies and horses is similar, pony myofibroblasts bring about greater wound contraction [36]. This difference is thought to be related to the milieu of the wound and the presence of proinflammatory mediators, such as interleukin-1 (IL-1), prostaglandin (PG) E_2, and tumor necrosis factor-α (TNFα), inhibiting contractility in chronically inflamed granulation tissue beds in horses [36].

Epithelialization concludes wound healing and results in a nonfunctional scar. Scars are devoid of adnexa, have reduced dermal projections, and have reduced tensile strength [37]. Fetal wounds heal without scarring, where tissue is regenerated rather than repaired [41]. In fetal wounds, factors present in adult wounds, such as basic FGF and TGF-β1, TGF-β2 and TGF-β3, are virtually absent [38,42]. Epithelialization is the slowest phase of wound healing, is inversely proportional to the rate of wound contraction after approximately 3 weeks, and is inhibited by persistent inflammation [37]. In horses, more epithelialization occurs as wound contraction is limited, resulting in a larger scar. Promising work in this field includes the application of platelet-rich plasma gel, which accelerated epithelialization and wound maturation in terms of the formation of organized interlocking collagen bundles in equine limb wounds [40]. The antipseudomonal drug silver sulfadiazine has antifungal and antimicrobial properties, and in other species, it increases the rate of epithelialization; however, it has not been shown to do this in horses [43].

Wounds of the trunk generally heal remarkably well. The inflammatory phase is more pronounced, and a chronic inflammatory cytokine profile is not usually a feature of trunk wounds [37]. Better blood perfusion, higher local temperatures, and the resident leukocyte population may be responsible for these differences [37]. Granulation tissue forms more slowly but takes less time to become healthy and organized compared that in with limb wounds [36]. Compared with distal limb wounds, TGFβ recedes more rapidly, fibroplasia is less profound, and the ECM and cells become organized sooner in trunk wounds [43]. This makes trunk wounds easier to manage and less prone to EGT that could harbor infection. Wound contraction is more pronounced and starts sooner in trunk wounds compared with distal limb wounds [43,44]. Resistance to wound contraction in the distal limb likely results from skin in this region being more rigidly adhered to the skeleton compared with trunk skin [37]. Increased tissue resistance to contraction leads to increased TGFβ levels and less differentiation and organization of fibroblasts within limb wounds compared with trunk wounds [45]. Pronounced wound contraction and slower epithelialization result in stellate trunk scars [37].

Wound evaluation

In a survey of horses that were presented to a number of veterinary schools, injury to the foot, forelimb, and hind limb were the most common sites of traumatic wounds [46]. More than 60% of these wounds were treated with debridement and second-intention healing, and 38% were sutured [46]. The lack of soft tissue protection and abundance of vulnerable synovial, tendon, ligament, and neurovascular structures make early and thorough evaluation of limb wounds critical. Types of lesions include lacerations from sharp objects, puncture wounds, and avulsions. Wound evaluation can usually be performed with sedation and local anesthesia. General anesthesia may be necessary to evaluate a wound fully but should be performed only when the patient is judged to be physiologically stable and the injuries are not likely to increase the risks of catastrophic failure during induction or recovery from general anesthesia.

Radiographs of traumatized areas should be performed in all cases of distal limb wounds, and stressed views of joints or contrast radiography should also be considered, especially when evaluating penetrating foot wounds (Fig. 1) [34]. Devitalized bone subject to the sequestrum formation may not be evident immediately after injury [47]. Multiple views and repeat radiographs in 10 to 14 days should be performed (Fig. 2). Sequestrum formation should be considered in wounds that become chronic nonhealing wounds and where bone is exposed [47].

Ultrasonography provides information about the integrity of soft tissue structures, fluid pocket accumulation, and radiolucent foreign material. Doppler imaging can assist in determining the arterial and venous integrity of the region [48].

Wounds should be clipped and cleaned with antiseptic preparations, such as povidone-iodine and chlorhexidine gluconate or diacetate. Both of these products are available as detergent scrubs (Betadine Surgical Scrub, Purdue Pharma LP, Stamford, Connecticut; Nolvasan Surgical Scrub, Fort Dodge

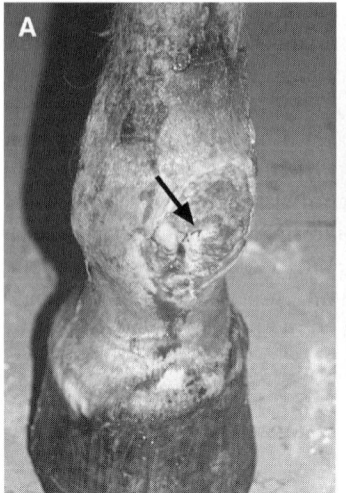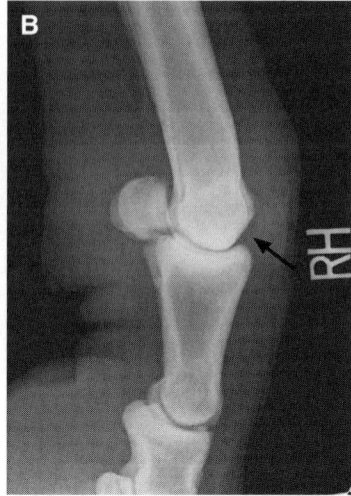

Fig. 1. (*A*) Five-day old fetlock wound on a 3-year-old Suffolk Punch gelding. This wound is the result of the horse falling in a carriage accident and abrading the dorsal surface of its hind fetlock joint on the road surface. The joint capsule in the area of the wound was abraded. The arrow points to two sutures that were placed as part of a reconstruction operation. (*Courtesy of* Dr. D.W. Richardson, DVM, DACVS, University of Pennsylvania, Kennett Square, PA.) (*B*) Flexed lateral-to-medial radiograph of the limb pictured in (*A*). The arrow points to the large defect in the dorsal sagittal ridge. Digital exploration of the wound was limited because of space limitations, and the defect in the sagittal ridge could not be fully appreciated by digital palpation. (*Courtesy of* Dr. D.W. Richardson, DVM, DACVS, University of Pennsylvania, Kennett Square, PA.)

Laboratories Wyeth, Madison, New Jersey) or solutions (Betadine Solution, Purdue Pharma LP; Nolvasan Solution, Fort Dodge Laboratories Wyeth). The detergent form provides effective removal of dirt and oils from the skin [49]. After the initial scrub, the area should be rinsed with sterile isotonic fluid, such a 0.9% saline solution. Lavage solutions should be dilute to avoid cytotoxicity [49]. Betadine Solution comes as 10% povidone-iodine and should be diluted to a 0.1% solution by adding stock solution (1 mL) to sterile diluent (100 mL). Chlorhexidine diacetate (Nolvasan Solution) comes as a 2% solution and should be made into a lavage solution by adding 2.5 mL per 100 mL of sterile diluent. Disadvantages of chlorhexidine include corneal irritation and possible inhibition of wound healing [50]. Disadvantages of povidone-iodine include dermal reactions, questionable residual activity, and reduced efficacy in the presence of organic matter [50]. Chloroxylenol products (Techni-care Surgical Scrub; Care-Tech Laboratories, St. Louis, Missouri) are supposed to be less irritating to tissue (Care-Tech data, 2006). In a study comparing the use of 4% chlorhexidine gluconate and 3% chloroxylenol as a surgical scrub in canine skin, the number of skin reactions was similar [51]. The investigators found that chlorhexidine gluconate was better able to reduce the number of colony-forming bacteria, regardless of the prescrub bacterial load, than chloroxylenol [51].

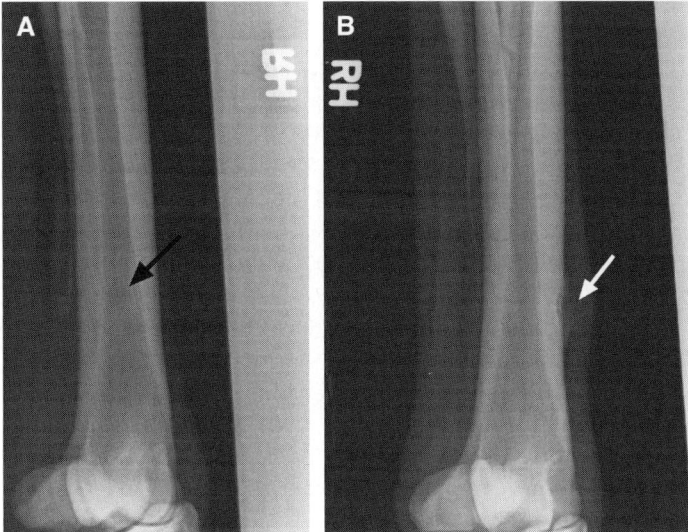

Fig. 2. (A) Dorsomedial-plantarolateral view of a 4-week-old wound on the dorsomedial aspect of the right hind third metacarpal of a 2-year-old Thoroughbred. The arrow points to a radiolucent area in the dorsomedial cortex. (*Courtesy of* Dr. D.W. Richardson, DVM, DACVS, University of Pennsylvania, Kennett Square, PA.) (B) Dorsolateral-plantaromedial view of the same limb pictured in (A). This view highlights the importance of multiple radiographic views, because the dorsomedial sequestrum (*arrow*) and periosteal reaction are much more obvious in this view. This horse was euthanized because of severe lameness, joint sepsis, and a grave prognosis for pasture soundness. (*Courtesy of* Dr. D.W. Richardson, DVM, DACVS, University of Pennsylvania, Kennett Square, PA.)

Sterile lubricant gel can be applied to the wounds to facilitate the removal of clipped hair during the cleansing process. Alcohol should be avoided because its desiccating action is cytotoxic [49]. Hydrogen peroxide should also be avoided because its exothermic reaction can cause thermal damage and it is cytotoxic [52]. Copious lavage should be performed with dilute solutions, such as 0.1% povidone-iodine or 0.05% chlorhexidine solution, which maintain antiseptic properties and minimize tissue toxicity. Pressures of greater than 8 psi and up to 70 psi dislodge adherent bacteria without forcing them deeper into tissue [47]. A 60-mL syringe with a 14-gauge needle can generate 8 psi, and a Water Pik (Water Pik, Fort Collins, Colorado) can generate up to 70 psi [47]. Sterile digital evaluation of the wound should be performed. Alternatively, a blunt sterile probe, such as a sterile teat cannula, can be used with extreme caution to palpate the wound gently [34].

The integrity of synovial structures should be assessed whenever wounds or dead space is near synovial structures. Knowledge of anatomy should enable the practitioner to prepare a sterile site distant to the lesion for synoviocentesis. This reduces the risk of introducing bacteria from the wound into a sterile synovial structure. A synovial fluid sample should be obtained for cytologic evaluation and microbiologic culture whenever possible. Sterile saline, balanced polyionic fluid, or mepivacaine can be used to test the integrity of the synovial structure. A sufficient volume should be used to obtain distention, and the limb should be manipulated through a range of motion to avoid overlapping tissue planes resulting in a false-negative finding. Repeatedly drying the wound with sterile gauze improves the ability to see fluid leakage. Before withdrawal of the needle, a small volume (250–500 mg) of amikacin can be deposited within the synovial structure if initial examination of the fluid suggests that it is not infected (ie, good viscosity and clear yellow color). A drop of normal synovial fluid should string between the forefinger and thumb approximately 2.5 to 5 cm before the string breaks [47]. If the synovial fluid appears turbid or the wound communicates with a joint or tendon sheath in question, the structure should be copiously lavaged. The decision whether to perform through-and-through lavage using needles with the horse standing or under general anesthesia or to lavage with arthroscopy is discussed in the article on septic arthritis, tenosynovitis, and infections of hoof structures elsewhere in this issue.

Samples for microbiologic culture should be obtained before antimicrobial administration. Debridement should be performed on cleaned wounds in a sedated horse with local anesthesia or with the horse under general anesthesia. If antimicrobials are to be used, they should be administered before wound debridement demonstrates that administration of antimicrobials is most efficacious at preventing SSIs when given at the time of induction of general anesthesia [53]. Necrotic, devitalized, or macerated tissue and organic debris should be removed. Lavage should be continued during this process. When there is little tissue to debride or the risk of disrupting a synovial structure is high, the wound must be considered contaminated [47]. Skin that is cool and unhealthy, even after debridement, is likely to contract and possibly to lose viability [48]. When this occurs, the devitalized tissue is a potential cause of continued inflammation and source of bacterial infection. Demarcation of healthy from devitalized tissue is not easy in a fresh traumatic injury. Tissue warmth and the bleeding at cut surfaces can be helpful factors in determining viable from nonviable tissue, but they are not precise indicators [47]. Re-evaluation of the wound every 24 or 48 hours is essential, and the possibility of the wound progressing to include vital or synovial structures should be considered [47]. Wounds in which infection is likely are better left to heal by second intention or delayed primary closure once the infection is sterilized; however, if economics permit, every attempt at debridement and surgical reconstruction of the wound should be attempted to maximize repair [46,47]. The application of Penrose and closed-suction drains reduces the accumulation of exudate that can harbor bacteria.

Chronic wounds should be considered to be infected. Chronic wounds in the distal limb can be the result of EGT (proud flesh), persistent infection, the presence of a foreign body, or self-trauma. EGT is more likely to develop when the limb is bandaged or cast [43]. Although bandaging and casting help with decreasing swelling and provide hemostasis, it is thought that the steep oxygen gradient created by bandaging increases angiogenesis and stimulates fibroplasia in addition to lowering wound pH and trapping inflammatory exudate [35]. Bandaging, with or without a splint, offers the advantage of protecting the wound from further trauma, restricting wound edge movement, preventing contamination with debris, and facilitating the application of topical therapy. The use of a silicone gel (CicaCare; Smith & Nephew, La Jolla, California) greatly helps in the prevention of EGT, and treated wounds contracted and healed more rapidly when compared with nonadherent traditional dressings on distal limb wounds [54]. Persistent infection warrants investigation in terms of whether the antimicrobials in use are appropriate and, if not being used, are necessary. The question should also be asked whether fungal or parasitic agents are involved [55]. Small wounds can become chronic granulating beds when the wounds become infected with *Habronema* spp or *Draschia* spp ("summer sores"; Fig. 3). Identification of larvae on a histologic section from a biopsy sample confirms a diagnosis of habronemiasis, which can be present even in horses regularly dewormed with ivermectin products. Topical applications of fenthion, corticosteroid, and dimethylsulfoxide mixtures [56] can usually avoid the need for surgical excision. All in-contact horses should be dewormed with ivermectin. These wounds are pruritic, some intensely so, making self-trauma a confounding factor for wound healing and infection. One differential diagnosis for pruritic progressive wounds is a fungal infection, such as cutaneous pythiosis [56]. Cutaneous pythiosis lesions present as progressive, suppurating, ulcerative, invasive wounds that can be intensely pruritic

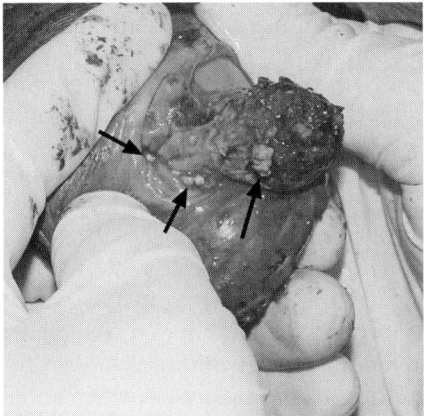

Fig. 3. Glans penis of a 15-year-old pony gelding with a chronic ulcerative and exudative wound. Histologic examination of a biopsy confirmed a diagnosis of cutaneous habronemiasis. The coagulated exudate (*arrows*) can be a feature of cutaneous habronemiasis and pythiosis. The lesion was successfully treated with topical fenthion/dimethylsulfoxide/dexamethasone and enteral ivermectin. (*Courtesy of* Dr. J. Joyce, DVM, Texas A&M University, College Station, TX.)

and the cause of self-mutilation [56,57]. This disease, also known as phycomycosis or Florida leeches, is traditionally thought of as a subtropical disease and is seen in the southern United States, but it should be a consideration for these types of lesions in horses with a history of standing in water and living in a warm climate. Diagnosis is based on clinical signs, such as the presence of "kunkers," and is confirmed with biopsy and immunoassays [57]. Kunkers are staghorn-coral–shaped coagula of necrotic vessels, dead eosinophils, and *Pythium* hyphae, usually within draining sinus tracts [57]. Treatment should include radical excision as soon as possible and systemic administration of amphotericin B and topical Phycofixer (Franck's Pharmacy, Ocala, Florida).

Evaluation of trauma to the head and neck should include a neurologic examination in addition to ophthalmic, oral, and endoscopic examinations. Cranial and cervical spinal radiographs may be indicated. Wounds to the head and neck can generally be evaluated in the standing horse with sedation. The effects of sedation may not be as expected in cases in which head trauma is encountered, and caution should be exercised. Phenothiazine tranquilizers produce hypotension, can lower seizure threshold, and last for several hours [58]. α_2-Adrenergic agonists, such as xylazine and detomidine, may reduce central venous blood pressure; however, in the case of xylazine, the effect is relatively short lived [58].

Wounds of the head tend to heal rapidly, given that the head is well supplied with blood. In cases of chronic wounds, however, the lack of soft tissue and skin mobility can make surgical debridement and reconstruction difficult. Cicatrix formation can be a cosmetic and functional problem, especially if lesions involve the palpebrae. Chronic and infected wounds on the head often signify the presence of a foreign body or a secondary process, such as neoplasia, fungal infection, or habronemiasis (Fig. 4). Repeat radiographs should be performed to look for sequestra. EGT rarely develops on the head. When EGT is presented with a nonhealing head wound, further diagnostic tests should include scrapings, culture, and biopsy. Rule-outs for these types of lesion include bone sequestrum, foreign body, cutaneous habronemiasis, pythiosis, and fibroblastic sarcoid (Fig. 5) [55].

Traumatic wounds to the trunk can pose severe complications in terms of penetrating the thoracic or abdominal cavity. Wounds to the trunk can result from impalement and blunt trauma as well as from fractured ribs in the case of the thorax. Penetration of the thoracic cavity requires emergency stabilization in terms of respiratory and circulatory collapse from pneumothorax or pneumomediastinum and hemothorax, respectively [59]. Packing of the wound and evacuation of the pneumothorax should be performed. Aspiration of gas from the pleural space should be performed using a large-gauge needle or cannula with a three-way stopcock adjacent to the cranial edge of the 12th to 15th ribs dorsally. Intensive care support and monitoring need to be used. The potential for a mixed population of bacteria inoculating accumulated fluid and devitalized tissue makes managing such wounds

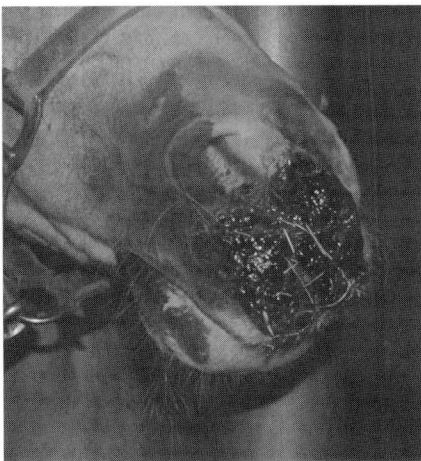

Fig. 4. Chronic nonhealing wound on the nose and upper lip of an 8-year-old Arabian gelding. Histologic examination of a biopsy of this lesion revealed it to be a squamous cell carcinoma. The extensive nature of this lesion made surgical debridement difficult. (*Courtesy of* Dr. J. Joyce, DVM, Texas A&M University, College Station, TX.)

a challenge. Drainage of fluid and debridement of devitalized tissue, lavage of closed spaces, and prolonged antimicrobial therapy are necessary when treating infections in the thoracic cavity (Fig. 6). Monitoring the patient with serial ultrasonography and radiography as well as with hematologic values, such as leukocyte count and fibrinogen, is invaluable.

Wounds to the axilla can cause subcutaneous emphysema. The horse often remains comfortable in spite of alarming subcutaneous gas accumulation. Packing of the wound with moist gauze and strict stall rest can

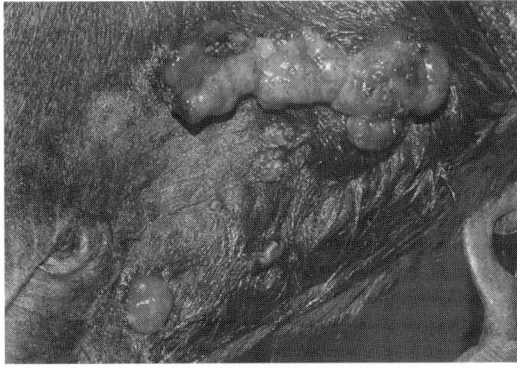

Fig. 5. Chronic nonhealing wound on the rostral aspect of the left cheek and lower lip of an 8-year-old gelding. Histologic examination of a biopsy confirmed a diagnosis of fibroblastic sarcoid. (*Courtesy of* Dr. J. Joyce, DVM, Texas A&M University, College Station, TX.)

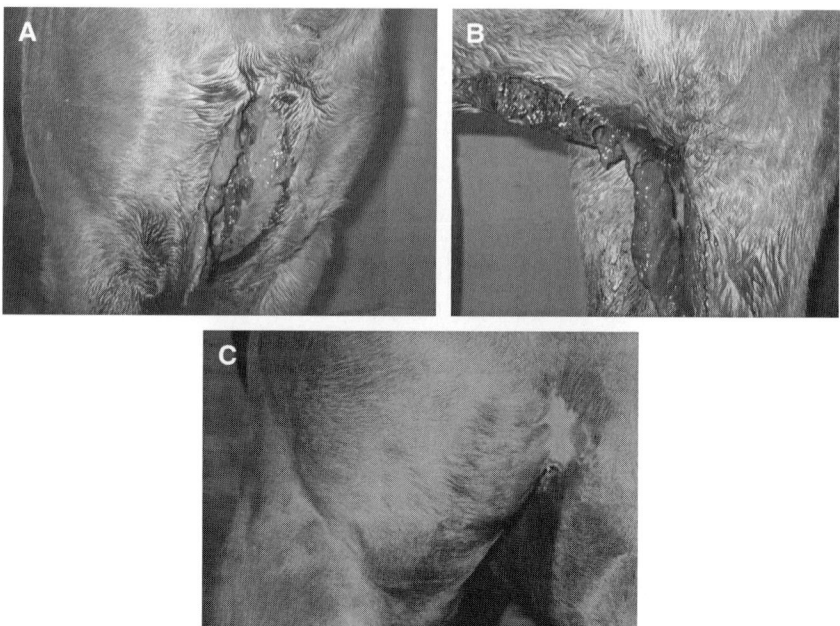

Fig. 6. A 3-year-old Quarter Horse mare with a right axilla wound. Cranial view (*A*) and lateral view (*B*). The wound was approximately 50 cm deep. Although the ribs and sternebrae could be palpated, the thoracic cavity had not been penetrated. The wound was treated with daily lavage with water and surgical scrub, and the horse was treated with systemic antimicrobials. The distal limb was kept clean and dry, and topical petroleum jelly was applied to prevent serum scald. The horse was stall confined and had extensive subcutaneous emphysema, which took approximately 8 weeks to resolve. (*C*) Cranial view of the wound several months later.

offset further emphysema until sufficient granulation prevents further aspiration of air (Fig. 7). This can take weeks; during that time, the skin overlying areas of subcutaneous emphysema should be monitored for normal texture and temperature. Although the subcutis rarely succumbs to infection provided that the wound is kept clean, the patient must be monitored for air dissecting to the mediastinum, which can cause pneumomediastinum and subsequent respiratory distress associated with pneumothorax. In warm climates, these horses may need protection from hot weather, because the emphysema acts as an insulating layer. Management of these wounds should include cleansing with 0.1% povidone-iodine or 0.05% chlorhexidine gluconate. Granulation tissue can be stimulated by hydrotherapy once or twice daily. Skin care to prevent scalding is important.

Penetrating wounds to the abdomen carry with them a guarded prognosis resulting from the ensuing peritonitis [60]. If the bowel is lacerated, the clinical picture is one of a horse that is obtunded or showing signs of colic, toxemia, tachycardia, and tachypnea. Fever is present if circulatory collapse is not advanced. The prognosis for horses with a lacerated bowel is so poor that

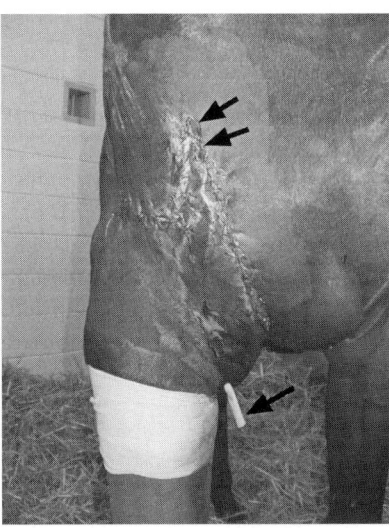

Fig. 7. A 4-year-old Thoroughbred mare with a right axilla wound. Primary closure of this wound was performed. A Jackson-Pratt closed-suction drain and a Penrose drain were placed. The Jackson-Pratt drain was removed after 3 days, and the Penrose drain (*arrow*) was removed after 5 days. The risks involved in primary closure of this kind of wound include sealing a dead space, leading to the accumulation of fluid and the development of infection. The advantage is the reduced amount of subcutaneous emphysema developing. The inverted "V" of skin was nonviable (*double arrow*). Dehiscence usually occurs and requires management similar to that described for the horse in Fig. 6. If sufficient granulation tissue develops, the further development of subcutaneous emphysema can be avoided. The distal limb was wrapped to reduce edema.

euthanasia is usually considered the best option. If a penetrating wound breaches the peritoneum without bowel damage, infections are usually mixed [60]. When wounds do not penetrate the peritoneal cavity, the wound and peritoneal fluid (collected from a distant site) should be monitored for any sign of infection. The contamination phase of peritonitis, generally considered to be the first 3 to 6 hours, involves inoculation of the peritoneum and the subsequent inflammatory response. If the infection is not eliminated, the peritoneal circulation results in the entire area becoming infected [60]. Progression of the inflammatory process results in exudate hindering bacterial clearance by phagocytes. In polymicrobial models of peritonitis, coliforms are the organisms that cause septicemia at this stage, and mortality is high [61]. In cases of postoperative septic peritonitis, the mortality rate was 56% [61]. In cases of abdominal wounds in which the peritoneum is involved, broad-spectrum antimicrobials should be used and therapy should be aggressive.

Wounds that involve partial thickness of the body wall generally heal well in terms of granulation and re-epithelialization but may require reconstructive surgery to repair an area of body wall weakness that may develop into a hernia. Belly bandages may offer support and reduce dead space and edema [62].

Cellulitis

Cellulitis is infection and inflammation of the subcutaneous tissues anywhere on the body, for example, after esophageal rupture or limb laceration. This section is devoted to the clinical syndrome of severe cellulitis, where a deep suppurative process dissects through tissue planes of one or more affected limbs, resulting in major tissue damage and a guarded prognosis.

The horse develops acute swelling and severe lameness, and the entire limb rapidly becomes two or three times its normal size and is hot and painful to the touch [63]. The horse may be febrile, with hyperfibrinogenemia and a normal white cell count or leukocytosis [63,64]. The skin becomes devitalized and suppurates or sloughs (see Fig. 7). Laminitis, bacteremia, and osteomyelitis are possible sequelae [63]. Counterirritant application can mimic the clinical signs of cellulitis but usually responds well to anti-inflammatory therapy and bandaging [63]. Radiographs should be performed to rule out bone-related causes of lameness and swelling. Ultrasonography can be used to locate areas of fluid accumulation to aspirate for culture and to evaluate blood flow with Doppler imaging [48]. Flow-phase scintigraphy can be helpful in determining the degree of blood flow movement to an affected limb (Fig. 8). Scintigraphy is better tolerated by the horse compared with Doppler imaging, because no direct pressure is applied to the painful limb. In a case series of nine racehorses with cellulitis, coagulase-positive *Staphylococcus* spp were identified as the causative organisms [64]. *S aureus* and *Staphylococcus intermedius* are the most common infecting organisms [63]. *S aureus* is capable of producing several toxins that are directly related to the pathogenesis of disease. Important toxins include leukocidin, toxin shock syndrome toxin-1 (TSST-1), exfoliative toxins, and hemolysins (α, β, δ, and γ) [65]. Leukocidin causes leukocyte degranulation and, with the other toxins, induces massive release of cytokines, directly damages endothelial cells, and increases cell sensitivity to cytokines [65]. The hemolysins are cytotoxic to erythrocytes, skin, and nerve cells; cause an increase in cell permeability; and activate the arachidonic acid cascade [66]. All these toxins can act as superantigens, which form a bridge between the major histocompatibility complex on macrophages and the T-cell receptor [66]. This results in heightened sensitivity to cytokines and T-cell multiplication, leading to a massive release of proinflammatory cytokines from macrophages and the proliferating T cells [66]. TSST-1 is one of the more potent toxins and, in vitro, is directly cytotoxic to endothelial cells [66]. These toxins have been identified in equine *S aureus* isolates [67]. Staphylococcal cellulitis resembles wound-associated toxin shock syndrome in human patients [65]. This syndrome in people may not be exclusively a staphylococcal manifestation, because *S pyogenes* is a recently recognized cause of necrotizing fasciitis [68]. Case reports exist that demonstrate that

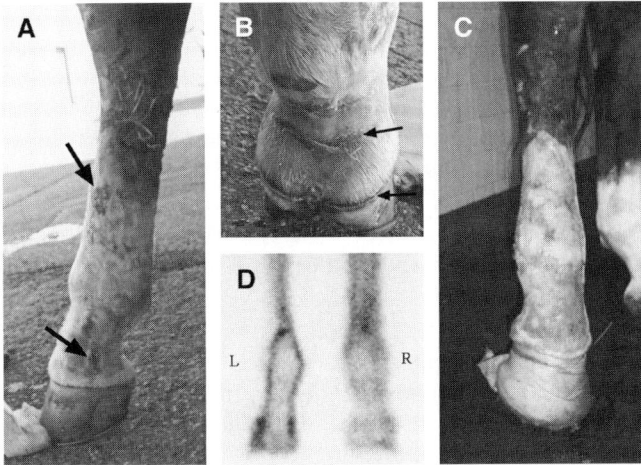

Fig. 8. An 18-year-old Quarter Horse mare with right hind limb cellulitis. The mare was reluctant to bear weight on the limb, which was hot and painful to the touch. Dorsomedial view (*A*) and plantar view (*B*). The arrows point to areas of skin that were starting to slough and to separation of the coronary band. (*C*) Dorsolateral view. Approximately 7 days after presentation, the mare started using the limb, but it was cold to the touch and did not bleed when pricked with a sterile needle. Ischemia, leading to tissue necrosis, was confirmed with flow-phase scintigraphy and was thought to be the reason for improved comfort on the limb. (*D*) Flow-phase scintigraphy of the hind limbs was performed. This image represents the plantar view minutes after intravenous injection of the radiopharmaceutical. The limb on the left shows the radiopharmaceutical flow through the plantar metatarsal and digital vessels. The limb on the right shows photopenia resulting from vascular thrombosis. The mare was euthanized. (*Courtesy of* Dr. B.M. Kraus, DVM, DACVS, University of Pennsylvania, Kennett Square, PA.)

Corynebacterium equi [69] and *Rhodococcus equi* [70] can be causes of cellulitis, and samples for culture and susceptibility testing should always be submitted if possible.

Aggressive therapy should be instituted, including broad-spectrum bactericidal antimicrobials, such as penicillin and gentamicin, until culture and susceptibility test results are available. The promotion of weight bearing and analgesia with nonsteroidal anti-inflammatory drugs (NSAIDs), hydrotherapy, and bandaging should be used [63]. Cellulitis is a severe disease in the horse, and aggressive therapy is necessary to reduce severe life-threatening complications, such as extensive tissue necrosis, laminitis, and widespread thrombosis. Horses that recover rarely regain the original contour of their limb and seem to be predisposed to recurrence [63].

Horses with ulcerative lymphangitis can present with clinical signs that resemble staphylococcal cellulitis. The causative agent is *Corynebacterium pseudotuberculosis*, a gram-positive pleomorphic rod, which is found to cause infection of cutaneous lymphatics and abscesses in the western United States. The incidence of ulcerative lymphangitis is seasonal and thought to be associated with horn fly activity [55]. The affected limb is swollen and painful, with palpable cording and nodule formation of the lymphatics. Abscesses develop, drain, and heal quickly, but more develop in adjacent areas. Ulcerative lymphangitis does not share the necrotizing nature that is so devastating in staphylococcal cellulitis but does produce some toxins, such as phospholipase D and sphingomyelinase, that damage endothelial cells and increase vascular permeability. The synergistic action of sphingomyelinase with the exotoxin of *R equi* in lysing erythrocytes in agar forms the basis of the synergistic hemolysis inhibition (SHI) test that is used to confirm infection [71]. Staining of smears of pus samples reveal gram-positive, pleomorphic, rod-shaped bacteria in abundance. Microbiologic culture confirms the diagnosis, and implementation of rapid treatment limits chronic lameness and disfigurement. Treatment should include systemic penicillin (eg, procaine penicillin G, 22,000–44,000 IU/kg, administered intramuscularly every 12 hours for up to 30 days, or potassium penicillin, 22,000 IU/kg, administered intravenously every 6 hours), NSAIDs, and wound care, bearing in mind that drainage is critical [55]. Although it is endemic on certain farms, appropriate hygiene and precautions should be observed so that no other animals come into contact with the purulent discharge draining from ruptured abscesses. Affected animals should be isolated, and good fly control should be practiced [71].

Myositis

Infectious diseases of the musculature can be bacterial, viral, or parasitic. Immune-mediated myositis is recognized in horses with a history of *Streptococcus equi* subsp *equi* infection. Two forms are recognized: IgA-mediated and IgG-mediated poststreptococcal myositis. These disease entities are beyond the scope of this review, which focuses on bacterial myositis.

Bacterial myositis is most commonly caused by a variety of *Clostridium* spp, such as *Clostridium septicum*, *Clostridium perfringens*, *Clostridium novyi*, *Clostridium chauvoei*, and *Clostridium sordelli*. *C perfringens* and *C septicum* are the most common bacteria isolated from horses [72]. Culture and sensitivity testing can still be valuable, because *Bacillus cereus* has been documented to cause a fulminant necrotizing infection after penetrating trauma in human patients [73,74]. *Gas gangrene* and *malignant edema* are terms applied to clostridial myositis and historically represent the pathologic features associated with specific organisms; however, mixed infections are common. Historical information pertinent to a case includes previous intramuscular injection as well as recent parturition, castration, or a puncture wound [75]. Intramuscular injection techniques had no influence on the development of disease [76], and the preparation was more likely to be associated with disease [75]. Colic, exertional myopathy, and laminitis may also be part of the history, because these are reported reasons for intramuscular medication administration [75]. Intramuscular injections of irritating substances with an alkaline pH or that lower redox potential are thought to create a suitable environment for clostridial spore germination [72]. There is limited evidence that spores are present in normal equine skeletal muscle [72], further supporting the hypothesis that a change in muscle milieu is responsible for germination. In one study of 37 horses with clostridial myonecrosis, most of the horses had received one or more of the following as intramuscular injections; flunixin meglumine, B vitamins, or procaine penicillin G [75]. Thirty-four of the 37 horses in that study received intramuscular flunixin meglumine. A number of these horses were being treated with flunixin meglumine for colic. In the human literature, although IM injections are not a feature, there seems to be an association between certain types of gastrointestinal disease and the development of clostridial myositis [77].

Clinical signs in horses can range from sudden death to delayed-onset muscle swelling and lameness (Fig. 9). Gas crepitation is often, but not always, present, and the skin overlying the region is taut and may be hot and discolored, progressing to cold and firm. Horses are often toxemic, febrile, obtunded, and showing signs of cardiovascular shock. Rapid progression to coma and death can occur. Ultrasonography is of limited use over the area of crepitus but is essential to identify deep necrotic areas.

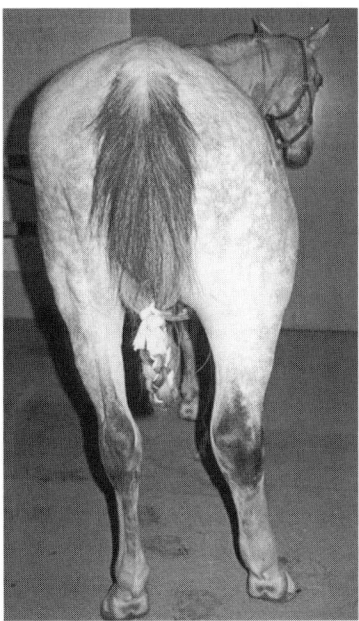

Fig. 9. Adult Thoroughbred with acute severe lameness and swelling of the right thigh area. This horse had clostridial myositis. Ultrasonography can be used to detect pockets of subcutaneous gas and to ensure that fasciotomies are performed in appropriate areas and at appropriate depths. Fasciotomy incisions should be a minimum of 2 cm in length and deep enough to reach gas pockets in the musculature. Incisions can be extended as necessary to facilitate massive debridement of necrotic muscle. (*Courtesy of* Dr. J. Hardy, DVM, PhD, DACVS, Texas A&M University, College Station, TX.)

Aspiration of foul-smelling gas and fluid from the site leads to a clinical diagnosis, and aspirates show numerous gram-positive rods when stained. Hematology shows hemoconcentration, leukocytosis with a left shift, and toxic changes in neutrophils, and serum levels of creatine kinase (CK) and aspartate aminotransferase (AST) are high compared with normal. Immune-mediated hemolytic anemia has been found in a few horses [78] but remains rare. The absolute absence of neutrophils in affected tissue perplexed earlier physicians examining gangrenous limbs. Now, we recognize a potent array of exotoxins produced during the log-phase growth period, including α-toxin, a phospholipase C, which is the most important. α-Toxin, along with the other exotoxins, inhibits leukocyte infiltration, increases vascular permeability and platelet aggregation, causes cell lysis, and can cause direct myocardial dysfunction [79].

Treatment of clostridial myositis should be aggressive and include antimicrobials, intravenous fluids, surgical debridement and fasciotomy, anti-inflammatory and/or analgesic therapy, and supportive care (Fig. 10). Intravenous fluids should be used to support circulating volume and offset any pigment nephropathy that may result from extensive muscle damage. When deciding on antimicrobial choice, bacterial killing and toxin production inhibition should be considered. In a mouse model of *C perfringens* gas gangrene, survival was poorest for penicillin-treated mice compared with those treated with tetracycline, chloramphenicol, clindamycin, rifampin, or metronidazole [80,81]. None of these antimicrobials were found to directly interfere with α-toxin activity. Further in vitro studies showed that

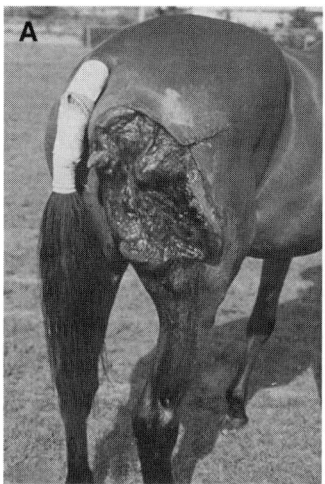
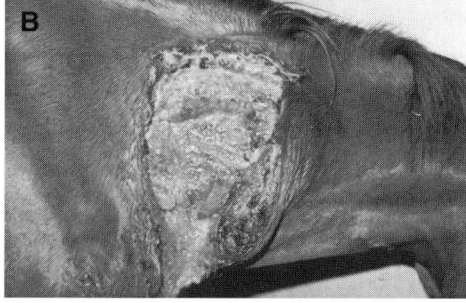

Fig. 10. Adult horses with a large wound that is the result of clostridial myonecrosis. Both horses had received an intramuscular injection in the affected sites. (*A*) Adult horse with a large wound on the hindquarters. (*B*) Adult horse that received an intramuscular injection in the left side of its neck and subsequently developed clostridial myonecrosis. (*Courtesy of* Dr. J. Hardy, DVM, PhD, DACVS, Texas A&M University, College Station, TX.)

penicillin was not as effective at bacterial killing, however, nor did it reduce α-toxin production as effectively as the above-mentioned drugs [81]. Metronidazole and rifampin are bactericidal drugs that also inhibit α-toxin production. Although penicillin has emerged over the years as the drug of choice for treating clostridial myositis, we need to review its role in terms of these data. Intravenous metronidazole alone may be the best choice [81]. Irritating intramuscular injections should be avoided if an intravenous alternative is readily available. Peek and colleagues [75] demonstrated that procaine penicillin G administered intramuscularly does not prevent clostridial myositis. Anecdotally, any intramuscular injections in the semitendinosus or semimembranosus muscles of horses with diarrhea should be avoided. Fasciotomy and debridement should be extensive and provide drainage, removal of all necrotic tissue, portals for vigorous lavage, and aeration. Intravenous fluids should be administered to improve cardiovascular status and prevent pigment nephropathy.

Infections with *C sordelli* carry the worst prognosis [75]. Infections with *C perfringens* carry a better prognosis provided that therapy is implemented quickly and aggressively, with a reported survival to the time of discharge from the hospital of 73% [75]. There is some supportive evidence that hyperbaric oxygen therapy has some benefit as an adjunctive treatment of necrotizing myositis in human patients [82].

Summary

SSIs and traumatic wound management remain challenging clinical scenarios. The prevention of SSIs involves meticulous surgical technique and aftercare. Traumatic wounds require thorough evaluation to assess the involvement of synovial structures and radiographs to check for fractures. Chronic wounds can require a biopsy and histologic evaluation to obtain a diagnosis, because many underlying pathologic processes grossly appear similar but different treatment regimens are required.

Early recognition and diagnosis of cellulitis and myositis enable the rapid aggressive intervention necessary for a positive outcome. Any delay in diagnosis and treatment increases the complication and mortality rates and makes these conditions difficult to treat successfully.

References

[1] Horan TC, Gaynes RP, Martone WJ, et al. CDC definitions of nosocomial surgical site infections, 1992: a modification of the CDC definitions of surgical wound infections. Am J Infect Control 1992;20:271–4.
[2] Roettinger W, Edgerton MT, Kurtz LD, et al. Role of inoculation site as a determinant of infection in soft tissue wounds. Am J Surg 1973;126:354–8.
[3] Grewe SR, Stephens BO, Perlino C, et al. Influence of internal fixation on wound infections. J Trauma 1987;27:1051–4.

[4] Elek SD, Conen PE. The virulence of *Staphylococcus pyogenes* for man: a study of the problems of wound infection. Br J Exp Pathol 1975;38:573–86.
[5] Vinh DC, Embil JM. Device-related infections: a review. J Long Term Eff Med Implants 2005;15:467–88.
[6] Trotter GW. Osteomyelitis. In: Nixon AJ, editor. Equine fracture repair. Philadelphia: WB Saunders; 1996. p. 359–66.
[7] Aricola CR, Campoccia D, Gamberini S, et al. Prevalence of *cna*, *fnbA* and *fnbB* adhesin genes among *Staphylococcus aureus* isolates from orthopaedic infections associated with different types of implant. FEMS Microbiol Lett 2005;246:81–6.
[8] Smeltzer MS, Gillaspy AF. Molecular pathogenesis of staphylococcal osteomyelitis. Poult Sci 2000;79:1042–9.
[9] Moore RM, Schneider RK, Kowalski J, et al. Antimicrobial susceptibility of bacterial isolates from 233 horses with musculoskeletal infection during 1979–1989. Equine Vet J 1992;24:450–6.
[10] Patti JM, Allen BL, McGavin MJ, et al. MSCRAMM-mediated adherence of microorganisms to host tissue. Annu Rev Microbiol 1994;48:585–617.
[11] Mohanty SS, Kay PR. Infection in total hip joint replacements. Why we screen MRSA when MRSE is the problem. Br J Bone Joint Surg 2004;86:266–8.
[12] Aricola CR, Campoccia D, Gamberini S, et al. Antibiotic resistance in exopolysaccharide-forming *Staphylococcus epidermidis* clinical isolates from orthopaedic implant infections. Biomaterials 2005;26:6530–5.
[13] Trostle SS, Peavey CL, King DS, et al. Treatment of methicillin-resistant *Staphylococcus epidermidis* infection following repair of an ulnar fracture and humeroradial joint luxation in a horse. J Am Vet Med Assoc 2001;218:554–9.
[14] Stewart PS. Mechanisms of antibiotic resistance in bacterial biofilms. Int J Med Microbiol 2002;292:107–13.
[15] Phillips TJ, Walmsley JP. Retrospective analysis of the results of 151 exploratory laparotomies in horses with gastrointestinal disease. Equine Vet J 1993;25:427–31.
[16] MacDonald DG, Morley PS, Bailey JV, et al. An examination of occurrence of surgical wound infection following orthopedic surgery (1981-1990). Equine Vet J 1994;26:323–6.
[17] Kaye KS, Schmit K, Pieper C, et al. The effect of increasing age on the risk of surgical site infection. J Infect Dis 2005;191:1056–62.
[18] Wong ES. Surgical site infections. In: Mayhall CG, editor. Hospital epidemiology and infection control. Baltimore (MD): Williams & Wilkins; 1996. p. 154–60.
[19] Wilson DA, Baker GJ, Boero MJ. Complications of celiotomy incisions in horses. Vet Surg 1995;24:506–14.
[20] Riou JP, Cohen JR, Johnson H Jr. Factors influencing wound dehiscence. Am J Surg 1992;106:573–7.
[21] Hill GE, Frawley WH, Griffith KE, et al. Allogenic blood transfusion increases the risk of postoperative bacterial infection: a meta-analysis. J Trauma 2003;54:908–14.
[22] Sorensen LT, Hemmingsen U, Kallehave F, et al. Risk factors for tissue and wound complications in gastrointestinal surgery. Ann Surg 2005;241:654–8.
[23] Dougherty SH, Fiegel VD, Nelson RD, et al. Effects of soil infection potentiating factors on neutrophils in vitro. Am J Surg 1985;150:306–11.
[24] Santschi EM. Diagnosis and management of surgical site infections and antimicrobial prophylaxis. In: Auer JA, Stick JA, editors. Equine surgery. 2nd edition. Philadelphia: WB Saunders; 1992. p. 54–60.
[25] Schneider RK, Bramlage LR, Moore RM, et al. A retrospective study of 192 horses affected with septic arthritis/tenosynovitis. Equine Vet J 1992;24:436–42.
[26] Schneider RK, Bramlage LR, Mecklenburg LM, et al. Open drainage, intra-articular and systemic antibiotics in the treatment of septic arthritis/tenosynovitis in horses. Equine Vet J 1992;24:443–9.

[27] Brumbaugh GW. Use of antimicrobials in wound management. Vet Clin North Am Equine Pract 2005;21:63–76.
[28] Snyder J, Pascoe J, Hirsch D. Antimicrobial susceptibility of microorganisms from equine orthopedics patients. Vet Surg 1987;16:197–201.
[29] Chambers HF. The aminoglycosides. In: Hardman JG, Limbird LE, Gilman AG, editors. Goodman & Gilman's the pharmacological basis of therapeutics. 10th edition. New York: McGraw-Hill; 2001. p. 1219–38.
[30] Sayegh AI, Moore RM. Polymethylmethacrylate beads for treating orthopedic infections. Compend Contin Educ Pract Vet 2003;25:788–96.
[31] Ingle-Fehr JE, Howard RD, Trotter GW, et al. Bacterial culturing of ventral median celiotomies for prediction of postoperative incisional complications in horses. Vet Surg 1997;26: 7–13.
[32] Wiley AM, Ha'eri GB. Routes of infection: a study of using tracer particles in the orthopedic operating room. Clin Orthop 1979;139:150–5.
[33] Smith MA, Ross MW. Postoperative infection with Actinobacillus spp in horses: 10 cases (1995–2000). J Am Vet Med Assoc 2002;221:1306–10.
[34] Stashak TS. Management of lacerations and avulsion injuries of the foot and pastern region and hoof wall cracks. Vet Clin North Am Equine Pract 1989;5:195–220.
[35] Kirsner RS, Eaglstein WH. The wound healing process. Dermatol Clin 1993;11:629–40.
[36] Van Den Bloom R, Wilmink JM, O'Kane S, et al. Transforming growth factor-β levels during second intention healing are related to the different course of wound contraction in horses and ponies. Wound Repair Regen 2002;10:188–94.
[37] Wilmink JM, Van Weeren PR. Second-intention repair in the horse and pony and management of exuberant granulation tissue. Vet Clin North Am Equine Pract 2005;21:15–32.
[38] Wilson DA. Cellular events of wound healing and their potential clinical applications. In: Proceedings of the American College of Veterinary Surgeons Annual Conference, Denver, CO. American College of Veterinary Surgeons; 2004. p. 134–6.
[39] Gomez JH, Schumacher J, Lauten SD, et al. Effects of 3 biologic dressings on healing of cutaneous wounds on the distal limbs of horses. Can J Vet Res 2004;68:49–55.
[40] Carter CA, Jolly DG, Worden CE, et al. Platelet-rich plasma promotes differentiation and regeneration during equine wound healing. Exp Mol Pathol 2003;74:244–55.
[41] Rowlatt U. Intrauterine wound healing in a 20 week old human fetus. Virchows Arch A Pathol Anat Histol 1979;381:353–61.
[42] Wilgus TA, Bergdall VK, Dipietro LA, et al. Hydrogen peroxide disrupts scarless fetal wound repair. Wound Repair Regen 2005;13:513–9.
[43] Berry DB, Sullins KE. Effects of topical applications of antimicrobials and bandaging on healing and granulation tissue formation in wounds of the distal aspect of the limbs in horses. Am J Vet Res 2003;64:88–92.
[44] Theoret CL, Barber SM, Moyana TN, et al. Expression of transforming growth factor $β_1$, $β_3$ and basic fibroblast growth factor in full-thickness skin wounds of equine limbs and thorax. Vet Surg 2001;30:269–77.
[45] Knottenbolt DC. Handbook of equine wound management. Liverpool (UK): WB Saunders; 2003.
[46] Baxter GM. Wound management. In: White NA, Moore JA, editors. Current techniques in equine surgery and lameness. 2nd edition. Philadelphia: WB Saunders; 1998. p. 72–80.
[47] Stashak TS. Equine wound management. Philadelphia: Lea & Febiger; 1991.
[48] Reef VB. Ultrasonographic evaluation of small parts. In: Equine diagnostic ultrasound. Philadelphia: WB Saunders; 1998. p. 480–547.
[49] Southwood LL, Baxter GM. Instrument sterilization, skin preparation, and wound management. Vet Clin North Am Equine Pract 1996;12:173–94.
[50] Sebben JE. Surgical antiseptics. J Am Acad Dermatol 1983;9:759–65.
[51] Stubbs WP, Bellah JR, Vermaas-Hekman D, et al. Chlorhexidine gluconate versus chloroxylenol for preoperative skin preparation in dogs. Vet Surg 1996;25:487–94.

[52] Higgins KR, Ashry HR. Wound dressings and topical agents. Clin Podiatr Med Surg 1995; 12:31–40.
[53] Kunin CM. Resistance to antimicrobial drugs—a worldwide calamity. Ann Intern Med 1993;118:557–61.
[54] Ducharme M, Celeste C, Theoret CL. Effect of a silicone gel dressing on exuberant granulation tissue formation in the horse. In: Proceedings of American College of Veterinary Surgeons Annual Conference, Denver, CO. American College of Veterinary Surgeons; 2004. p. 22.
[55] Rees CR. Disorders of the skin. In: Reed SM, Bayly WM, Sellon DC, editors. Equine internal medicine. 2nd edition. St. Louis (MO): WB Saunders; 2004. p. 667–720.
[56] Rees CA, Craig TM. Cutaneous habronemiasis. In: Robinson NE, editor. Current therapy in equine medicine 5. St. Louis (MO): WB Saunders; 2003. p. 195–200.
[57] Poole HM, Brashier MK. Equine cutaneous pythiosis. Compend Contin Educ Pract Vet 2003;25:229–36.
[58] Muir WW. Standing chemical restraint in horses: tranquilizers, sedatives, and analgesics. In: Muir WW, Hubbell JA, editors. Equine anesthesia: monitoring and emergency therapy. St. Louis (MO): Mosby; 1991. p. 247–80.
[59] Holcombe SJ, Laverty S. Thoracic trauma. In: Auer JA, Stick JA, editors. Equine surgery. 2nd edition. Philadelphia: WB Saunders; 1999. p. 382–6.
[60] Dickinson C. Peritonitis. In: Reed SM, Bayly WM, Sellon DC, editors. Equine internal medicine. 2nd edition. St. Louis (MO): WB Saunders; 2004. p. 941–9.
[61] Hawkins JF, Bowman KF, Roberts MC, et al. Peritonitis in horses: 67 cases (1985–1990). J Am Vet Med Assoc 1993;203:284–8.
[62] Hardy J, Rakestraw PC. Postoperative care and complications associated with abdominal surgery. In: Auer JA, Stick JA, editors. Equine surgery. 2nd edition. Philadelphia: WB Saunders; 1999. p. 294–306.
[63] Evans AG, White SD. Bacterial diseases. In: Smith BP, editor. Large animal medicine. 3rd edition. St. Louis (MO): Mosby; 2002. p. 1208–9.
[64] Markel MD, Wheat JD, Jang SS. Cellulitis associated with coagulase-positive staphylococci in racehorses: nine cases (1975–1984). J Am Vet Med Assoc 1986;189:1600–3.
[65] Long MT. Mechanisms of establishment and spread of bacterial and fungal infections. In: Reed SM, Bayly WM, Sellon DC, editors. Equine internal medicine. 2nd edition. St. Louis (MO): WB Saunders; 2004. p. 59–72.
[66] Dinges MM, Orwin PM, Schlievert PM. Exotoxins of Staphylococcus aureus. Clin Microbiol Rev 2000;13:16–34.
[67] Sato H, Matsumori M, Tanabe T, et al. A new type of staphylococcal exfoliative toxin from Staphylococcus aureus isolated from a horse with phlegmon. Infect Immun 1994;62:3780–5.
[68] Barnham MR, Weightman NC, Anderson AW, et al. Streptococcal toxic shock syndrome: a description of 14 cases from North Yorkshire, UK. Clin Microbiol Infect 2002;8:174–81.
[69] Etherington WG, Prescott JF. Corynebacterium equi cellulitis associated with Strongyloides penetration in a foal. J Am Vet Med Assoc 1980;177:1025–7.
[70] Perdrizet JA, Scott DW. Cellulitis and subcutaneous abscesses caused by Rhodococcus equi infection in a foal. J Am Vet Med Assoc 1987;190:1559–61.
[71] Aleman MR, Spier SJ. Corynebacterium pseudotuberculosis infection. In: Smith BP, editor. Large animal medicine. 3rd edition. St. Louis (MO): Mosby; 2002. p. 1078–84.
[72] Vengust M, Arroyo LG, Weese JS, et al. Preliminary evidence for dormant clostridial spores in equine skeletal muscle. Equine Vet J 2003;35:514–6.
[73] Darbar A, Harris IA, Gosbell IB. Necrotizing infection due to Bacillus cereus mimicking gas gangrene following penetrating trauma. J Orthop Trauma 2005;19:353–5.
[74] Dryden MS. Pathogenic role of Bacillus cereus in wound infections in the tropics. J R Soc Med 1987;80:480–1.
[75] Peek SF, Semrad SD, Perkins GA. Clostridial myonecrosis in horses (37 cases 1985–2000). Equine Vet J 2003;35:86–92.

[76] Brown CM, Kaneene JB, Walker RD. Intramuscular injection techniques and the development of clostridial myonecrosis or cellulitis in horses. J Am Vet Med Assoc 1988;193:668–70.
[77] Stevens DL, Musher DM, Watson DA, et al. Spontaneous, nontraumatic gangrene due to *Clostridium septicum*. Rev Infect Dis 1990;12:286–96.
[78] Weiss DJ, Moritz A. Equine immune-mediated hemolytic anemia associated with *Clostridium perfringens* infection. Vet Clin Pathol 2003;32:22–6.
[79] Rood JI, McClane BA, Songer JG, et al, editors. The clostridia. Molecular biology and pathogenesis. San Diego (CA): Academic Press; 1997.
[80] Stevens DL, Maier KA, Mitten JE. Effect of antibiotics on toxin production and viability of *Clostridium perfringens*. Antimicrob Agents Chemother 1987;31:213–8.
[81] Stevens DL, Maier KA, Laine BM, et al. Comparison of clindamycin, rifampin, tetracycline, metronidazole, and penicillin for efficacy in prevention of experimental gas gangrene due to *Clostridium perfringens*. J Infect Dis 1987;155:220–8.
[82] Stevens DL, Bryant AE, Adams K, et al. Evaluation of therapy with hyperbaric oxygen for experimental infection with *Clostridium perfringens*. Clin Infect Dis 1993;17:231–7.

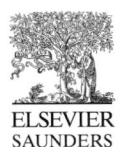

Septic Arthritis, Tenosynovitis, and Infections of Hoof Structures

Joel Lugo, DVM, MS, Earl M. Gaughan, DVM*

J.T. Vaughan Large Animal Hospital, Department of Clinical Sciences, College of Veterinary Medicine, Auburn University, Auburn, AL 36849, USA

Infection of synovial compartments and the structures within a horse's foot can be devastating to soundness, athletic careers, and even life for affected animals. Joint and tendon sheath sepsis disrupts normal function in the short term because of associated pain and inflammation. If unsuccessfully treated, long-term function is affected because of degenerative joint disease and fibrous tissue restriction of tendon and joint capsule motion. Unfortunately, these infections are quite common as a result of the anatomy and exposed nature of the distal limbs of horses. Early diagnosis and aggressive treatment can often result in satisfactory and normal return to function and athleticism, however.

Pathogenesis

An accurate medical history is essential to understand completely the etiopathogenesis of a case of septic synovitis. Signalment information can often give some insight into how an organism likely arrived in a synovial compartment. Younger foals typically are affected with septic synovitis, primarily septic arthritis, after systemic distribution of bacteria from a site distant to the affected joint. Foals with a primary nidus of infection are known to develop septic arthritis secondary to bacteremia. The most common sites of primary infection seeding joints seem to be the lungs and umbilical remnant tissues [1]. Therefore, it is wise to investigate thoroughly these tissues and the systemic health of a foal diagnosed with septic arthritis [1]. The most common avenue of bacterial delivery to synovial compartments of adult horses is through a wound.

---

* Corresponding author.
 E-mail address: gaughem@auburn.edu (E.M. Gaughan).

A thorough examination of any traumatic injury to the distal limb of a horse is essential for early detection of synovial contamination. Lacerations and puncture wounds are the most common avenues of bacterial delivery to a synovial structure. Therefore, when these types of wounds are near to or associated with a joint or tendon sheath, close inspection is required to determine the tissues involved. Wounds that lacerate or abrade the skin and subcutaneous tissues overlying synovial compartments can be frustrating to assess completely immediately after wounding. Occasionally, delayed contamination of a synovial compartment can occur if the capsule is damaged, such that necrosis and sloughing of overlying capsular tissue occurs over several days after wounding. Although rare, this type of synovial exposure should not be overlooked with wounds that disrupt superficial tissues over a joint or tendon sheath.

Diagnosis

The physical examination of a horse suspected of having septic synovitis should be thorough and should evaluate all appropriate body systems and tissues. Lameness resulting from septic synovitis is expected to be severe. With infection that is contained within a closed synovial compartment, the pressure and inflammation of the septic process can result in grade 4 to 5 (toe touching to non–weight-bearing) lameness. This is common secondary to puncture wounds and small synovial penetrations from other wounds. Severe lameness is also observed as an open synovial wound heals by second intention before the septic process has resolved. This particular situation may follow a misleading presentation. Horses with open joints and tendon sheaths may be comfortable if the synovial compartment is draining. Horses may also be comfortable if they are receiving higher doses of phenylbutazone. The observed lameness may be completely attributable to the wound and the tissue disruption rather than to the infection until the contaminated structure begins to close and entrap the septic inflamed fluid. Thus, it is possible that a horse with septic synovitis may not initially demonstrate the more severe grades of lameness commonly associated with this disease. This can be true for several days after injury.

Careful local examination of wounded or suspected infected tissues is indicated. Palpation of affected joints and tendon sheaths typically reveals swelling, which can be edema in perisynovial tissues and effusion within the synovial compartment. Other classic signs of inflammation are also normally present. Regional heat is often palpable, and erythema can be detected when hair is removed. Palpation and assessment of range of motion are often associated with an avoidance response indicating pain.

When suspected synovial sepsis is associated with a wound, careful cleaning is important in the acute stages. Restraint appropriate for close manipulative examination is essential. This typically requires sedation and often local anesthesia. At times, general anesthesia may be necessary to facilitate a complete assessment of tissue injury and contamination. Xylazine with butorphanol or detomidine is usually sufficient for sedation, and regional local anesthesia can make the examination easier. Sterile lavage solutions are recommended for wound cleaning to avoid any complicating factors from other sources of contamination. Clean tap water can also be helpful if the limb has marked gross contamination. Aggressive wound cleansing and removal of foreign material should be completed. The addition of disinfectants at this stage of evaluation is often used but may not be necessary. The removal of gross contaminants is most important to allow deeper assessment of the wound and underlying synovial structures. Manual palpation with a sterile gloved hand or the fingers can help to assess the depth of a wound as well as to identify intrasynovial tissue exposure. With appropriate restraint and local anesthesia, a wounded limb can be assessed with the horse standing in a weight-bearing position and with the affected limb held in the examiner's hand as palpation and manipulations are completed. Whenever an open synovial compartment is confirmed, aggressive treatment should be initiated. If any doubt exists, other diagnostic measures should be pursued and the suspect synovial structure considered infected until proven otherwise. One such method is to use a sterile surgical probe as an extension of the fingers. Malleable probes can be used to investigate punctures, smaller wounds, and the depths of larger wounds inaccessible to sterile fingers. If uncertainty remains when using a probe, radiographs can be made with a probe in place to determine the location of the probe and the likely tissues involved in a wound.

Perhaps the most convincing evidence that a synovial compartment has been opened after wounding is to place a sterile solution in the synovial space and confirm communication with the wound. This is accomplished in the same manner as routine synoviocentesis. The greatest challenge after wounding is to identify a location for needle placement that is sterile and does not increase the risk of synovial contamination. A site of unwounded normal skin over the "opposite" side of a joint from a wound is preferred. This is often difficult to identify and may depend on the timing after occurrence of the injury. With delay of hours to days, a wound site can become swollen and the subcutaneous space contaminated, such that passing a hypodermic needle could result in synovial contamination of an otherwise normal joint or tendon sheath. This should obviously be avoided and efforts concentrated on resolving the cellulitis before synoviocentesis is performed in the region. During this period, the synovial space should otherwise be treated as if infected, with administration of systemic antimicrobials and anti-inflammatory medications.

If an appropriate site can be identified, the overlying skin should be aseptically prepared and a hypodermic needle (21- to 14-gauge) placed in the suspected joint or tendon sheath. If at all possible, an aliquot of synovial fluid should be obtained from any synovial space under suspicion. This is often not possible, because the synovial fluid may be drained from an open structure and is not available for aspiration. If synovial fluid can be obtained, however, a nucleated cell count and measurement of total solids can be used to confirm infection. Synovial fluid can also be quickly assessed for total protein content with a refractometer. Total protein concentrations of 3.5 mg/dL or greater (normal ≤ 2.5 mg/dL) have been associated with septic synovial fluid. Total protein concentrations of 4.0 mg/dL or greater have been considered to indicate sepsis with more sensitivity than total synovial white blood cell counts [2]. Joint and tendon sheath fluid white blood cell counts greater than 30,000 cells/μL are typically associated with synovial sepsis. Some cases may present with lower cell counts if substantial deposits of fibrinous material are present, however. Absolute proof of synovial sepsis is dependent on locating and identifying a microorganism from the tissues in question. Therefore, cytologic identification of bacteria in synovial fluid and within synovial white blood cells is of great assistance. Culture and identification of the infecting microorganism(s) represent the ultimate confirmation of sepsis and are also tremendously helpful in orienting appropriate therapy. Positive culture and sensitivity results are substantially enhanced by placing synovial fluid in blood culture media and incubating for 24 hours before plating samples versus directly plating synovial fluid [1]. Blood culture incubation of infected synovial fluid samples can increase the odds of obtaining a positive culture from 40% to 80% compared with culturing synovial fluid directly onto agar plates [1]. Most often, there is a minimal period of empiric antimicrobial treatment while synovial fluid cultures are pending.

After synovial fluid has been obtained, a volume of sterile irrigation fluid (balanced polyionic fluid or saline) sufficient to distend the synovial compartment should be injected under pressure. Placing an intravenous extension set on the needle can assist with this procedure by accommodating for some motion on the part of the horse. If the injected fluid distends the synovial compartment without communication with the wound site, the joint or tendon sheath can be assumed to be closed at the time of examination. Again, it should be recalled that this assessment can change with time in rare cases. If the injected fluid becomes evident at the wound site (appears as drips of fluid under pressure), it must be interpreted that the synovial compartment is open, contaminated, and, for treatment purposes, infected (Fig. 1). This technique has been the most useful for acute-phase interpretation and assessment of wounds near joints and tendon sheaths in relation to penetration of the synovial space. Careful observation is often required to detect the exit of injected fluid.

Imaging techniques can be used to assess wounds associated with joints and tendon sheaths further. Plain radiography can occasionally reveal evidence of an open synovial compartment. The presence of gas densities in these spaces is not normal and can be interpreted as air that has entered a joint space. Care must be exercised if radiographs are made after synoviocentesis, because air can be present and lead to false interpretation. It seems

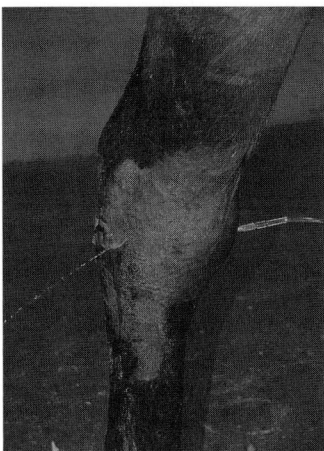

Fig. 1. Sterile polyionic fluid injected into a joint distant from a wound egresses from the wound site, indicating an open contaminated synovial compartment.

that this radiographic sign is rare, and it may be more likely in large spaces than in smaller joints and tendon sheaths.

Positive-contrast radiography has great potential to assist in obtaining an early diagnosis of synovial cavity communication with a wound site. Positive-contrast material can be administered in two ways. It can be injected into a wound to determine if the underlying synovial space is opened. Alternately, the contrast media can be placed directly into a suspected joint, bursa, or tendon sheath, and communication between the wound track and synovial structure can be determined. Perhaps the most common use of positive-contrast material is its direct injection into a tract or injection via a small catheter placed in a tract (fistula). This is more useful with a puncture or small exit wound than with wide laceration trauma. The resulting fistulogram can provide useful information as to the depth and direction of a wound and whether or not the wound communicates with the suspected synovial compartment. A 14- or 16-gauge intravenous catheter or small animal urinary catheter can work well to access this type of wound tract for injection of contrast material. A volume sufficient to allow backflow from the catheter is usually enough for a diagnostic study. Radiographs should be taken as soon as possible after injection, and any excess contrast material should be cleaned from the hair and skin before exposure so as to avoid artifacts and poor images. Any evidence of communication between the wound and synovial structure should be taken seriously as an indication to institute treatment of septic synovitis (Fig. 2).

Radiographs can reveal other abnormalities indirectly associated with septic disease of synovial structures. Soft tissue swelling, loss of joint space, and lysis or erosion of periarticular bone may be seen on radiographs of

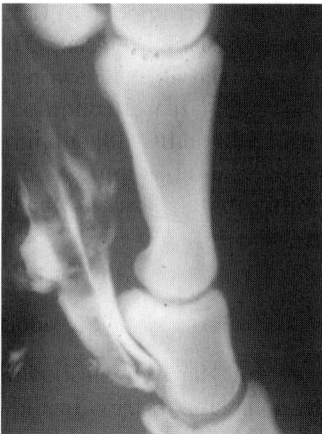

Fig. 2. Positive-contrast material injected into an open tract indicates an open digital tendon sheath.

infected joints. Signs of septic osteitis or osteomyelitis of bone associated with joints are perhaps the most consistent radiographic signs from survey films that infectious synovitis is present [1]. Septic tenosynovitis alone is rarely associated with specific findings from survey films.

Ultrasonography of joint spaces and tendon sheaths can provide useful information. Normal synovial fluid has a uniform anechoic appearance. The dark image is typically clear of echogenic material. With sepsis, synovial fluid can appear to contain echogenic particles and strands of material. This is likely consistent with the accumulation of fibrin, inflammatory debris, and foreign material. The absence of this flocculent material does not rule out a septic process when infection is highly considered for an affected joint or tendon sheath.

Nuclear scintigraphy is not commonly used in the diagnosis of septic synovitis. Some rare cases that do not demonstrate typical signs may benefit from scintigraphy. Vascular and soft tissue phase scintigraphy may offer some advantage for horses with unusual presentations by demonstrating increased uptake of radiopharmaceutic agent at sites of inflammatory change. Perhaps nuclear scintigraphy could be used to monitor an affected horse as tissues respond to treatment; however, final resolution remains in question. A return to a normal baseline image may indicate resolution of inflammation and, likely, the infectious component of the disease as well.

The growing presence and use of three-dimensional imaging of equine limbs may have an impact on the diagnosis of synovial diseases. Soft tissue abnormalities may be better visualized with MRI, and subtle bone lesions may be more readily identified with CT. To date, no distinct advantage of these imaging modalities over radiography and ultrasonography for diagnosis of septic arthritis and tenosynovitis in horses has been described. Injury and abnormalities of the navicular region, including the navicular bursa, have been recently characterized using MRI, however, and there seems to be promise of gaining more insight into the nature of these injuries in the horse using this type of imaging [3].

An early accurate assessment and diagnosis of septic synovitis are necessary to achieve a successful outcome. Whether considering a foal with hematogenous origin septic arthritis or an adult horse with an infected synovial structure secondary to wounding, time is an essential factor influencing final success. The described diagnostic efforts are indicated and recommended. In the absence of these, or if indications are not absolutely convincing, it is wise to consider a suspect joint, tendon sheath, or bursa as infected until proven otherwise and to institute aggressive treatment as soon as possible. Delay in doing so can be costly to tissue disruption, destruction, soundness, and possibly life. Open synovial compartments seem to respond much better to aggressive treatment before the establishment of frank sepsis. It is possible to prevent infection after wounding if these aggressive treatment efforts are initiated as soon as possible. Again, an early and accurate diagnosis is the key.

Treatment

The aim in treating septic arthritis and tenosynovitis is eradication of the bacterial load, removal of any foreign material, elimination of inflammatory mediators and free radicals, pain relief, and restoration of the normal synovial environment so as to promote tissue healing. These objectives are achieved by appropriate administration of antimicrobial drugs, joint lavage, surgical debridement, anti-inflammatory drugs, and a postinfection rehabilitation program. Early recognition and aggressive treatment are essential to eliminate infection and obtain a successful outcome.

Antimicrobial drugs

Judicious use of antimicrobial drugs for the management of infected or contaminated synovial structures requires knowledge of the most likely organisms responsible for the infection and an understanding of the mechanism of action and spectrum of activity for each antimicrobial. For example, injuries to equine joints are more likely to have a mixed bacterial population consisting of *Enterobacter* spp, *Streptococcus* spp, *Staphylococcus* spp, *Pseudomonas* spp, and anaerobes [2]. Septic arthritis after surgery or intra-articular injection is mainly caused by *Staphylococcus* spp [4]. The goal of therapy is to achieve antimicrobial concentrations above the minimum inhibitory concentration (MIC) in the infected tissue without producing toxic effects to the animal [1]. Efficacy of an antimicrobial depends on the physiochemical properties of the drug and the biologic properties of the target bacteria. Factors at the site of infection, such as pH, bacterial load, phases of bacterial growth, and the presence or absence of oxygen, influence the activity of the antimicrobial [5].

Antimicrobials are classified by their pharmacologic properties into concentration-dependent and time-dependent categories [5]. This is clinically important when administering antimicrobials by local methods, such as intravenous or intraosseous regional perfusion or intra-articular medication, in which concentration-dependent drugs are more beneficial. With concentration-dependent drugs, the higher the concentrations achieved in the tissue, the greater is the killing effect [5]. Otherwise, time-dependent antimicrobials do not have a greater killing effect by increasing the concentration in the tissue. In general, aminoglycosides, fluoroquinolones, and metronidazole are considered concentration-dependent, whereas β-lactams, macrolides, and vancomycin are considered time-dependent [5].

The route of antimicrobial administration is important. Combinations of systemic and local administration of antimicrobials are recommended for the treatment of horses with septic arthritis and tenosynovitis [1]. Intravenous administration of broad-spectrum antimicrobials must be initiated as soon as the diagnosis of a septic condition is presumed after obtaining a sample for culture. The intravenous route provides a faster onset of action and maximizes penetration of a drug into the synovial structures compared with the oral or intramuscular route [5]. Systemic antimicrobial therapy is particularly necessary for foals with septic arthritis so as to treat bacteremia and prevent hematogenous dissemination of the causative organism to other tissues. Selection of an antimicrobial depends on its efficacy against the contaminating organism, safety for the animal, and expense of the drug. The clinician should administer broad-spectrum antimicrobials initially and then make adjustments according to clinical progression, culture, and antimicrobial sensitivity. Broad-spectrum coverage is important, because synovial fluid cultures are positive in only 40% to 64% of horses suspected of having an infected synovial structure [6]. Furthermore, in many cases, other infecting organisms may not be isolated by culture but remain present, infecting the synovial structure. This is particularly important in synovial infections caused by penetrating wounds, where mixed bacterial infections are common [2].

Traditionally, the most common antimicrobials used to treat horses with septic arthritis or tenosynovitis are a β-lactam agent (eg, sodium or potassium penicillin, cephazolin) combined with an aminoglycoside (eg, gentamicin, amikacin). When administered systemically, these antimicrobials distribute well into extracellular fluid, reaching high concentrations in synovial fluid [7–10]. This antimicrobial combination is a good initial choice, because the antimicrobial spectrum is effective for the most common isolates causing musculoskeletal infections in horses [4,11]. Other antimicrobials that have been clinically effective or have been shown to enter the synovial fluid at therapeutic concentrations in clinically normal joints include tetracycline, trimethoprim-sulfonamide combinations, metronidazole, ticarcillin sodium, ceftiofur sodium, and vancomycin [1,12]. It is important to avoid the routine use of ticarcillin and vancomycin, however, and to use them only as a last resort. This is necessary to prevent the development of more resistance by the bacteria.

Aminoglycosides are still considered the drugs of choice for treatment of orthopedic infections in horses. The duration of sustained antimicrobial effectiveness is concentration dependent and has an excellent post-antimicrobial effect, which refers to the ability to suppress bacterial growth after exposure to the antimicrobial [5]. The larger the drug tissue and serum concentration, the greater is the bactericidal effect. A single daily dose of gentamicin (6.6 mg/kg administered intravenously) is more beneficial than the conventional thrice-daily dosing (2.2 mg/kg administered intravenously every 8 hours) [13]. Godber and colleagues [13] demonstrated that a single daily dose of gentamicin reached the targeted antimicrobial tissue concentration, prolonged the post-antimicrobial effect, and lowered the risk for nephrotoxicity in normal adult horses. Nevertheless, the pharmacokinetic properties of aminoglycosides are altered in hypoxic neonatal foals [14]. Therefore, in neonates, serum aminoglycoside peak and trough concentrations should be measured to adjust the dose and dose interval [14]. Although aminoglycosides have been good antimicrobials for treating musculoskeletal infections in horses, the emergence of multiple antimicrobial-resistant organisms has created great concern in human and veterinary medicine [15]. Methicillin-resistant *Staphylococcus aureus* has been isolated in orthopedic infections in horses. The antimicrobial spectrum of *S aureus* has revealed resistance to most aminoglycosides, including amikacin and gentamicin [15]. Therefore, judicious use of antimicrobials and evaluation of new antimicrobial alternatives are required for future success in treating equine synovial sepsis.

Enrofloxacin is used for horses with refractory septic arthritis and osteomyelitis or when long-term administration of antimicrobials is required. The use of enrofloxacin is considered extralabel because enrofloxacin is not currently approved for use in horses. It has been widely used, however, because of its broad-spectrum bactericidal effect, relatively safety, and ease of administration [16]. Similar to aminoglycosides, enrofloxacin is a concentration-dependent antimicrobial drug and has a good post-antimicrobial effect [5]. A single daily intravenous dose of 5.5 mg/kg or oral dose of 7.5 mg/kg administered every 24 hours or 4.0 mg/kg administered every 12 hours penetrates tissues adequately and would attain concentrations high enough in the tissue fluids to treat infections caused by susceptible bacteria [17]. A study evaluating the effects of injectable enrofloxacin demonstrated that long-term administration using 5.5 mg/kg administered intravenously once daily was safe in adult horses [16]. Enrofloxacin is not recommended for use in foals because it may cause cartilage lesions and lameness in neonates [18,19]. Furthermore, enrofloxacin inhibits cell proliferation, induces morphologic changes, decreases total monosaccharide content, and alters small proteoglycan synthesis at the glycosylation level in equine tendon cell cultures [20]. These effects are more pronounced in juvenile tendon cells than in adult equine tendon cells [20]. Therefore, the use of fluoroquinolones is not without risk. Tendonitis and spontaneous tendon rupture have been reported in people during or after therapy with fluoroquinolones [20]. The oral route of administration is preferable in horses requiring long-term antimicrobial administration because of the relative ease of administration compared with the intravenous route. An oral gel formulation made from the injectable cattle product was shown to produce blood levels sufficient to resolve infections caused by a variety of common equine pathogens and did not cause any detrimental effect in normal adult horses [21].

Imipenem-cilastin, cefotaxime, and amoxicillin have been studied as potential alternatives for the treatment of septic arthritis in horses [22,23]. Cefotaxime is a third-generation cephalosporin. It has a broad spectrum of activity, having bactericidal activity against many gram-positive and gram-negative aerobic bacteria. Based on a pharmacokinetic study, a dose of 25 mg/kg administered every 6 hours reached therapeutic concentrations within 30 minutes of intravenous administration for cefotaxime-susceptible organisms in the synovial fluid of horses [22]. Because the drug concentration falls below the targeted MIC (<1 µg/mL) 6 hours after injection, administration every 6 to 8 hours was recommended [22]. Amoxicillin is a class of penicillin with a better gram-negative spectrum [23]. Errecalde and coworkers [23] investigated the pharmacokinetics of amoxicillin at a dose of 40 mg/kg administered intravenously in normal horses and horses with experimental arthritis. The rate of penetration from serum to synovial fluid was greater in arthritic animals compared with normal animals, indicating better penetration in these cases. In contrast, the rate of disappearance from synovial fluid was more rapid in normal horses compared with arthritic horses, indicating persistence of the drug in the diseased joint [23]. Pharmacokinetic studies of imipenem-cilastin indicated that a dose of 10 to 20 mg/kg administered by slow intravenous infusion every 6 hours achieve antimicrobial concentrations that are effective for most susceptible pathogens and do not cause any adverse effects in normal horses [24].

Oral antimicrobial administration is generally preferred when long-term administration is required. Oral administration is not recommended in the acute phase of infection, because gastrointestinal tract absorption may be erratic; thus, serum and tissue concentrations may be lower than needed. Exceptions include the use of metronidazole tablets for the treatment of anaerobic infections, especially for treatment of *Bacteroides fragilis* infections. We routinely prescribe oral antimicrobials, such as trimethoprim-sulfonamide combinations or enrofloxacin, for 10 to 14 days after resolution of clinical signs and discharge from the hospital.

Nonsteroidal anti-inflammatory drugs

When bacteria invade synovial structures, a severe inflammatory response develops. Inflammatory mediators, free radicals, and destructive enzymes released by the inflamed synovium and neutrophils induce a vicious cycle of inflammation and tissue destruction [1]. Breakdown products of the inflammatory cells, such metalloproteinases, oxygen free radicals, and cytokines, in turn, cause synovitis and cartilage degradation, leading to joint effusion, severe lameness, and, eventually, osteoarthritis [25]. Nonsteroidal anti-inflammatory drugs (NSAIDs) may help to diminish the inflammatory process, minimize cartilage destruction, and provide analgesia, which is important for these horses to prevent support limb laminitis. Phenylbutazone (4.4–8.8 mg/kg administered once daily), ketoprofen (2.2 mg/kg administered two or three times a day), and flunixin meglumine (1.1 mg/kg administered two times daily) are commonly used to reduce synovial inflammation in horses [26]. These drugs can suppress induced synovial membrane prostaglandin E_2 (PGE_2) production without detrimental effects on synovial membrane viability and function [27]. In experimentally induced synovitis in horses, phenylbutazone was more effective than ketoprofen for reducing lameness, joint temperature, synovial fluid volume, and synovial fluid PGE_2 [28]. Selective cyclooxygenase 2 inhibitors are currently under investigation and seem promising at reducing the toxic side effects observed with the currently used NSAIDs [27,29].

Administration of intravenous dimethyl sulfoxide (DMSO) solution has been advocated by one of the authors (EMG) as an adjunctive therapy to reduce synovial inflammation. DMSO is a free radical scavenger, it is antiseptic and analgesic, and it may inhibit chemotaxis of inflammatory mediators [30]. In addition, some evidence suggests that DMSO can boost the effects of other drugs [31]. The most commonly used dose is 0.25 to 1 g/kg of body weight administered intravenously up to a 10% solution, with a maximum duration of treatment of 5 days [32]. This dose is safe in awake and anesthetized horses, but higher DMSO concentrations (>10% solution) can cause hemolysis and should be avoided [32]. Hyaluronan (HA) and polysulfated glycosaminoglycans may also be used to alleviate signs of synovial inflammation in horses with induced nonseptic synovitis and may have beneficial effects in horses with septic joints [33]. One study of infected joints in horses demonstrated that a single intra-articular injection of HA after joint lavage significantly reduced lameness, joint circumference, synovial fluid white blood cells (WBCs), and proteoglycan loss from articular cartilage [34]. In another study, intrathecal administration of sodium hyaluronate in a collagenase-induced tendonitis model demonstrated some beneficial effect in tendon healing and prevention of adhesion formation [35]. The intra-articular use of these drugs in the acute stage of infection should be avoided, however, because the immunosuppressive properties may enhance the risk of infection recurrence [36]. Until the risk of infection after administration via the local and systemic routes is investigated further, these drugs should be used after signs of infection have resolved. The authors usually recommend a series of systemic injections (HA or polysulfated glycosaminoglycans) 3 to 4 weeks after discharge from the hospital.

Our clinical impression is that these agents can be used to help resolve the synovitis and capsulitis that occurs after infection and can help to prevent adhesion formation in the case of septic tenosynovitis.

Regional perfusion

Regional perfusion can be used to achieve high local concentrations of antimicrobials in a selected region of the limb, particularly in areas of ischemic tissue [37]. The antimicrobial is injected into a superficial vein proximal to the site of infection (intravenous; Fig. 3) or into the medullary cavity of a bone in a similar location (intraosseous). For both techniques, a tourniquet is placed proximal and distal to the site of infection so as to occlude the superficial venous system. As the perfusate is infused, it distends the venous system, allowing the antimicrobial to diffuse into the tissues. Experimental and clinical investigations have demonstrated the beneficial value of these techniques as adjunctive therapy for orthopedic infections in horses [38]. Local antimicrobial concentrations can reach 25 to 100 times the MIC for most common equine pathogens [37–41]. This suggests that administration of concentration-dependent antimicrobials, such as aminoglycosides, by regional perfusion should have an excellent bactericidal effect and should improve treatment efficacy. A high ratio of peak concentration (C_{max}) to MIC is associated with a greater bactericidal effect and a longer post-antimicrobial effect [5]. Amikacin and gentamicin are usually the drugs of choice to infuse by regional perfusion [37–40]. Other antimicrobials agents that have been anecdotally used include potassium penicillin, ampicillin, cefotaxime, ceftiofur, chloramphenicol, and enrofloxacin. The use of enrofloxacin, which is another concentration-dependent antimicrobial, for regional perfusion is currently under investigation; however, until further results are reported, it should be used with caution. A single dose of enrofloxacin of 1.5 mg/kg diluted in saline (60 mL) and regionally perfused into the cephalic vein achieved concentrations 10 times the MIC for the most common

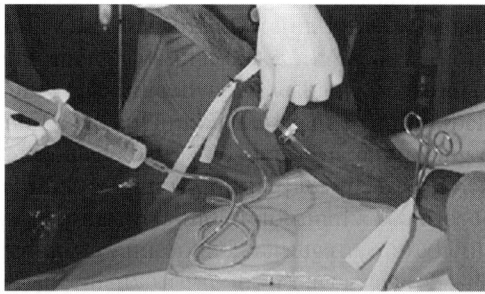

Fig. 3. Intravenous regional limb perfusion in a 4-week-old foal with septic arthritis. The foal is in lateral recumbency; tourniquets are placed above or below the hock, and a catheter is placed in the saphenous vein for perfusion.

organisms causing equine orthopedic infections in the midcarpal synovial fluid, bone marrow, and interstitial tissue of the third metacarpal bone. A higher dose or extravasation of the antimicrobial solution caused mild to moderate perivascular cellulitis, however. Fluoroquinolones at high concentrations are toxic to chondrocytes [19].

The decision to use the intravenous or intraosseous route of administration depends on the target tissue to be treated (joint versus bone), the presence of periarticular edema, access to a peripheral vein, availability of equipment, and the clinician's preference. Both procedures can be performed with a horse standing or under general anesthesia. Two studies have been published comparing the pharmacokinetic effects of amikacin delivered by intraosseous or intravenous infusion [39,40]. One study compared the two techniques using an infusion of amikacin (500 mg) in the digital vein or medullary cavity of the third metacarpal bone [39]. No significant differences were found with the time to C_{max} or elimination half-life between methods in synovial fluid samples in the distal interphalangeal joint, metacarpophalangeal joint, or digital flexor tendon sheath [39]. Each technique can produce a mean C_{max} ranging from 5 to 50 times that of the recommended serum C_{max} for therapeutic efficacy. The second study compared the two techniques of regional perfusion for delivery of antimicrobials in the tibiotarsal joint [40]. Results of this study demonstrated that intravenous infusion of amikacin at a rate of 1 g diluted in sterile saline (60 mL) produced the highest concentration of amikacin in the tibiotarsal joint compared with intraosseous infusion, which was performed in the distal portion of the tibia (mean ± standard error [SE]: 701.8 ± 366.8 µg/mL versus 203.8 ± 64.5 µg/mL, respectively) [40]. Our opinion is that intravenous administration is technically easier and faster to perform, special equipment is not required, and the vein can be catheterized at a location distal to the surgical site. Nevertheless, when there is severe soft tissue swelling or edema or when veins are not easily accessed, intraosseous perfusion is probably the best choice. Significantly higher concentrations of antimicrobials can be achieved with intra-articular administration than those obtained with regional intravenous or intraosseous perfusion [41]. Therefore, intra-articular administration of antimicrobials may be more effective for the treatment of septic synovitis. For further discussion on regional perfusion, the reader is referred to the article by Cruz and colleagues in this issue.

Technique for intravenous regional perfusion

In most of the initial studies on regional perfusion, the procedure was performed with the horse under general anesthesia [37,38,42]; however, the technique can be readily performed with the horse standing. The horse is sedated with a combination of detomidine and butorphanol, and a tourniquet is placed proximal and distal to the targeted area and infusion site. For perfusion of the distal limb (distal metacarpus or tarsus to foot), the digital vein is used. The cephalic vein in the forelimb or the saphenous vein in the hind limb can be used to perfuse the region distal to the distal third of the radius or tibia, including the carpus and tarsus, respectively. Any other superficial vein that is exposed after the tourniquet is in place can be used, however (see Fig. 1). After aseptic preparation of the site, a 23-gauge butterfly catheter is inserted into the selected vein and the antimicrobial solution is slowly infused over 5 to 15 minutes. For larger vessels, such as the cephalic or saphenous vein, a 20-gauge, 1-in intravenous catheter can be placed. The catheter can be used to prevent extravasation of the drug during perfusion and the associated complications. After infusion, the catheter is removed, pressure is applied for a few minutes over the venipuncture site, and the tourniquet is maintained in place for 30 minutes. The procedure is repeated every 24 hours for 3 to 5 days or as needed. We have used intravenous regional perfusion as the only route for antimicrobial administration in several horses affected with septic arthritis after open injuries to joints. Resolution of the infection was achieved. Regional perfusion was performed every 24 to 36 hours for a total of seven times with amikacin or enrofloxacin.

Technique for intraosseous perfusion

This technique can be performed with the horse standing or under general anesthesia [43]. After the horse is sedated and restrained in stocks, the site is clipped and prepared as for aseptic surgery. Regional nerve blocks and local infiltration of anesthetic drugs are used to desensitize the region. A 1-cm stab incision is made through the skin, subcutaneous tissue, and periosteum on the most readily accessible aspect of the bone. The soft tissue is retracted, and a 3.2- to 4.0-mm (3.2 mm in foals) unicortical hole is drilled through the cortex. A special cannulated screw is then inserted after tapping the hole to the specific screw diameter. The cannulated screw is not always necessary, however, because infusion can be performed by introducing the male end of a catheter extension set into the unicortical hole. Regional perfusion is performed as described for the intravenous technique. After the procedure, the skin over the cortical hole or cannulated screw is sutured and bandaged.

Intrasynovial antimicrobials

Intra-articular administration of antimicrobials is an effective and inexpensive method for treating septic arthritis. Advantages of intra-articular administration include achievement of high concentrations of the drug in the synovial structure, the ability to use cost-prohibitive drugs in small doses, and the reduction of systemic toxic effects. Administration of a single 150-mg dose of gentamicin or ceftiofur provides high and sustained concentrations above the MIC (≤ 2 µg/mL) for the most common equine bacterial pathogens for at least 24 hours [44,45]. A recent investigation compared intra-articular and bone gentamicin concentrations after intra-articular and intravenous regional limb perfusion in horses [41,45]. The C_{max} of gentamicin in synovial fluid was significantly higher (800 times) with intra-articular administration than with regional perfusion and remained 6 times higher 24 hours after treatment. The bone gentamicin concentration remained higher than the MIC for only 8 hours using both techniques, and no significant difference was observed between methods [41].

In clinical cases, antimicrobials are usually injected through a hypodermic needle into a joint or tendon sheath each day for 3 to 5 days or are injected at the end of a joint lavage procedure. Recently, equine clinicians have advocated the use of an indwelling catheter, intravenous administration sets, or specialized pumps to administer antimicrobials into a joint more frequently (two to three times per day) or continuously [46–48]. Lescun and colleagues [47] developed a method for continuous infusion of gentamicin into the tarsocrural joint by using an infusion catheter. The infusion catheter consists of flow control tubing connected to a balloon infuser (Flow Control Tubing; Mila International, Erlanger, Kentucky) by the use of an extension set with a T-shaped connector. Most of the catheters functioned well for the 5-day infusion period, and continuous intra-articular infusion of gentamicin (0.17 ± 0.02 mg/kg/h) resulted in antimicrobial concentrations greater than 100 times the MIC of 2 to 4 μg/mL [47]. Complications with the infusion method occurred in 7 of 24 horses and were primarily associated with failure of the infuser balloon and blockage of the catheter [47]. In a second part of the study, investigators evaluated the effects of continuous infusion of gentamicin on synovial membrane and articular cartilage [46]. Continuous infusion of gentamicin produced mild but transient inflammatory changes in the articular cartilage and synovium [46].

Intra-articular administration of antimicrobials and joint lavage may be all that is necessary to resolve septic arthritis in adult horses, but this is not recommended in foals. Systemic administration of antimicrobials is essential to treat bacteremia and prevent the hematogenous dissemination of organisms. Appropriate antimicrobial selection can lead to a dramatic response in eliminating the infection. Aminoglycosides, particularly gentamicin and amikacin, are routinely chosen because of their efficacy against the most common equine pathogens. Many other antimicrobials have been used to treat septic joints; however, it is essential that antimicrobials be evaluated for potential inflammatory effects on the synovium and articular cartilage before their clinical use. High tissue concentrations of some antimicrobials (eg, enrofloxacin) may damage the synovium and are toxic to chondrocytes [19]. The addition of antiseptic solutions to lavage fluids used to treat infected synovial structures was not more effective than lavage with a balanced electrolyte solution alone [49,50]. Furthermore, the use of chlorhexidine and povidone iodine ($\geq 0.1\%$ solution) is too irritating to the joint and tendon sheaths for safe use [51–53].

Repositol antimicrobials

Another effective method for local antimicrobial delivery is the use of antimicrobial-impregnated nonbiodegradable implants [54]. The most common nonbiodegradable matrix implant is polymethylmethacrylate (PMMA), which is a type of bone cement. Antimicrobials are incorporated evenly within the matrix and are released by diffusion. These types of implants are characterized by rapid release of the antimicrobial in the first 24 hours, followed by slow and prolonged release thereafter [54]. Numerous studies have reported that heat-stable antimicrobials (stable up to 100°C) are eluted from the PMMA in concentrations that exceed the MIC of the most common equine bacterial pathogens [54]. In horses, PMMA impregnated with gentamicin sulfate, tobramycin sulfate, amikacin sulfate, and cefazolin has been used successfully in the treatment of open fractures and joint infections [55]. In another report, gentamicin-impregnated PMMA beads were used in the treatment of 12 horses with septic synovitis [56]. Selected cases had been refractory to standard treatments (lavage, debridement, joint drainage, and systemic antimicrobials) or had evidence of osteomyelitis adjacent to a synovial cavity [56]. Eleven of the 12 horses survived, and 6 returned to full athletic use [56]. Recently, the same authors reported the use of gentamicin-impregnated PMMA beads for the treatment of infections involving the tarsometatarsal and distal intertarsal joints in 11 horses [57]. After a 7- to 8-mm tract was drilled through the joint to stimulate ankylosis [57], 5 to 10 beads were placed into the tract drilled across the affected joint and were left in place for 14 days [57]. In this report, 81% of these horses survived and 7 returned to athletic use [57]. In our experience, antimicrobial-impregnated PMMA beads are better to use when horses have developed chronic refractory septic arthritis or osteomyelitis or when ankylosis of a joint can be stimulated (eg, distal tarsal joint). It is important to recognize that implantation of beads can produce a marked inflammatory reaction and cartilage erosion that can lead to progressive joint damage [58]. Another disadvantage is that PMMA beads are nonbiodegradable and a second operation is necessary to remove the implants from the joint. In some clinical cases, however, PMMA beads have been left in place for years with no obvious problem.

Antimicrobial-impregnated PMMA beads can be prepared in the surgical room at the time of implantation or ahead of time and sterilized with ethylene oxide [54]. Beads can be fabricated by hand or by injecting the material into a mold. The PMMA hardens within 5 to 10 minutes. When it becomes like clay, the material is made into beads or cylinders and is implanted into the joint through an arthrotomy. Usually, antimicrobial powder or liquid (1–2 g) is mixed with the PMMA polymer (1:10 or 1:5 ratio) and shaped as desired [54]. Different studies have found that the addition of more antimicrobial powder or the type of antimicrobial used can alter the mechanical strength of the implant [59,60]. In the treatment of septic joints, mechanical strength is not an issue, however, and high concentrations can be used if there is no effect on polymerization. The beads can be placed on suture material or surgical wire to facilitate implantation and retrieval from the surgical site. Factors that influence the antimicrobial C_{max} and the length of time concentrations remain above the MIC after impregnated PMMA bead implantation depend on the brand of the PMMA polymer, the amount of antimicrobial mixed, the elution properties of the antimicrobial used (aminoglycosides > ceftiofur), and the amount of fluid flowing past the implants [54]. Antimicrobial elution is related to surface area; therefore, more rapid elution of the antimicrobial occurs from small rough beads than from large smooth beads, because smaller beads have a larger surface area per volume [59]. Several antimicrobials elute from PMMA, including gentamicin, amikacin, ceftiofur, fluoroquinolones, metronidazole, and clindamycin [59,61]. Elution of metronidazole is dependent on the dose, and combinations of metronidazole and gentamicin sulfate in PMMA resulted in higher rates of elution compared with elution of metronidazole or amikacin alone [61]. Unfortunately, tetracycline and chloramphenicol do not tolerate the polymerization process [59]. If the infection does not resolve, implantation of new PMMA beads with the same or different antimicrobials every 7 to 10 days should be considered.

Because PMMA impregnated with antimicrobials has been effective in eliminating infection, there have been multiple investigations to develop biodegradable matrix implants. The main advantage of this type of delivery system is that the entire volume of antimicrobial can be slowly released while the material degrades. The most common materials investigated include collagen, plaster of Paris, hydroxyapatite, polylactide-polyglycolide, and polypropylene fumarate cross-linked with a methylmethacrylate monomer (a type of bone cement) [54]. Many of these materials are still under investigation and are not yet being used in clinical studies. In addition, biocompatibility studies need to be performed in vitro and in vivo before placement of these biodegradable implants into joints. Potentially dangerous release of large amounts of antimicrobials or induction of a severe inflammatory response may occur during degradation of these implants [54]. Cook and coworkers [62] investigated the use of a biodegradable drug delivery system (50:50 DL-lactide-glycolide copolymers and poly(DL) lactide impregnated with gentamicin) for the release of gentamicin in synovial explants from the cadavers of four adult horses. This investigator concluded that gentamicin released at high concentrations for 10 days resulted in the elimination of infection, with no adverse effect on synovial HA production or synovial morphology and viability [62]. The only available in vivo study on biodegradable implants in horses was reported by Summerhays and colleagues [63] in 2002. Gentamicin-impregnated collagen sponges were used to treat eight horses with traumatically induced synovial sepsis. The antimicrobial-impregnated collagen sponges were introduced into the joints through the arthroscopic cannula after arthroscopy and joint lavage. Seven of the eight horses responded well to treatment, were sound at follow-up, and had no long-term effect secondary to implantation of the collagen sponges [56]. Presently, gentamicin-impregnated collagen sponges are only available in Europe and are not approved for use in the United States. The use of biodegradable implants is an area of extensive research, and their use is likely to increase in the near future. For further discussion on repositol antimicrobials, the reader is referred to the article by Cruz and colleagues in this issue.

Lavage

Synovial lavage and drainage are essential in horses with septic joints and tendon sheaths. The goals of joint lavage are removal of debris and foreign material, debridement of contaminated or devitalized tissue, and elimination of inflammatory mediators [12,25]. A number of techniques have been described, including through-and-through lavage via hypodermic needles, open incisions with or without drains, and lavage under arthroscopic guidance. The decision to use any of these techniques is based on the cause (induced by trauma versus hematogenous spread), duration of the infection, and severity of clinical signs. In acute cases and for joints that do not have multiple compartments, through-and-through needle lavage may be effective in eliminating infection. If infection is well established, there are large fibrin clots in the joint, or the joint has multiple compartments (eg, stifle, hock), however, the lavage fluid may totally bypass the infected area and the infection persists. Joint lavage through needles can be performed with a standing horse using sedation and local anesthesia, although it is usually easier and more effective with the horse under general anesthesia. Three to 5 L of fluid is recommended for routine lavage. After the lavage procedure, antimicrobials are injected into the joint and the limb is bandaged to reduce inflammation and to protect the surgical sites. Systemic anti-inflammatory drugs should be administered as well.

Arthroscopic surgery is a valuable tool in the management of synovial contamination and infection. Arthroscopy offers several advantages, including improved visibility; lavage of a larger area of the synovial structure; and identification and removal of foreign material, fibrin, and devitalized tissue. The benefits of arthroscopic exploration and lavage of contaminated joints were demonstrated in a retrospective study by Wright and colleagues [64]. In that report, 41 of 121 affected horses that had arthroscopic surgery had intra-articular foreign material that was identified during surgery and was predicted to be present before surgery in only 6 of those horses [64]. Furthermore, osteochondral lesions were identified in 51 horses and recognized before surgery in only 25 cases [64]. Tenoscopic-assisted lavage and debridement are effective for the treatment of open injuries of the digital flexor tendon sheath [65]. At the conclusion of arthroscopy or tenoscopy, the instrument portals can be primarily closed or enlarged for continued decompression and drainage of the synovial compartment.

The fluid of choice for synovial lavage is a sterile balanced electrolyte solution [1]. The addition of antiseptics, such as chlorhexidine or povidone iodine, into the lavage solution causes irritation to the joints and has not proven to be more effective than a balanced electrolyte solution alone [50]. The addition of DMSO to lavage solutions has been used by many equine clinicians. Lavage or intra-articular administration of DMSO (10% up to 40% solution) has been used experimentally and clinically to treat septic arthritis in horses [1]. As previously mentioned, the free radical scavenging and anti-inflammatory properties of DMSO may help in decreasing the inflammation inside a joint. One of the authors (EMG) routinely adds DMSO as a 1% to 10% solution to the lavage fluid. Nevertheless, a recent in vitro study demonstrated that exposure of DMSO to cartilage explants at concentrations greater than 5% suppresses equine articular cartilage metabolism (decreases proteoglycan synthesis and lactate metabolism) in normal joints [66]. In another study, daily exposure of 10% DMSO to equine cartilage explants resulted in detrimental effects on cartilage proteoglycan synthesis and caused chondrocyte death in a time-dependent manner (>3 days of exposure) in normal joints [67]. This effect has not been demonstrated in cases of synovial sepsis.

In chronic or refractory cases with established inflammation, open incisions are recommended for decompression and removal of inflammatory debris [68]. An arthrotomy permits extensive lavage and constant joint drainage by leaving the incision open. Arthrotomies are typically performed under general anesthesia. One or two 3- to 5-cm incisions can be made into a joint at locations that allow adequate drainage of fluid and removal of fibrin [68]. Arthrotomy incisions can be left open and protected by a sterile bandage, which should be changed daily. For sites that are difficult to bandage, such as the stifle region, a stent bandage can be sutured in place. Once an infection resolves, the incisions can be closed. Complications include premature closure of an incision site or, in contrast, the formation of exuberant granulation tissue attributable to chronic infection [69]. Arthrotomy was more effective for treating experimentally induced septic arthritis than arthroscopy and synovectomy because it provided better drainage [69].

After surgical drainage is established and initial lavage and debridement are performed, daily assessment and medical management are essential for successful treatment. In horses with an established infection, daily lavage and intra-articular administration of antimicrobials are typically performed until lameness and synovial fluid cytology improve. The decision to repeat the joint lavage is based on clinical examination of the patient. If drainage ceases, joint distention occurs, lameness recurs, or the synovial fluid nucleated cell count remains high (>30,000 cells/μL), the joint should be retreated with local therapy and lavage, and this should be repeated until complete resolution of the infection. If clinical improvement occurs, joint lavage can be discontinued, followed by discontinuation of local antimicrobial therapy. In some instances, a single lavage procedure may clear the infection; however, the need for multiple lavage procedures is more typical.

Rehabilitation

Capsulitis and articular degeneration can be detrimental consequences of septic arthritis in horses [49]. Furthermore, infection of the digital tendon sheath can result in severe adhesion formation and fibrosis, which can lead to chronic pain or mechanical lameness [1,35]. After elimination of an infection, physical therapy and medical management of the patient are critical to return a joint or tendon sheath to full athletic potential and minimize damage to the synovium and articular cartilage or to prevent the formation of adhesions.

Physical therapy

Early passive range-of-motion exercises should be initiated as soon as an infection is eliminated. This is particularly important after a tendon sheath infection so as to minimize the formation of adhesions. Passive joint flexion may improve circulation, reduce edema, improve the range of motion of the joint, and break down fibrinous adhesions. Exercise should be restricted, however, so as to minimize damage to affected articular cartilage. After a joint infection has resolved, several weeks of stall rest and passive joint motion are suggested. A progressively increasing exercise program, the length of which depends on the severity of the infection and damage to the synovial structures, should then be instituted. It is difficult to convince owners and trainers to rest a horse for 4 to 6 months. Rest is essential for healing of affected cartilage, subchondral bone, or tendon. For horses with mild infection and articular damage, we usually recommend 4 weeks of stall rest, followed by 4 weeks of stall rest and hand walking, followed by 4 weeks of turnout or swimming. For horses with severe infections, we usually recommend 3 to 4 months of stall rest with passive joint motion. If available, swimming physiotherapy can provide excellent exercise and passive joint motion. Otherwise, horses affected with septic tendon sheaths undergo a more intensive controlled exercise program minimizing the amount of total stall confinement and gradually increasing the amount of exercise. Walking exercise is recommended as soon as an affected horse is comfortable enough to walk freely and willingly.

Pharmaceutic management

Intra-articular administration of HA, polysulfated glycosaminoglycans, or corticosteroids is not routinely used during the acute stage of infection, but these pharmaceutic agents can be of benefit after resolution of the infection. The anti-inflammatory and chondroprotective properties of these agents may be beneficial during the healing process of the synovial compartment and may help to reduce the capsulitis or adhesion formation usually observed after joint or tendon sheath infections. One of the authors (JL) recommends intra-articular medication with HA and corticosteroids 6 weeks after resolution of the infection. More research in this area is necessary to increase the number of horses that can return to full athletic performance after synovial infections.

Hoof structures

Wounding of the coffin joint can and should be approached as for other joints. The other, almost unique, synovial structure within the equine foot is the navicular bursa. The navicular bursa is structured and responds similarly to joint and tendon sheath tissues in that it is a synovial compartment. The main difference is the relatively isolated and protected location of the navicular bursa. The navicular bursal location renders it difficult to reach and assess for potential contamination.

The navicular bursa is most commonly wounded by puncture from the solar surface of the foot. The bursa can also be opened from heel bulb lacerations that wound deeply into the heel region; however, this is far less common than puncture trauma. The nature of puncture wounds can make certain diagnosis of navicular involvement difficult. The keratinized tissue of the sole and frog is quite elastic and may not reveal the exact location of acute puncture wounds. It is recommended that radiographic images be made of any foot with a penetrating foreign body while the foreign body is in place. It is helpful for a veterinarian to be able to evaluate a foot before a nail or other foreign body has been removed. At least two radiographic projections are necessary to assess the location of the foreign body. With more chronic cases, purulent exudate and/or distortion of the solar tissues can make identification of a tract easier. Positive-contrast studies of penetrating tracts or bursal tissues can also be helpful in diagnosing septic bursitis. As with other synovial structures, early diagnosis is the key to success. Delays of greater than 24 hours seem to result in more challenging treatment requirements and a decreasing prognosis for soundness as treatment delays increase.

The basic tenets of treatment are the same as for septic synovitis in any other location. The challenging location of the navicular bursa makes physical treatment difficult. Traditionally, the "street nail" procedure has been used to open the palmar or plantar aspect of the navicular bursa for drainage, debridement, and lavage. This procedure is effective, although modifications to the procedure also seem to accomplish the same goals successfully. Reviews of septic navicular bursitis have indicated a poor prognosis for success of the street nail procedure [70]. This may be attributable to a number of factors, however, including the dimensions of the open ventral approach. When only the soft tissue structures of the foot and navicular bursa are involved, the traditional street nail approach can be abbreviated to expand the wound site for drainage and lavage. This can reduce the magnitude of the soft tissue disruption and perhaps improve clinical results. The arthroscopic approach for navicular bursa lavage has been described [71].

This seems to be a serviceable procedure for lavage and some visual inspection of the bursal anatomy. Some cases require continuous drainage for resolution of the septic process, however. It has been demonstrated from clinical cases that open drainage can be beneficial and can also provide a ready portal for repeated lavage.

Deep penetrating trauma that does not involve the synovial structures of the foot can reach the distal phalanx. Subsolar abscesses that are refractory to routine care and deep puncture wounds should be considered candidates for developing septic pedal osteitis. This can be a difficult diagnosis in the early stages; however, with time and loss of bone, radiographic assessment can be used to assess bone involvement accurately. Local lysis and loss of uniform osseous density as seen on a 60° dorsoventral projection of the distal phalanx are the diagnostic signs for septic pedal osteitis (Fig. 4).

Treatment of septic pedal osteitis should be based on removal of the diseased bone. It is unlikely that systemic, regional, or local antimicrobial therapy alone can resolve the septic process in the distal phalanx. The locally involved bone may be devitalized and antimicrobial penetration limited, such that clinical signs can abate during antimicrobial use only to return when antimicrobials are discontinued. Debridement of the infected bone is necessary. This can be accomplished from a solar approach or through the hoof wall. The ventral approach has some advantages in that ventral drainage is achieved and the solar aspect of the foot can be fit to a treatment plate shoe for easy access and wound management. Debridement of the distal phalanx can be performed under general anesthesia or with local anesthesia and standing restraint. A distal limb tourniquet is highly recommended to maintain visibility of the surgical site. Debridement can be performed with a curette or powered instruments. An interface between diseased and

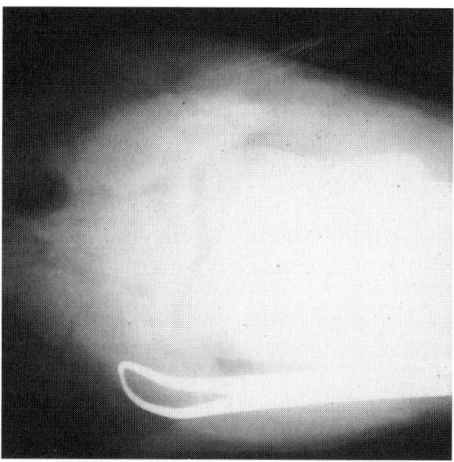

Fig. 4. The local lysis of bone is consistent with septic pedal osteitis.

normal bone is typically apparent based on color and texture. Debridement can be stopped once hard and lighter colored bone is exposed. A treatment plate shoe is usually placed to allow repeated wound cleaning after surgery. The treatment plate is recommended until second-intention healing and keratinization of the solar tissues are complete. The prognosis for future soundness is good if the insertion of the deep digital flexor tendon and the distal interphalangeal joint are not affected [72].

Summary

Septic arthritis, tenosynovitis, bursitis, and septic diseases of the distal limbs of horses can be successfully treated, and affected horses can return to athletic work. These results are most likely after early accurate diagnosis and aggressive targeted treatment. In some instances, protracted rehabilitation programs may also be required. If treatment is not pursued aggressively through diagnostic and therapeutic efforts, affected horses can have debilitating and life-threatening complications. Therefore, timing and early success with treatment are essential to return a horse to normal.

References

[1] Bertone AL. Infectious arthritis. In: McIlwraith CW, Trotter GW, editors. Joint disease in the horse. Philadelphia: WB Saunders; 1996. p. 397–408.
[2] Schneider RK, Bramlage LR, Moore RM, et al. A retrospective study of 192 horses affected with septic arthritis/tenosynovitis. Equine Vet J 1992;24:436–42.
[3] Dyson S, Murray R, Schramme M, et al. Magnetic resonance imaging of the equine foot: 15 horses. Equine Vet J 2003;35:18–26.
[4] Snyder JR, Pascoe JR, Hirsh DC. Antimicrobial susceptibility of microorganisms isolated from equine orthopedic patients. Vet Surg 1987;16:197–201.
[5] Dowling PM. Antimicrobial therapy. In: Bertone JJ, Hospool LJI, editors. Equine clinical pharmacology. St. Louis (MO): WB Saunders; 2004. p. 13–47.
[6] Madison JB, Sommer M, Spencer PA. Relations among synovial membrane histopathologic findings, synovial fluid cytologic findings, and bacterial culture results in horses with suspected infectious arthritis: 64 cases (1979–1987). J Am Vet Med Assoc 1991;198:1655–61.
[7] Bertone A, Caprile K, Davis D. Serum and synovial of gentamicin administered chronically to horses with experimentally-induced septic arthritis [abstract]. Vet Surg 1990;19:57.
[8] Brown MP, Gronwall RR, Pattio N, et al. Pharmacokinetics and synovial fluid concentrations of cephapirin in calves with suppurative arthritis. Am J Vet Res 1991;52:1438–40.
[9] Brown MP, Mayo MB, Gronwall RR. Serum and synovial fluid concentrations of ampicillin trihydrate in calves with suppurative arthritis. Cornell Vet 1991;81:137–43.
[10] Firth EC, Klein WR, Nouws JF, et al. Effect of induced synovial inflammation on pharmacokinetics and synovial concentration of sodium ampicillin and kanamycin sulfate after systemic administration in ponies. J Vet Pharmacol Ther 1988;11:56–62.
[11] Moore RM, Schneider RK, Kowalski J, et al. Antimicrobial susceptibility of bacterial isolates from 233 horses with musculoskeletal infection during 1979–1989. Equine Vet J 1992;24:450–6.
[12] Bertone AL, McIlwraith CW, Jones RL, et al. Comparison of various treatments for experimentally induced equine infectious arthritis. Am J Vet Res 1987;48:519–29.

[13] Godber LM, Walker RD, Stein GE, et al. Pharmacokinetics, nephrotoxicosis, and in vitro antibacterial activity associated with single versus multiple (three times) daily gentamicin treatments in horses. Am J Vet Res 1995;56:613–8.
[14] Green SL, Conlon PD. Clinical pharmacokinetics of amikacin in hypoxic premature foals. Equine Vet J 1993;25:276–80.
[15] Hartmann FA, Trostle SS, Klohnen AA. Isolation of methicillin-resistant Staphylococcus aureus from a postoperative wound infection in a horse. J Am Vet Med Assoc 1997;211: 590–2.
[16] Bertone AL, Tremaine WH, Macoris DG, et al. Effect of long-term administration of an injectable enrofloxacin solution on physical and musculoskeletal variables in adult horses. J Am Vet Med Assoc 2000;217:1514–21.
[17] Giguere S, Sweeney RW, Belanger M. Pharmacokinetics of enrofloxacin in adult horses and concentration of the drug in serum, body fluids, and endometrial tissues after repeated intragastrically administered doses. Am J Vet Res 1996;57:1025–30.
[18] Egerbacher M, Edinger J, Tschulenk W. Effects of enrofloxacin and ciprofloxacin hydrochloride on canine and equine chondrocytes in culture. Am J Vet Res 2001;62:704–8.
[19] Beluche LA, Bertone AL, Anderson DE, et al. In vitro dose-dependent effects of enrofloxacin on equine articular cartilage. Am J Vet Res 1999;60:577–82.
[20] Yoon JH, Brooks FL Jr, Khan A, et al. The effect of enrofloxacin on cell proliferation and proteoglycans in horse tendon cells. Cell Biol Toxicol 2004;20:41–54.
[21] Epstein K, Cohen N, Boothe DE, et al. Pharmacokinetics, stability, and retrospective analysis of use of an oral gel formulation of the bovine injectable enrofloxacin in horses. Vet Ther 2004;5:155–67.
[22] Orsini JA, Moate PJ, Norman T, et al. Cefotaxime kinetics in plasma and synovial fluid following intravenous administration in horses. J Vet Pharmacol Ther 2004;27:293–8.
[23] Errecalde JO, Carmely D, Marino EL, et al. Pharmacokinetics of amoxicillin in normal horses and horses with experimental arthritis. J Vet Pharmacol Ther 2001;24:1–6.
[24] Orsini JA, Moate PJ, Boston RC, et al. Pharmacokinetics of imipenem-cilastatin following intravenous administration in healthy adult horses. J Vet Pharmacol Ther 2005;28:355–61.
[25] Meijer MC, van Weeren PR, Rijkenhuizen AB. Clinical experiences of treating septic arthritis in the equine by repeated joint lavage: a series of 39 cases. J Vet Med A Physiol Pathol Clin Med 2000;47:351–65.
[26] Moses VS, Bertone AL. Nonsteroidal anti-inflammatory drugs. Vet Clin North Am Equine Pract 2002;18:21–37.
[27] Moses VS, Hardy J, Bertone AL, et al. Effects of anti-inflammatory drugs on lipopolysaccharide-challenged and -unchallenged equine synovial explants. Am J Vet Res 2001;62:54–60.
[28] Owens JG, Kamerling SG, Stanton SR, et al. Effects of ketoprofen and phenylbutazone on chronic hoof pain and lameness in the horse. Equine Vet J 1995;27:296–300.
[29] Soraci AL, Tapia O, Garcia J. Pharmacokinetics and synovial fluid concentrations of flurbiprofen enantiomers in horses: chiral inversion. J Vet Pharmacol Ther 2005;28:65–70.
[30] Ali BH. Dimethyl sulfoxide: recent pharmacological and toxicological research. Vet Hum Toxicol 2001;43:228–31.
[31] Williams RE Jr. Dimethyl sulfoxide (DMSO). A review of the literature. NC Med J 1966;27: 237–43.
[32] Lin HC, Johnson CR, Duran SH, et al. Effects of intravenous administration of dimethyl sulfoxide on cardiopulmonary and clinicopathologic variables in awake or halothane-anesthetized horses. J Am Vet Med Assoc 2004;225:560–6.
[33] Kawcak CE, Frisbie DD, Trotter GW, et al. Effects of intravenous administration of sodium hyaluronate on carpal joints in exercising horses after arthroscopic surgery and osteochondral fragmentation. Am J Vet Res 1997;58:1132–40.
[34] Brusie RW, Sullins KE, White NA II, et al. Evaluation of sodium hyaluronate therapy in induced septic arthritis in the horse. Equine Vet J Suppl 1992;11:18–23.

[35] Gaughan EM, Nixon AJ, Krook LP, et al. Effects of sodium hyaluronate on tendon healing and adhesion formation in horses. Am J Vet Res 1991;52:764–73.
[36] Gustafson SB, McIlwraith CW, Jones RL. Comparison of the effect of polysulfated glycosaminoglycan, corticosteroids, and sodium hyaluronate in the potentiation of a subinfective dose of Staphylococcus aureus in the midcarpal joint of horses. Am J Vet Res 1989;50:2014–7.
[37] Whitehair KJ, Adams SB, Parker JE, et al. Regional limb perfusion with antibiotics in three horses. Vet Surg 1992;21:286–92.
[38] Murphey ED, Santschi EM, Papich MG. Regional intravenous perfusion of the distal limb of horses with amikacin sulfate. J Vet Pharmacol Ther 1999;22:68–71.
[39] Butt TD, Bailey JV, Dowling PM, et al. Comparison of 2 techniques for regional antibiotic delivery to the equine forelimb: intraosseous perfusion vs. intravenous perfusion. Can Vet J 2001;42:617–22.
[40] Scheuch BC, Van Hoogmoed LM, Wilson WD, et al. Comparison of intraosseous or intravenous infusion for delivery of amikacin sulfate to the tibiotarsal joint of horses. Am J Vet Res 2002;63:374–80.
[41] Werner LA, Hardy J, Bertone AL. Bone gentamicin concentration after intra-articular injection or regional intravenous perfusion in the horse. Vet Surg 2003;32:559–65.
[42] Whithair KJ, Bowersock TL, Blevins WE, et al. Regional limb perfusion for antibiotic treatment of experimentally induced septic arthritis. Vet Surg 1992;21:367–73.
[43] Mattson S, Boure L, Pearce S, et al. Intraosseous gentamicin perfusion of the distal metacarpus in standing horses. Vet Surg 2004;33:180–6.
[44] Mills ML, Rush BR, St. Jean G, et al. Determination of synovial fluid and serum concentrations, and morphologic effects of intraarticular ceftiofur sodium in horses. Vet Surg 2000;29: 398–406.
[45] Lloyd KC, Stover SM, Pascoe JR, et al. Synovial fluid pH, cytologic characteristics, and gentamicin concentration after intra-articular administration of the drug in an experimental model of infectious arthritis in horses. Am J Vet Res 1990;51:1363–9.
[46] Lescun TB, Adams SB, Wu CC, et al. Effects of continuous intra-articular infusion of gentamicin on synovial membrane and articular cartilage in the tarsocrural joint of horses. Am J Vet Res 2002;63:683–7.
[47] Lescun TB, Adams SB, Wu CC, et al. Continuous infusion of gentamicin into the tarsocrural joint of horses. Am J Vet Res 2000;61:407–12.
[48] Hogan P. How to treat synovial sepsis using a modified indwelling extension set tubing. In: Proceedings of the 50th Annual Convention of the American Association of Equine Practitioners. Lexington (KY): American Association of Equine Practitioners; 2004. p. 224–6.
[49] Bertone AL. Infectious arthritis. In: Ross MW, Dyson SJ, editors. Lameness in the horse. St. Louis (MO): WB Saunders; 2003. p. 598–604.
[50] Bertone AL, McIlwraith CW, Powers BE. Effect of four antimicrobial lavage solutions on the tarsocrural joint of horses. Vet Surg 1986;15:305–15.
[51] Anderson MA, Payne JT, Kreeger JM, et al. Effects of intra-articular chlorhexidine diacetate lavage on the stifle in healthy dogs. Am J Vet Res 1993;54:1784–9.
[52] Bertone AL, McIlwraith CW, Jones RL, et al. Povidone-iodine lavage treatment of experimentally induced equine infectious arthritis. Am J Vet Res 1987;48:712–5.
[53] Baird AN, Scruggs DW, Watkins JP, et al. Effect of antimicrobial solution lavage on the palmar digital tendon sheath in horses. Am J Vet Res 1990;51:1488–94.
[54] Streppa HK, Singer MJ, Budsberg SC. Applications of local antimicrobial delivery systems in veterinary medicine. J Am Vet Med Assoc 2001;219:40–8.
[55] Holcombe SJ, Schneider RK, Bramlage LR, et al. Use of antibiotic-impregnated polymethyl methacrylate in horses with open or infected fractures or joints: 19 cases (1987–1995). J Am Vet Med Assoc 1997;211:889–93.
[56] Butson RJ, Schramme MC, Garlick MH, et al. Treatment of intrasynovial infection with gentamicin-impregnated polymethylmethacrylate beads. Vet Rec 1996;138:460–4.

[57] Booth TM, Butson RJ, Clegg PD, et al. Treatment of sepsis in the small tarsal joints of 11 horses with gentamicin-impregnated polymethylmethacrylate beads. Vet Rec 2001;148: 376–80.
[58] Farnsworth KD, White NA, Robertson JT. The effect of implanting gentamicin-impregnated polymethylmethacrylate beads in the tarsocrural joint of the horse. Vet Surg 2001;30:126–31.
[59] Buchholz HW, Elson RA, Heinert K. Antibiotic-loaded acrylic cement: current concepts. Clin Orthop 1984;190:96–108.
[60] Lautenschlager EP, Marshall GW, Marks KE, et al. Mechanical strength of acrylic bone cements impregnated with antibiotics. J Biomed Mater Res 1976;10:837–45.
[61] Ramos JR, Howard RD, Pleasant RS, et al. Elution of metronidazole and gentamicin from polymethylmethacrylate beads. Vet Surg 2003;32:251–61.
[62] Cook VL, Bertone AL, Kowalski JJ, et al. Biodegradable drug delivery systems for gentamicin release and treatment of synovial membrane infection. Vet Surg 1999;28:233–41.
[63] Summerhays GE. Treatment of traumatically induced synovial sepsis in horses with gentamicin-impregnated collagen sponges. Vet Rec 2000;12:184–8.
[64] Wright IM, Smith MR, Humphrey DJ, et al. Endoscopic surgery in the treatment of contaminated and infected synovial cavities. Equine Vet J 2003;35:613–9.
[65] Frees KE, Lillich JK, Gaughan EM, et al. Tenoscopic-assisted treatment of open digital flexor tendon sheath injuries in horses: 20 cases (1992–2001). J Am Vet Med Assoc 2002; 220:1823–7.
[66] Matthews GL, Engler SJ, Morris EA. Effect of dimethylsulfoxide on articular cartilage proteoglycan synthesis and degradation, chondrocyte viability, and matrix water content. Vet Surg 1998;27:438–44.
[67] Smith CL, MacDonald MH, Tesch AM, et al. In vitro evaluation of the effect of dimethyl sulfoxide on equine articular cartilage matrix metabolism. Vet Surg 2000;29:347–57.
[68] Schneider RK, Bramlage LR, Mecklenburg LM, et al. Open drainage, intra-articular and systemic antibiotics in the treatment of septic arthritis/tenosynovitis in horses. Equine Vet J 1992;24:443–9.
[69] Bertone AL, Davis DM, Cox HU, et al. Arthrotomy versus arthroscopy and partial synovectomy for treatment of experimentally induced infectious arthritis in horses. Am J Vet Res 1992;53:585–91.
[70] Honnas CM, Crabill MR, Mackie JT, et al. Use of autogenous cancellous bone grafting in the treatment of septic navicular bursitis and distal sesamoid osteomyelitis in horses. J Am Vet Med Assoc 1995;206:1191–4.
[71] Wright IM, Phillips TJ, Walmsley JP. Endoscopy of the navicular bursa: a new technique for the treatment of contaminated and septic bursae. Equine Vet J 1999;31:5–11.
[72] Gaughan EM, Ducharme NG, Rendano VT. Surgical treatment of septic pedal osteitis: 9 horses (1980–1987). J Am Vet Med Assoc 1989;195:1131–4.

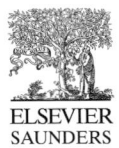

Osteomyelitis in Horses

Laurie R. Goodrich, DVM, MS, PhD

College of Veterinary Medicine, Colorado State University, 300 West Drake Road, Fort Collins, CO 80523, USA

There are few complications in orthopedic surgery more dreaded than infection. This is especially true when sepsis is associated with implants because of the difficulty, time, and monetary investment associated with treatment. In the horse, these concerns are especially magnified because of the large expense incurred with treatment. Furthermore, because of the ongoing ambulation required in the horse, early implant removal may result in a catastrophic outcome. It has been reported that the overall postoperative infection rate in equine musculoskeletal surgery is approximately 10% [1]. Of those cases considered clean-contaminated in the same study, a 53% infection rate was found [1]. This rate is much higher than those experienced by orthopedic surgeons operating on human patients [2], and this fact alone should alert equine orthopedic surgeons to the growing need to understand the pathophysiology of osteomyelitis and the current growing armamentarium of diagnostic and therapeutic options.

Within the past decade, research in the area of orthopedic infection has revealed compelling data regarding the nature of bacterial growth on bone and implants. Because of an improved understanding of the pathophysiology of osteomyelitis, diagnostic techniques and treatment options have also become more sophisticated. The goal of this article is to review the current literature on the pathophysiology of osteomyelitis as well as current diagnostic and treatment techniques. Some of the diagnostic and treatment options are not readily available at this time but should be considered in management of the disease as progress in the areas of diagnosis and treatment continues. Traditional treatments are only briefly reviewed.

Definition

Osteomyelitis is an inflammatory process accompanied by bone destruction and caused by an infecting microorganism(s) [2,3]. The infection can be

E-mail address: laurie.goodrich@colostate.edu

limited to a single portion of bone or can involve several regions, such as the marrow, cortex, periosteum, and surrounding soft tissue, in addition to the synovial structures at the ends of the bone [4,5]. If only bone is infected, it is classified as osteitis, and if bone marrow is involved, it is correctly termed *osteomyelitis*.

In general, the sources of infection can be divided into hematogenous, traumatic, and iatrogenic [4]. Hematogenous infections are almost exclusively seen in foals as a result of sepsis, and, most often, they occur in a joint, epiphysis, or physis. Traumatic infections are usually secondary to a laceration or puncture wound and can infect the bone, joint, tendon sheath, or bursa. Finally, iatrogenic infections are most often secondary to surgical procedures with or without implants. Osteomyelitis associated with implants presents the greatest treatment challenges.

Pathophysiology

Bacterial colonization requires the adherence of bacteria to bone or substrata and subsequent permanent attachment [6]. In most tissues, host defense systems naturally eliminate transient bacterial colonization unless (1) the inoculum exceeds threshold levels, (2) host defense is impaired, (3) tissue surfaces are traumatized, (4) a foreign body is present, or (5) the surface or tissue has low cellularity [6,7]. Bone or cartilage in a traumatized state is an example in which many of these apply. The smooth articular surface of joints and the surfaces of bone are unique in that they have low cellularity. Furthermore, these surfaces do not have a protective layer. Traumatized tissue and normal bone and cartilage have surfaces that resemble surfaces in nature that have evolved an affinity for bacteria. The presence of a biomaterial enhances infectivity, decreases effectiveness of host defense mechanisms, and alters bacterial phenotypic behavior and susceptibility to antimicrobials [8].

Bacteria colonize on the surface of bone, cartilage, or implants by way of direct contamination, spread of local wound infection, or hematogenous seeding. A conditioning film of glycoproteinaceous material spontaneously forms when exposed to a biologic environment [6,7]. Bacteria anchor to the nutrient-rich substratum, proliferation occurs within the polysaccharide slime, and a biofilm layer forms. The "biofilm slime" layer is formed by bacterial extracapsular exopolysaccharides that bind to surfaces or participate in cell-to-cell aggregation and promote tissue adhesion and microcolony formation within the infected tissue [9]. Biofilm formation follows a developmental progression consisting of four main stages: reversible attachment, irreversible attachment, growth and differentiation, and dissemination (or detachment). The extracellular polymeric slime that forms the matrix of biofilm within which the individual cells live is the hallmark feature of biofilms. In the dissemination phase, cells within the biofilm are released to colonize new surfaces through a number of different processes. Motile bacteria, such as *Pseudomonas aeruginosa*, swim out of specialized "fruiting body-like" microcolonies into the surrounding fluid or move along surfaces by gliding or twitching motility [10]. Nonmotile species, such as *Staphylococcus aureus*, seem to use fluid-borne dispersal and detach as large multicellular aggregates encased in slime or roll along surfaces using viscoelastic tethers [10].

Being attached to a surface and encased within a matrix allows bacteria obvious advantages with regard to maintaining homeostasis and a defense. Other advantages include undertaking cooperative metabolism based on complex intercellular signaling systems and the ability to use horizontal gene transfer to protect against environmental challenges [10,11]. It is this biofilm substance that makes the treatment of osteomyelitis a true challenge. The promotion of additional bacterial adherence is probable and likely to result in syntropic interactions. Unfortunately, the surface colonization in biofilm is a survival strategy that is often successful because of its impenetrability, and thus resistance to antimicrobials [12–14]. Studies suggest that biofilm also prevents inflammatory molecules and phagocytic cells from effectively penetrating the biofilm matrix, and the inflammatory response is often more damaging to the host tissue than the biofilm [10]. In fact, the release of inflammatory proteases may be beneficial to biofilm bacteria by promoting host cell lysis and the subsequent release of cellular contents as a nutrient source for the bacteria.

Unfortunately, surface colonization in biofilms is a survival strategy that is often successful, because bacteria can logarithmically multiply and the infection can become a "multispecied consortia of bacteria" within the adhesive biofilm layer [15]. This results in a formidable challenge to the clinician to medicate and cure the infection before the devastating effects of osteomyelitis lead to the patient's demise.

Organisms commonly associated with osteomyelitis

It is important to be familiar with the organisms most commonly cultured in osteomyelitis so that patients can be placed on the appropriate antimicrobial drug for prophylaxis or treatment before the results of culture and sensitivity testing become available. In cases of hematogenous osteomyelitis in foals, enteric gram-negative organisms are most commonly isolated [5]. This is not the most common bacterial isolate in adult osteomyelitis, however.

In a study analyzing bacterial culture and susceptibility results from 233 horses with osteomyelitis, septic arthritis, or tenosynovitis, 91% of the bacteria were aerobic or facultatively anaerobic and 9% were anaerobic [16]. The most common bacterial group isolated was Enterobacteriaceae (29%), followed by non-β-hemolytic streptococci (13%), coagulase-positive staphylococci (12%), β-hemolytic streptococci (9.4%), and coagulase-negative staphylococci (7.3%) [16]. The rest of the organisms were other gram-negative (15.8%), other gram-positive (2.3%), and miscellaneous (2.6%) bacteria [16]. These findings were similar to an earlier study, where 147 bacterial isolates were cultured from 60 equine orthopaedic patients [17]. Multiple bacteria were often identified in osteomyelitis cases that developed subsequent to surgical fracture repair; therefore, broad-spectrum antimicrobial coverage is indicated as prophylaxis in any procedure that requires surgical implants [8].

Antibacterial sensitivity patterns can vary according to geographic location; therefore, patterns should be established for every laboratory. Although empiric antibacterial selection should be used only until culture and sensitivity results are available, knowledge of sensitivity patterns can be crucial in the early treatment of osteomyelitis [5,8]. Table 1 reveals common bacterial isolates from osteomyelitis and their likely sensitivities. This table should be considered a rough guide to the commonly cultured organisms and their sensitivity patterns. Each laboratory should establish its own sensitivity patterns for bacteria, however.

Table 1
A summary of recent studies reporting common sensitivity patterns of organisms found in various types of bone infections

Population of horses	Problem	Most common organism(s) cultured	Antibiotic most likely to be effective[a]
Foals	Hematogenous osteomyelitis/physitis	Enterobacteriaceae	Amikacin, Cefotaxmine, Moxalactam
Adults	Septic arthritis secondary to injection of surgery	Staphylococci	Amikacin
Adults	Septic arthritis attributable to a wound	Often mixed	
		Enterobacteriaceae	Amikacin
		β-*Streptococcus*	Cephalothin
		Staphylococcus haemolyticus	Amikacin
		Non *staphylococcus haemolyticus*	Amikacin
Adults	Osteomyelitis attributable to a wound	Enterobacteriaceae	Amikacin
Adults	Osteomyelitis attributable to an implant infection/ fracture repair	Often mixed	
		Enterobacteriaceae	Amikacin
		non-β-*Streptococcus*	Chloramphenicol, trimethoprim-sulfonamides
		Coagulase-positive *Staphylococcus*	Amikacin
		β-*Streptococcus*	Cephalothin

[a] Sensitivity patterns from Moore RM, Schneider RK, Kowalski J, et al.
Data from Antimicrobial susceptibility of bacterial isolates from 233 houses with musculoskeletal infection during 1979–1989. Equine Vet J 1992;24:450–6.

Clinical findings and diagnosis

Clinical findings can vary according to the severity or duration of infection. The horse may begin with a slight increase in lameness compared with that observed previously, and the lameness may worsen rapidly. Local swelling often appears in the area of a wound or surgical incision. Furthermore, a painful response to digital palpation can usually be elicited. The incision line may produce local drainage, and granulation tissue can appear along the drainage site. Few systemic signs are associated with osteomyelitis, except for a febrile response. Leukocytosis, along with hyperfibrinogenemia, may be present, but these symptoms are never diagnostic for a bone infection. Septic arthritis or osteomyelitis is almost always associated with a moderate to severe lameness and joint effusion, except in the case of an open draining joint.

A good physical examination should be performed, paying special attention to the area of concern to determine whether heat, pain, or swelling accompanies the lameness. Detailed digital palpation that carefully attempts to localize the pain and swelling can be helpful in localizing the site of infection and determining the most appropriate site for aspiration, radiography, or ultrasonography.

Many imaging techniques are available for diagnosing osteomyelitis. Several modalities, such as MRI, CT, and biomarker analysis, have been used more recently and have become useful tools in the sometimes difficult task of establishing a diagnosis of osteomyelitis. The overall diagnostic accuracy using imaging modalities is approximately 80% to 90% [18]. Radiographic diagnosis remains the most commonly used modality to determine whether osteomyelitis is present. Unfortunately, radiology is somewhat insensitive to bony changes that occur early in the disease process of osteomyelitis. The infection must cause 50% to 70% bone demineralization to observe bone lysis on plain radiographs. Furthermore, this amount of bone loss may take up to 21 days to be detected [18]. As infection progresses, radiographic lucencies associated with areas of demineralization and bone lysis become more evident. These areas can form sequestra, and an envelope of demineralized bone and periosteal proliferation called an involucrum can form around the sequestra. If implants are present, radiolucencies are often seen along the margins (Fig. 1).

Scintigraphy using technetium (99m-Tc) is an emerging technology used to aid in the diagnosis of osteomyelitis (Fig. 2) [19]. It can be used to detect osteomyelitis several months before radiography [20]. Although scintigraphy is a sensitive indicator of bone turnover, it does not distinguish between bone turnover attributable to infection, recent trauma, or fracture development. It is thus not helpful in cases in which recent implantation or trauma has occurred. Furthermore, false-positive results can also occur in young foals, in which physeal development is still taking place. White blood cell labeling is an emerging technology in veterinary medicine. Indium-111 is used

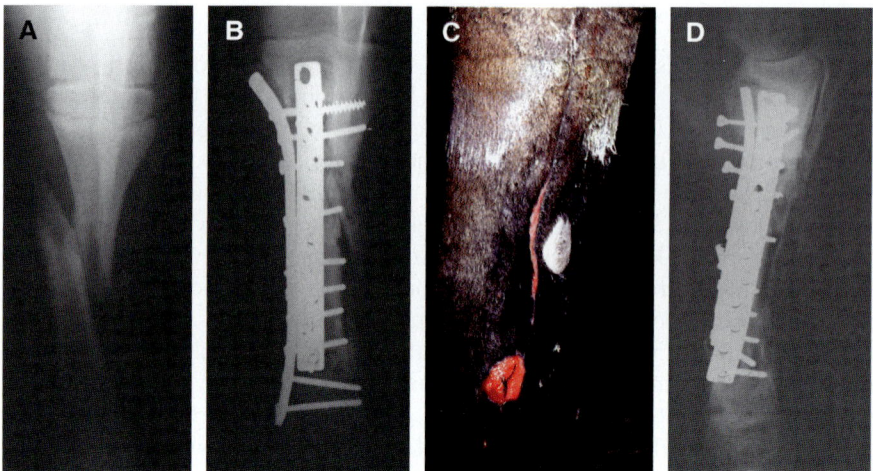

Fig. 1. Radiographic and gross examples of the progression of osteomyelitis. A middiaphyseal oblique fracture (*A*) repaired with two dynamic compression plates (*B*), subsequent resulting drainage associated with osteomyelitis (*C*), and radiolucencies around plates and screws associated with severe bacterial infection and osteolysis (*D*). (*Courtesy of* Dr. Alan Nixon, BVSc, MS, DACVS, Ithaca, NY.)

to label and reinject a patient's white blood cells to observe whether "pooling" (an indication of infection) is present. This is available at a few referral institutions and can be of great benefit in younger animals and when implants are present or recent trauma has taken place [19]. Another area in which scintigraphy has proven diagnostic is osteomyelitis associated with tooth root infections [21]. Scintigraphy was used to determine the presence or absence of disease and revealed the approximate area of tooth root

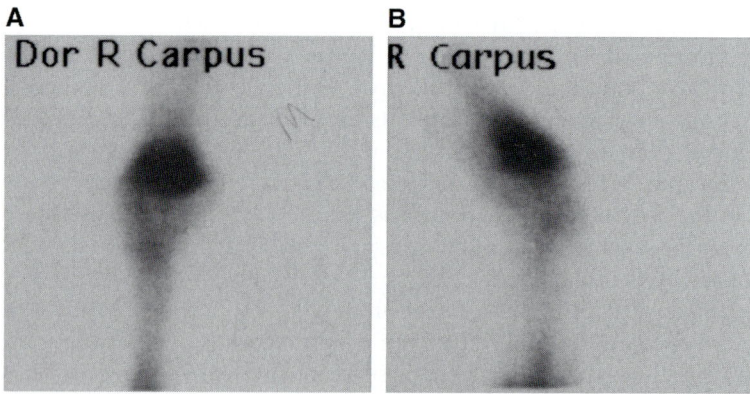

Fig. 2. Nuclear scintigraphy of osteomyelitis of the distal radius in a 4-year-old horse. Anteroplanar view (*A*) and lateral view (*B*).

involvement [21]. A more recent scintigraphic approach to diagnosing osteomyelitis consists of using 99m-Tc–labeled ciprofloxacin (99m-Tc-CIPRO). This method can be used to distinguish infection from other causes of inflammation [22,23]. Ciprofloxacin binds to bacterial DNA gyrase. Advantages of 99m-Tc-CIPRO scintigraphy for detecting infection include high specificity and no blood handling as well as the fact that minimal time, technical skills, and laboratory equipment are needed for radionuclide preparation and scanning [24]. A recent study in rabbits revealed that 99m-Tc-disodium hydroxymethylene diphosphonate (HDP) and 99m-Tc-CIPRO had higher uptake ratios in infected fractures than noninfected fractures [24]. Although 99m-Tc-CIPRO was better than 99m-Tc-HDP for diagnosing infections, it was also associated with a higher rate of false-positive results [24].

CT scanning can be used to determine the extent of bony involvement in osteomyelitis [25]. CT can reveal purulent material within the medullary cavity; adjacent soft tissue abscesses; intraosseous gas; decreased density of bone; or the presence of soft tissue masses, abscesses, or foreign bodies. CT is an alternate imaging modality to diagnose osteomyelitis in the horse, especially in areas in which radiographic interpretation is difficult, such as the head (Fig. 3). CT can also be used to identify sequestra in cases of chronic osteomyelitis. Contrast material can be used to delineate abscesses in necrotic tissue that are not delineated from the surrounding tissue [25].

MRI has also been used for evaluating bone and joint infections. MRI is a complex imaging method that aligns the protons within tissues along the axis of a magnetic field and then records the motion of the protons as they return to their natural state [25]. Each tissue has its own unique signal characteristics. MRI is particularly helpful for diagnosing lytic areas within the medullary cavity because of the distinct changes that it can reveal within soft tissues and fat. In a study of human patients, MRI was superior in

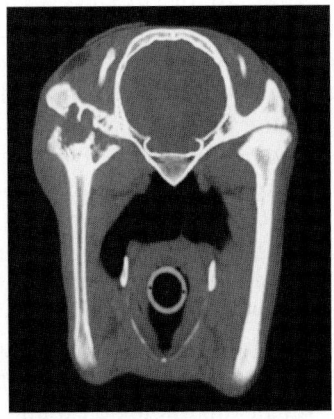

Fig. 3. CT scan of a skull. The left temporomandibular joint has severe osteomyelitis.

sensitivity (97%) and specificity (92%) to 99m-Tc phosphate bone scanning for the detection of osteomyelitis. MRI can be used to detect changes, such as lytic areas, much earlier in the course of disease than other imaging modalities because it provides greater definition of the medullary cavity. The signal changes seen on MRI, however, may be nonspecific, and anything that causes edema or hyperemia, such as fractures, tumors, and inflammatory processes, causes signal changes similar to those seen with osteomyelitis. Furthermore, because of the strong magnetic field, MRI should not be used with metallic implants [25]. Although MRI is good for detailing medullary involvement, it does not reveal cortical bone involvement like CT.

Ultrasonography can be an extremely helpful addition to other imaging modalities [26]. Ultrasonography may be more accurate than radiography for diagnosing infection, because small accumulations of fluid around implants are easier to detect. In one study, ultrasonography was used to diagnose osteomyelitis correctly in 30 of 32 cases, but radiography was used successfully in only 10 of 32 cases [26]. Imaging fluid pockets in perpendicular planes coincides with irregular bony echoes; this allows location and aspiration of the infected fluid so that the organisms associated with the infection can be determined.

Deep aspiration of fluid accumulations should follow ultrasonographic determination of location. A white blood cell count of the aspirated fluid can be used to determine the serous or purulent nature of the aspirate. A diagnostic culture of the aspirated fluid should be performed for aerobic and anaerobic bacteria [5]. Recent literature suggests that fluid should be inoculated directly into broth, particularly commercial culture vials, to enhance bacterial growth and decrease culture turnaround time [27–29]. Alternatively, aspirated fluid can be placed on a swab and put into transport medium, which stabilizes the local pH and minimizes the growth of contaminate bacteria, such as anaerobes, but does not possess the growth enhancement characteristics of broth. In the absence of fluid accumulations on ultrasonography examination, a draining tract should be prepared aseptically and a swab inserted. The swab should be processed as described previously. In cases of septic arthritis or osteomyelitis, the synovial fluid should be aspirated and a white blood cell count, cytology, and total protein content measured. If the synovial fluid white blood cell count is greater than 30,000 cells/µL and the total protein concentration is more than 3.5 to 4.0 g/dL, infection is present [4,30,31]. Cytology consistent with sepsis usually reveals mostly neutrophils; occasionally, bacteria are observed on direct smears. Synovial fluid should also be cultured in an attempt to determine the bacterial cause accurately.

In cases in which a diagnosis of infection is still suspected but is not confirmed after these diagnostic procedures, a Michelle trephine can be used to obtain a sample of bone for histopathologic examination as well as culture and sensitivity testing. This may result in an accurate diagnosis and a definitive bacterial culture, thereby aiding the clinician in determining appropriate local and systemic antimicrobial treatment.

Currently, serum biomarkers are being evaluated for their use in the diagnosis of osteomyelitis. Various biochemical markers of bone metabolism, including osteocalcin (OC), bone-specific alkaline phosphatase (BS-ALP), and deoxypyridinoline (DPYR), have been evaluated [32]. OC is a specific product of osteoblasts and is associated with bone mineralization [33,34]. A fraction of an OC molecule is released into the blood during the incorporation of OC into bone during bone formation. BS-ALP is an osteoblast enzyme that is thought to play a role in the formation and mineralization of bone matrix [35,36]. DPYR is a molecule associated with bone resorption [33]. When bone is resorbed, collagen is degraded and DPYR is released into the blood. In a recent study evaluating these biochemical markers in rabbits with and without osteomyelitis, measurement of OC, BS-ALP, and DPYR serum concentrations could predict the presence of osteomyelitis with 96% accuracy at 4 weeks [32]. The use of these biomarkers for determining the presence of infection in the horse may be extremely useful, economic, and accurate. Future studies in the horse are indicated to determine if their accuracy in the diagnosis of osteomyelitis is similar to that in the rabbit.

An emerging trend in the study of orthopedic implant infection is the use of molecular assays, such as confocal microscopy and real-time polymerase chain reaction (PCR)–based techniques, to examine bacterial characteristics of biofilm [10]. Authors of some reports claim that PCR-based analyses for bacteria can be used to identify microorganisms in samples in which standard microbiologic culture techniques have failed [37,38]. Some criticism exists, however, that PCR may be too sensitive an assay and may yield false-positive results when no active infection persists but DNA from nonviable bacteria may still be present [10]. Real-time PCR tests are currently being developed to detect bacterial RNA that only exists in live bacteria, thus eliminating false-positive results [10].

Traditional treatments of osteomyelitis

Systemic antimicrobial therapy

The traditional systemic therapy for osteomyelitis involves appropriate intravenous antimicrobial drugs, together with improving the wound environment [39]. Before the advent of local and more innovative therapies, systemic antimicrobials were the cornerstone of therapy for osteomyelitis. Local therapy may eventually supplant systemic therapy. Systemic antimicrobials alone are often ineffective for treating horses with severe or chronic osteomyelitis or synovial infections [4]. Broad-spectrum antimicrobials should be used as prophylaxis before orthopedic surgery or to treat osteomyelitis until results of culture and sensitivity patterns are known. Two studies analyzing the sensitivity patterns of common bacteria cultured from horses with osteomyelitis revealed that the combination of cephalosporin and amikacin provides the broadest coverage [16,17].

Penicillin and gentamicin in combination are commonly used to treat osteomyelitis until definitive culture and sensitivity results are known. Benefits of the combination are that it provides a broad spectrum of activity, is not cost-prohibitive, and has minimal side effects. Furthermore, the increased bacterial kill and reduced renal toxicity of once-daily dosing of gentamicin make it more efficacious than administering doses two or three times a day [40]. Amikacin is often similarly administered at this frequency. Oral antimicrobials are often used as follow-up therapy after the infection has been controlled with parenteral antimicrobials. In general, parenteral antimicrobials are recommended for a minimum of 7 to 10 days or until the osteomyelitis is controlled. To prevent relapses, oral antimicrobials are commonly instituted after that time because of their ease of administration, cost, and relative efficacy after the infection has been abated. Oral antimicrobials are usually continued for approximately 1 month or longer, depending on the response to therapy, specific drainage techniques, and severity of infection [41]. More studies are needed to determine proper timing for discontinuation of antibiotics after resolution of infection.

The duration of prophylactic antimicrobial administration still remains controversial [42,43]. For routine orthopedic procedures, prophylactic antimicrobials should only be given 1 hour before surgery and up to 24 hours after surgery [44]. No difference has been noted if antimicrobials are continued for 3 days or stopped 24 hours after surgery [44]. Nevertheless, antimicrobial therapy is extended if implants are used or the surgery is considered clean-contaminated.

Curettage and implant removal

Osteomyelitis is often considered a surgical disease. Thorough debridement of bone and soft tissue to remove necrotic debris, purulent material, and avascular bone is imperative for successful treatment [39]. Necrotic bone acts as a chronic focus of inflammation and encourages purulent drainage until removed. Granulation tissue often forms around necrotic bone, prevents resorption by isolating the bone from a healthy vascular supply, and impedes healing [45]. Wound debridement should be combined with appropriate stabilization of unstable fractures or removal of metallic implants. Stable fractures can heal in the face of infection. Determining whether bone is viable may be challenging. The decision to retain or discard a bone fragment should be based on its size, importance to stability, and extent of detachment from periosteum and surrounding soft tissues [5]. At the time of debridement, affected tissue should be obtained for culture and sensitivity testing to assist the clinician in choosing the most appropriate antimicrobial drug.

Bone graft

Bone grafts have been used in bone surgery for several decades to augment bone repair, speed healing of complicated fractures, and promote healing of nonunions and infected fractures. Autogenous bone grafts can serve two major functions in treating osteomyelitis: they have osteogenic potential, and they can provide mechanical support [46–49]. Bone grafts assist healing in cases with osteomyelitis by three different mechanisms: osteogenesis, osteoinduction, and osteoconduction. Cancellous bone has osteogenic potential because it has a much greater volume of viable cells compared with cortical bone. These cells begin forming new bone when implanted into debrided defects. The osteoinduction capabilities of cancellous bone are attributable to the mesenchymal precursor cells that differentiate into preosteoblasts and then into osteoblasts [50]. Proteins, such as bone morphogenetic protein (BMP) and transforming growth factor-β (TGFβ), are secreted from the graft and induce the migration of additional cells as well as the differentiation of mesenchymal cells within the graft. This osteoinduction occurs within the first weeks of bone grafting [51]. The osteoconductive capabilities of cancellous bone include ingrowth of capillaries, perivascular tissue formation, and osteoprogenitor cell migration [49,50]. Cancellous bone provides a scaffold that mechanically supports the tissue. In contrast to osteoinduction, osteoconduction lasts for several months with cancellous grafts and may last for many months to years with cortical bone grafts, depending on their size [51]. The benefits of cancellous bone grafts in treating osteomyelitis are numerous and, in the horse, there are abundant sources of autogenous bone in the ilium, sternum, and proximal tibia [51].

Recently, the fourth coccygeal vertebra has been reported as an alternative site of bone graft collection in the horse [52]. The authors of this study also quantitated the amount of osteogenic cells and the percentage of osteoprogenitor cells within the osteogenic population of the fourth coccygeal vertebra, tibial periosteum, sternum, and tuber coxae [52]. The tuber coxae, coccygeal vertebra, and periosteum were the best sites for osteogenic harvest, and the tuber coxae and periosteum yielded the greatest population of osteoprogenitor cells [52]. Another report described the technique of harvesting cancellous bone from the proximal humerus in horses; however, one of eight horses sustained a catastrophic fracture on recovery, deeming this site inadequate for cancellous bone collection [53].

Innovative treatments of osteomyelitis in the horse

The use of antimicrobial-impregnated polymethylmethacrylate (AIPMMA) implants for prevention and treatment of osteomyelitis in horses has drastically improved the success rate. Several case reports in horses testify to the strides that have been made in managing osteomyelitis [54–57]. In the 1980s, many studies reported the successful prevention and treatment of osteomyelitis using

AIPMMA [58,59]. Since then, a steady increase in the use of AIPMMA in human and animal patients has occurred [54].

Implantation of AIPMMA results in high local concentrations of antimicrobials for prolonged periods [60,61]. The slow local elution of antimicrobials can result in concentrations in wound fluid of up to 200 times that obtainable with systemic administration of the same antimicrobial. Antimicrobial concentrations above the minimum inhibitory concentration (MIC) can last for up to 80 days after implantation [43,62,63]. The distinct advantage of this form of preventative and treatment is that serum concentrations do not reach toxic levels, despite high wound concentrations of antimicrobials after bead implantation [43,60,62]. Furthermore, this method of treatment reduces, and sometimes eliminates, the need for systemic therapy. The resulting decrease in the risk of drug toxicity and the drastic decrease in costs incurred with this disease in the horse are noteworthy. Although variable, successful treatment responses of 80% for treatment of horses with osteomyelitis have been reported for this form of local antimicrobial therapy, which is a substantial improvement compared with systemic treatment responses [55,60]. Prophylactic use in people has resulted in as much as a 34% decrease in infection rates [60,64].

Antimicrobials are eluted from polymethylmethacrylate (PMMA) in a bimodal pattern [54]. Rapid elution of the antimicrobial usually takes place within the first 24 hours [60,65]. The subsequent elution rate is slower and, depending on the antimicrobial and bone cement used, detectable amounts of drug may be released weeks to months after implantation.

There are many factors that affect the elution rate of antimicrobials from PMMA. Those factors include the type and porosity of PMMA, surface area of the bead, volume of fluid surrounding the cement, antimicrobial concentration placed in the PMMA, and diffusion properties of each antimicrobial [54,60,65]. Antimicrobial elution rates of AIPMMA are directly proportional to surface area. Therefore, placing small rough beads in wounds is preferred over smooth beads, because small rough beads have a large surface area per volume and a sphere has the greatest surface area per volume. AIPMMA is most effective when formed into spheres before implantation.

The amount of antimicrobial placed into bone cement is directly proportional to the amount eluted. Therefore, the maximal concentration of antimicrobial should be used in the implants to achieve the highest local antimicrobial concentrations. If the "undefined" maximum concentration of an antimicrobial is surpassed during AIPMMA preparation, it seems to prolong, or inhibit, the "setup" time and lower the quality of the bone cement. Therefore, concentrations previously reported to elute successfully are best to use. A rule of thumb that the author currently uses is 5% of the weight of the PMMA (ie, amikacin, 0.5 g, for PMMA, 10 g).

The combination of antimicrobials in PMMA may also enhance or inhibit elution of the antimicrobial. For example, in a study in which tobramycin and oxacillin were combined in PMMA, the elution of oxacillin was increased but that of tobramycin was decreased compared with when they were used separately [59]. This is not the case for all antimicrobial combinations. Therefore, the clinician beginning to use AIPMMA should be familiar with the antimicrobial combinations documented to elute successfully.

Culture results are sometimes used to determine antimicrobial selection, but organisms have often not yet been cultured or AIPMMA is being used prophylactically. In these situations, a broad-spectrum antimicrobial that has high water solubility, low tissue toxicity, and is stable at temperatures up to 100°C is chosen [66–68].

Gentamicin-impregnated PMMA has been the focus in much of the literature because of gentamicin's broad-spectrum bactericidal activity as well as its water-soluble and heat-stable characteristics. Although this remains a good antimicrobial choice, there are now many different antimicrobials that reportedly have good elution rates from PMMA [69–71]. Table 2 lists some antimicrobials that are reportedly viable options to use in PMMA. Amikacin's broader coverage and greater efficacy in treating equine orthopedic infections compared with gentamicin have made it a popular antimicrobial choice [16].

It should be noted that liquid antimicrobial preparations are efficacious in PMMA. Powdered formulations of antimicrobials were previously

Table 2
Antibiotics and their combinations that may be appropriate for use with polymethylmethacrylate

Antibiotics that elute well from PMMA	Antibiotics that have minimal elution from PMMA	Antibiotic combinations that elute well from PMMA	Antibiotic combinations that have a negative effect on elution
Amikacin	Ceftiofur (<MIC for 10 days)	Vancomycin/ Amikacin	Tobramycin/Oxacillin
Gentamicin	Polymixin B[a]	Cefazolin/Amikacin	
Tobramycin	Tetracycline[a]	Cefazolin/ Metronidazole	
Amoxicillin	Chloramphenicol[a]	Metronidazole/ Gentamicin	
Ciprofloxacin			
Imipenem			
Amoxicillin			
Ticarcillin			
Cefazolin			
Clindamycin			
Vancomycin			
Erythromycin			
Metronidazole			
Fluoroquinolones			

Abbreviation: PMMA, polymethylmethacrylate.
[a] Not sufficiently heat stable to retain activity during the exothermic hardening process.

reported to be superior to liquid formulations [54]. Elution was optimized when a crystalline formulation rather than a fine powder was used, however [72].

Preparation of AIPMMA is easy and can be performed at or before surgery or implantation or sterilized and stored for later use. PMMA is a high-density plastic formed by combining a fluid monomer and powdered polymer (Fig. 4). When an antimicrobial is added, the antimicrobial becomes suspended in the cement as it hardens [60]. Elution rates vary according to the various brands of PMMA. Common brands used with reportedly good elution rates are Surgical Simplex P (Howmedica, Rutherford, New Jersey), Palacos (Richards Medical, Philadelphia, Pennsylvania), and Zimmer (Warsaw, Indiana). Typically, polymer (10 g) is placed into a plastic mixing bowl, and liquid monomer is added according to manufacturer's directions, along with the crystalline form of antimicrobial. The components are thoroughly mixed until the mixture becomes pasty (Fig. 5). The mixture is placed into a bead mold (Instrument and Mold Facility, University of Vermont, Burlington, Vermont) with a suture in the center (Figs. 6 and 7), or the cement is mixed into beads or molded into cylinders by hand (Fig. 8). The approximate time to hardening is 5 to 10 minutes. Implants not used immediately can be gas-sterilized for storage. A potential loss in antimicrobial potency from steam autoclaving makes ethylene oxide gas the preferred sterilization method [73,74]. Gas-sterilized beads should be aerated for approximately 24 hours at room temperature before use.

It is important to note that the addition of amounts greater than 10% of the PMMA (ie, any microbial at a rate of >4.5 g to PMMA, 40 g) weakens the biomechanical properties of PMMA. The compressive and tensile strengths are inferior when large amounts of the antimicrobial are used,

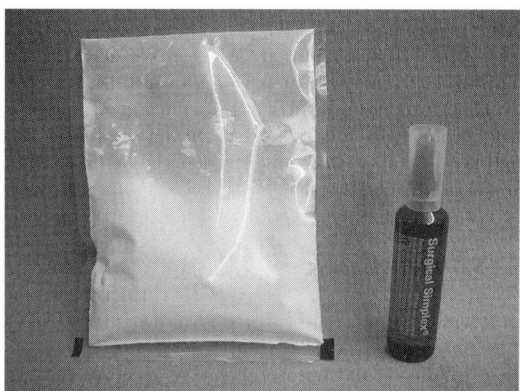

Fig. 4. PMMA. The powder (polymer) usually comes packaged in 40-g packets. The fluid (monomer) is most often packaged in a glass vial. (*From* Goodrich LR, Nixon AJ. Treatment options for osteomyelitis. Equine Vet Educ 2004;16:271; with permission.)

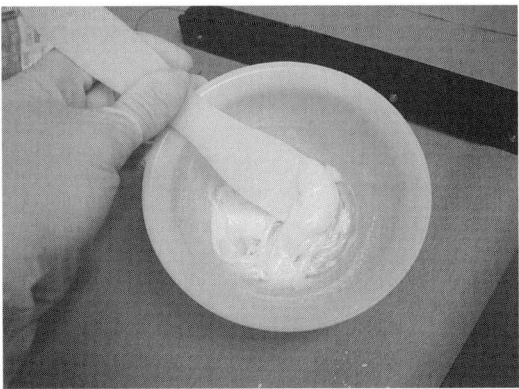

Fig. 5. Polymer, monomer, and antibiotic are mixed until the consistency is paste-like. (*From* Goodrich LR, Nixon AJ. Treatment options for osteomyelitis. Equine Vet Educ 2004;16:271; with permission.)

which is important to remember when the PMMA is used to lute a plate or metal implant [73,74].

Some controversy exists regarding the removal of AIPMMA implants. Some surgeons prefer to remove the implants, whereas others suggest that beads only be removed if they become infected. Figs. 9 and 10 are photographs of implants placed at the time of fracture repair and 2 years later, respectively. No complications were associated with the beads, the mare was sound, and removal of the implants was not necessary. The author only anticipates removal of beads if they are placed in an infected wound that is healing by second intention (Fig. 11). If removal is anticipated at the time of bead placement, the surgeon should be aware that many small beads attached to a suture may be easier to remove compared with beads placed randomly into a wound.

Few complications have been associated with the use of AIPMMA. Allergic reactions have not been reported. The most significant complications

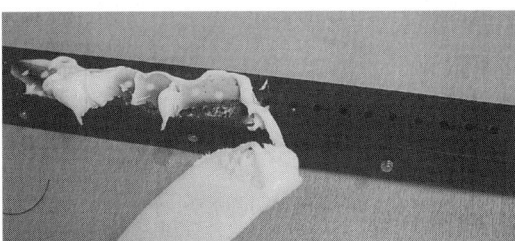

Fig. 6. Spatula is used to smear the paste-like AIPMMA into the bead mod that has a suture placed in it. (*From* Goodrich LR, Nixon AJ. Treatment options for osteomyelitis. Equine Vet Educ 2004;16:271; with permission.)

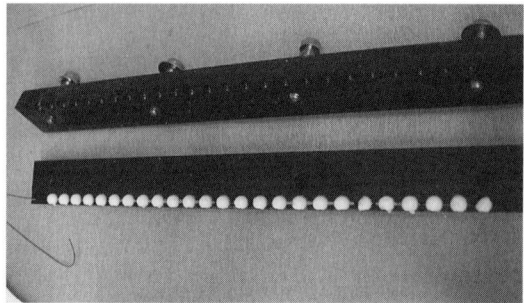

Fig. 7. Once the AIPMMA is hardened, the mold can be unscrewed and multiple beads on a suture can be placed into a wound or along a plate (*From* Goodrich LR, Nixon AJ. Treatment options for osteomyelitis. Equine Vet Educ 2004;16:271; with permission.)

have been soft tissue damage during removal and the formation of fibrous connective tissue complicating removal. Furthermore, AIPMMA should not be placed in joints because of its abrasive nature [75]. The widespread use of AIPMMA by orthopedic surgeons represents the general belief that the benefits from high local levels of antimicrobials and minimal systemic side effects outweigh the minimal risk of complications associated with these implants.

In conclusion, AIPMMA is invaluable in treating and preventing bone infections. Infection rates in people with grade III open fractures decreased from 42.9% to 8.7% with the addition of AIPMMA [60]. AIPMMA implants should never be used as the sole treatment of bone infections but should always be used in addition to adequate surgical debridement. Proper use of AIPMMA can mean greater surgical success in preventing and managing osteomyelitis, decreased cost, and fewer episodes of systemic toxicosis.

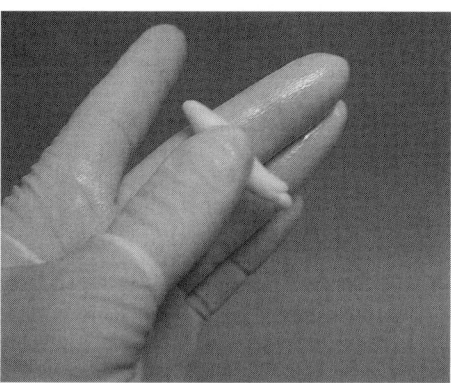

Fig. 8. AIPMMA can be molded into cylinders or spheres by hand. (*From* Goodrich LR, Nixon AJ. Treatment options for osteomyelitis. Equine Vet Educ 2004;16:271; with permission.)

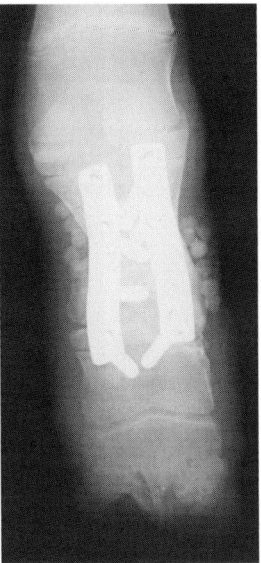

Fig. 9. Open fracture in a 5-month-old filly was repaired with two dynamic compression plates (DCP) plates and multiple strands of amikacin-impregnated PMMA beads.

Furthermore, the use of AIPMMA facilitates improved management of dead space and is more convenient than long-term parenteral administration of antimicrobials.

Plaster of Paris (POP) has been used for decades for local delivery of antimicrobials in cases of orthopedic infection. Its advantages are many and

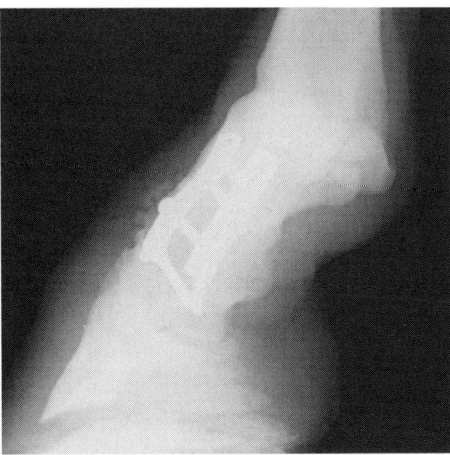

Fig. 10. Two years later, the fracture is healed and the beads can be visualized. The mare is sound, and the beads seem to be quiescent. Removal is not necessary.

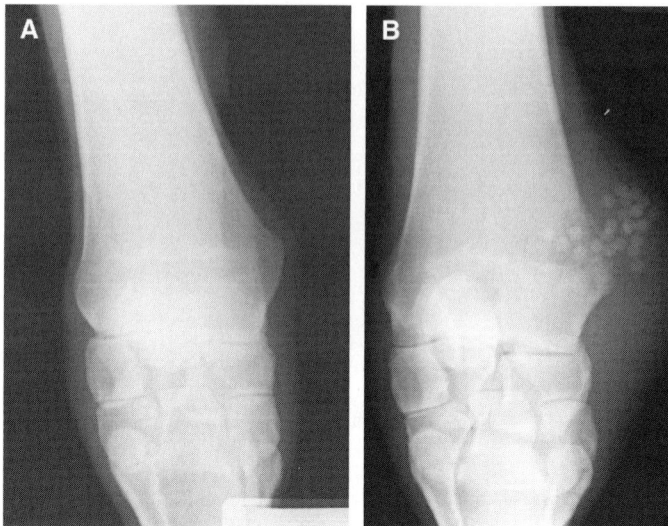

Fig. 11. (*A*) Radiograph of the osteomyelitic lesion from Fig. 2. (*B*) Bone was debrided, the wound was packed with a string of antibiotic-impregnated beads, and the beads were subsequently removed 14 days later.

include bioabsorbability, biocompatibility, availability, and affordability [76–79]. Studies assessing the elution of antimicrobials from POP reveal that antimicrobial release actually surpasses that of PMMA in the first 24 to 48 hours of implantation [70]. Elution rapidly drops below the MIC after 48 hours, however [77]. Therefore, POP's greatest efficacy in preventing and treating osteomyelitis is within the first 2 days. If long-term elution is desired, PMMA remains a more viable option, or a combination of POP and PMMA could be considered.

In a recent publication by Santschi and McGarvey [77], the process of preparing POP beads was described. Calcium sulfate hemihydrate was first weighed into aliquots and dried by baking for 4 hours at 200°C [77]. Twenty grams of dried calcium sulfate hemihydrate was then combined with gentamicin sulfate, 5 mL, and phosphate-buffered saline (PBS), 3 mL, in a mixing bowl. The POP-gentamicin slurry was then poured into a 200-mL syringe and injected into a bead mold with a number 2 polydiaxonon suture (PDS) suture in place [77]. The bead mold mixing vessel, stirrer, and PBS were all chilled in a freezer before making the beads. The beads were then gas-sterilized with ethylene oxide and stored at room temperature for 5 months before use [77]. Neither gas sterilization nor storage negatively affected the elution of antimicrobials [77], which was consistent with other reports [70,78,80].

The major technical disadvantage of using these beads is the necessity of preparing, sterilizing, and aerating them before surgery. The POP high antimicrobial elution rate in the first 48 hours and the complete absorption of the beads, combined with their purported osteoconductive and osteoinductive capabilities, make these beads an attractive alternative to AIPMMA, however [76].

Intense research to find other biodegradable materials that effectively deliver antimicrobials to bone is being conducted, and various materials have shown promise in equine models of osteomyelitis [81–86]. Some of these materials include hydroxyapatite (HAP), β-tricalcium phosphate (β-TCP), polylactic acid (PLA), polyglycolic acid (PGA), and polylactide-co-glycolide (PLGA). The advantages that these materials bring include prolonged systemic antimicrobial therapy for 4 to 6 weeks, biocompatibility, excellent mechanical properties, and positive effects on new bone formation [87]. Although promising for the future treatment of osteomyelitis, these materials presently remain unavailable or cost-prohibitive for use in the equine patient.

Intravenous and intraosseous regional limb perfusion

The use of regional limb perfusion to treat osteomyelitis in the limbs of horses has proven to be an effective, affordable, and convenient route of antimicrobial drug delivery [88–90]. This procedure has been increasingly used by equine orthopedic surgeons to treat and prevent bone and synovial infections. The technique uses an extracorporeal circuit, such as an isolated artery or vein, that supplies an area of tissue to which the antimicrobial is administered. Alternatively, the medullary space in the bone can be used utilizing a cannulated bone screw [4] or a commercial device specially manufactured to deliver fluids to human neonates (Fig. 12). Intravenous or intraosseous antimicrobials are delivered under pressure distal to a tourniquet [91,92]. As perfusate enters the venous system, it distends the vasculature, which promotes perfusate diffusion into local tissues [93].

Regional limb perfusion was first used to deliver antineoplastic drugs that resulted in toxic side effects when given systemically [94]. Extrapolating that principle to treat orthopedic infections has resulted in tissue antimicrobial

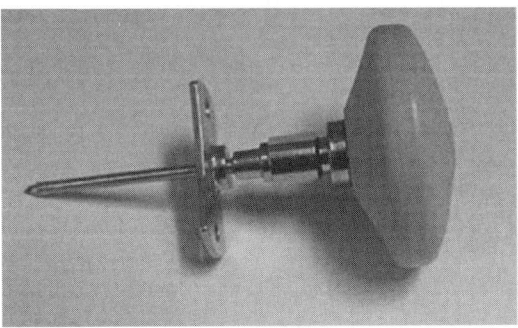

Fig. 12. Bone canula available from Cook (Bloomington, Indiana), which was originally manufactured to administer fluids to pediatric patients.

concentrations well above the MIC [88–90,93,95]. This is imperative when treating infected tissues, such as bone, where the inflammatory process causes vascular thrombosis, necrosis, and a biofilm layer that inhibits delivery of systemically administered antimicrobials [96,97].

An Esmarch or pneumatic tourniquet is applied to the affected limb proximal to the infection site to occlude the superficial vascular system. The antimicrobial solution is then injected through a catheter or butterfly needle under pressure. The antimicrobial should be diluted in saline (30–60 mL) to facilitate an increase in pressure via a volume effect and to minimize local tissue toxicity. Injection under pressure distends the venous vasculature, allowing diffusion into the tissue distal to the tourniquet. A subtraction radiography study by Whitehair and colleagues [88] showed that perfusate injected into the medullary cavity of the metacarpus exited through the epiphyseal vein and entered the adjoining synovial venous system. Figs. 13 through 16 exemplify the technique and the tissue perfusion that occurs when radiopaque dye is injected under pressure. The tourniquet should be maintained for a minimum of 30 minutes to allow complete diffusion of the antimicrobial solution.

Mattson and coworkers [98] used 99m-Tc pertechnetate and scintigraphic imaging to show that horses regionally perfused using a vein or an intramedullary cavity had no difference in limb perfusion. Butt and colleagues [99] confirmed these findings by comparing antimicrobial concentrations in

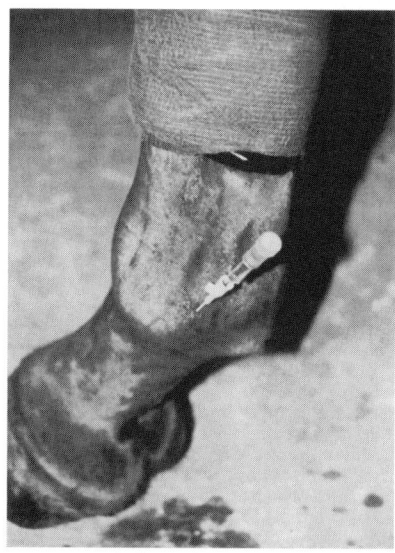

Fig. 13. Esmarch bandage is used as a tourniquet to restrict blood flow. A 20-gauge catheter in the palmar digital vein is used for infusion of antibiotic solution. (*From* Palmer SE, Hogan PM. How to perform regional limb perfusion in the standing horse. In: Proceedings of the 45th Annual American Association of Equine Practitioners Convention. Albuquerque (NM); 1999. p. 126; with permission.)

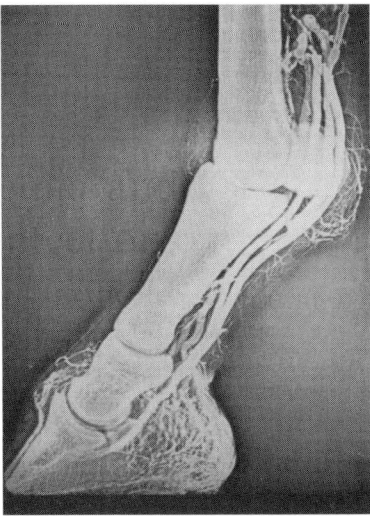

Fig. 14. Xeroradiograph taken 1 minute after injection of radiopaque dye. The dye is beginning to exit the vascular space and diffuse into the vascular tissue. (*From* Palmer SE, Hogan PM. How to perform regional limb perfusion in the standing horse. In: Proceedings of the 45th Annual American Association of Equine Practitioners Convention. Albuquerque (NM); 1999. p. 126; with permission.)

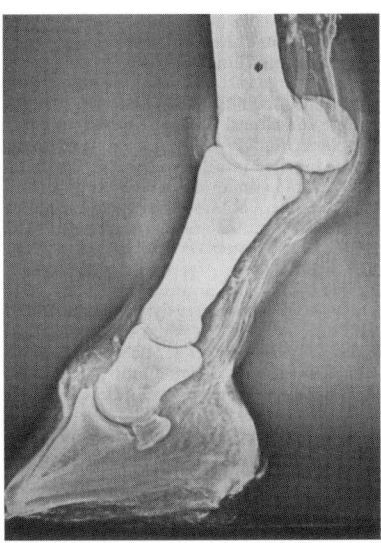

Fig. 15. Xeroradiograph taken 10 seconds after injection of a 40-mL solution of radiopaque dye under pressure. Excellent diffusion of the venous and arterial vessels is occurring. (*From* Palmer SE, Hogan PM. How to perform regional limb perfusion in the standing horse. In: Proceedings of the 45th Annual American Association of Equine Practitioners Convention. Albuquerque (NM); 1999. p. 126; with permission.)

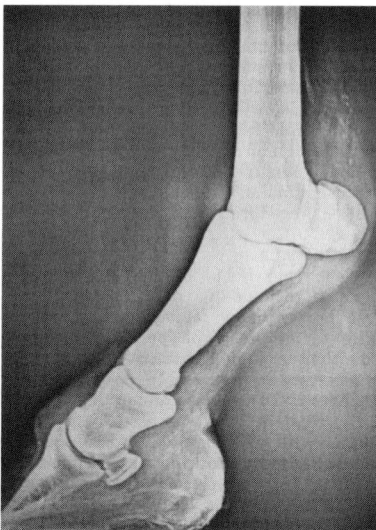

Fig. 16. Xeroradiograph taken 15 minutes later demonstrating the soft tissue diffusion of dye throughout the tissues distal to the tourniquet. Most of the dye has completely diffused out of the vessels. (*From* Palmer SE, Hogan PM. How to perform regional limb perfusion in the standing horse. In: Proceedings of the 45th Annual American Association of Equine Practitioners Convention. Albuquerque (NM); 1999. p. 126; with permission.)

joints of limbs perfused via an intravenous or intramedullary route. In a recent study, however, amikacin concentration in the tibiotarsal joint was compared after amikacin (1 g) was diluted in lactated Ringer's solution (56 mL) and administered by intravenous or intraosseous regional perfusion (distal portion of the tibia) [95]. In this study, intravenous perfusion resulted in an amikacin concentration up to three times higher in the synovial fluid compared with intraosseous perfusion [95].

Because veins are more accessible and an intravenous catheter is easier to maintain and less invasive than an intramedullary device, intravenous regional perfusion is more commonly used than the intramedullary route. Intramedullary regional perfusion is a logical alternative when vessel morbidity associated with limb swelling and infected tissues is a problem, however.

Higher concentrations of antimicrobials are reached in the horse using regional perfusion than using systemic dosing with drugs like cefazolin, ampicillin, amikacin, and potassium penicillin [89,99]. No local toxic effects were reported [89,99]. To date, the only reported local toxic effect associated with regional perfusion was with intravenous administration of enrofloxacin (G.A. Perkins, DVM, DACVIM, personal communication, 2003). It is theorized that concentrated doses of the vehicle in this antimicrobial can be detrimental to tissues. A study recently reporting on the local concentrations of regionally administered enrofloxacin did not report an associated toxicity, however [100].

Appropriate dose rates for most of the common locally administered antimicrobials have not been established. This remains one of the unknowns associated with this technique. Some authors use one third of a systemic daily dose of gentamicin and amikacin, whereas others use a single systemic dose for ampicillin sodium and potassium penicillin [89,90]. A dose of cefazolin based on the approximate weight of the perfused limb was used in another study [101]. Still other clinicians recommend diluting one systemic dose with saline at a rate of 30 or 60 mL before administration [4]. Many of the uncertainties regarding dosage come from unknown pharmacokinetics of regional drug delivery, and more clinical trials are necessary. The most conclusive equine studies on this subject to date are those by Mattson and coworkers [98] and Werner and colleagues [102]. In the study by Werner and colleagues [102], antimicrobial concentrations in joint fluid and subchondral bone were compared after administration of gentamicin, 1 g, by intra-articular injection or regional limb perfusion (1 g in 20 mL). No difference was noted in subchondral bone antimicrobial concentrations [102]. Furthermore, concentration of gentamicin in subchondral bone remained above the MIC for up to 8 hours when administered by regional intravenous perfusion. Alternatively, in the study by Mattson and coworkers [98], gentamicin, 2.2 mg/kg, was administered in sterile saline (0.9% NaCl) at a rate of 1 mL/kg and injected, under pressure, into the midmetacarpal bone with a tourniquet applied at the proximal metacarpus [98]. Using this technique, gentamicin concentrations attained in the bone reached

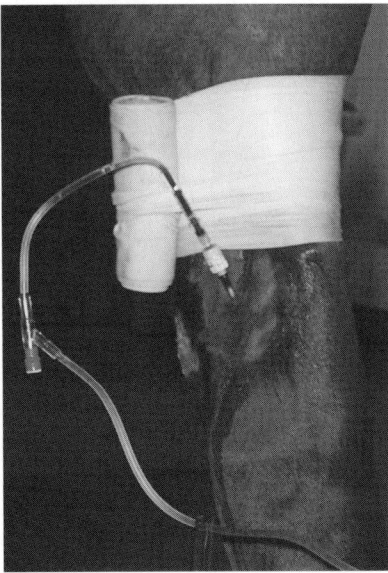

Fig. 17. Standing and minimally sedated patient receiving regional limb perfusion through a catheter in the cephalic vein.

two to six times the MIC for up to 36 hours for some locations of the metacarpal bone. The authors recommended using this dose once every 36 hours to allow the antimicrobial concentrations to drop below the level at which adaptive resistance of bacteria can take place.

In both regional limb perfusion techniques, clinicians need to attain adequate and constant tourniquet pressures, preferably using a pneumatic tourniquet, because inappropriate tourniquet application can lead to inadequate concentrations of antimicrobials in the target tissues. This technique can be performed in an anesthetized or standing horse. Earlier reports claimed that general anesthesia was necessary [4]; however, the author has

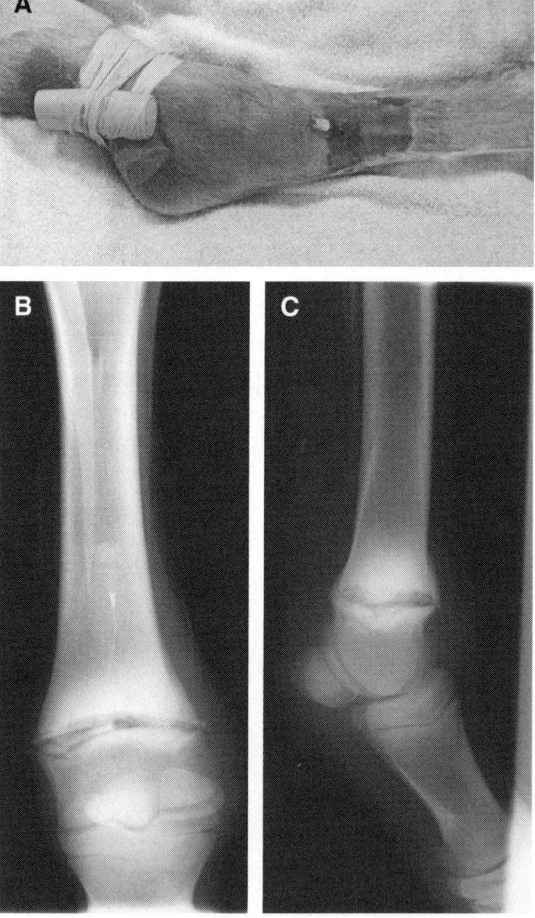

Fig. 18. Hind limb of a moderately sedated foal receiving regional limb perfusion through the saphenous vein distal to an Esmarch tourniquet (*A*) and anteroposterior (*B*) and lateral (*C*) radiographs of the limb receiving the local perfusion. The distal physis has moderate physitis.

performed repeated administration of intravenous and intraosseous regional perfusion in standing horses with minimal objection from the patients. Figs. 17 and 18 show intravenous regional limb perfusion being performed with sedation only in an adult standing horse with osteomyelitis and in a recumbent sedated foal with physitis, respectively.

For a discussion on treatment of joint infections, the reader is referred to the article on septic arthritis, tenosynovitis, and infections of hoof structures as well as to the article on new antimicrobials, systemic distribution, and local methods of antimicrobial delivery elsewhere in this issue.

Summary

Antimicrobial delivery systems, such as AIPMMA, antimicrobial-impregnated POP, intravenous or intraosseous regional limb perfusion, and fenestrated intra-articular drains have revolutionized the prevention and treatment of osteomyelitis. Only a decade ago, osteomyelitis in the horse often resulted in exorbitant costs and, sadly, the demise of the patient after an extended treatment period. New reports surface monthly about antimicrobial compatibility with these delivery systems and use of proper doses, which requires clinicians to search the current literature on a regular basis. These advances have contributed a great deal to our ability to treat diseases that once ended promising equine careers.

References

[1] MacDonald DG, Morley PS, Bailey JV, et al. An examination of the occurrence of surgical wound infection following equine orthopaedic surgery (1981–1990). Equine Vet J 1994;26: 323–6.
[2] Lew DP, Waldvogel FA. Osteomyelitis. Lancet 2004;364:369–79.
[3] Lew DP, Waldvogel FA. Osteomyelitis. N Engl J Med 1997;336:999–1007.
[4] Baxter GM. Instrumentation and techniques for treating orthopedic infections in horses. Vet Clin North Am Equine Pract 1996;12:303–35.
[5] Trotter GT. Osteomyelitis. In: Nixon AJ, editor. Equine fracture repair. Philadelphia: WB Saunders; 1996. p. 359–66.
[6] Gristina AG, Oga M, Webb LX, et al. Adherent bacterial colonization in the pathogenesis of osteomyelitis. Science 1985;228:990–3.
[7] Gristina AG, Naylor PT, Myrvik QN. Mechanisms of musculoskeletal sepsis. Orthop Clin North Am 1991;22:363–88.
[8] Goodrich LR, Nixon AJ. Treatment options for osteomyelitis. Equine Vet Educ 2004;16: 267–80.
[9] Savage DC, Fletcher M, editors. Bacterial adhesion: mechanisms and physiological significance. New York: Plenum Press; 1985.
[10] Stoodley P, Kathju S, Hu FZ, et al. Molecular and imaging techniques for bacterial biofilms in joint arthroplasty infections. Clin Orthop 2005;437:31–40.
[11] Davies DG, Parsek MR, Pearson JP, et al. The involvement of cell-to-cell signals in the development of a bacterial biofilm. Science 1998;280:295–8.
[12] Borriello G, Werner E, Roe F, et al. Oxygen limitation contributes to antibiotic tolerance of Pseudomonas aeruginosa in biofilms. Antimicrob Agents Chemother 2004;48:2659–64.

[13] Fux CA, Wilson S, Stoodley P. Detachment characteristics and oxacillin resistance of Staphylococcus aureus biofilm emboli in an in vitro catheter infection model. J Bacteriol 2004;186:4486–91.
[14] Mah TF, Pitts B, Pellock B, et al. A genetic basis for Pseudomonas aeruginosa biofilm antibiotic resistance. Nature 2003;426:306–10.
[15] Dankert J, Hogt AH, Feijen J. Biomedical polymers: bacterial adhesion, colonization and infection. CRC Crit Rev Biochem 1986;2:219–301.
[16] Moore RM, Schneider RK, Kowalski J, et al. Antimicrobial susceptibility of bacterial isolates from 233 horses with musculoskeletal infection during 1979–1989. Equine Vet J 1992; 24:450–6.
[17] Snyder JR, Pascoe JR, Hirsh DC. Antimicrobial susceptibility of microorganisms isolated from equine orthopedic patients. Vet Surg 1987;16:197–201.
[18] Wegener WA, Alavi A. Diagnostic imaging of musculoskeletal infection.Roentgenography; gallium, indium-labeled white blood cell, gammaglobulin, bone scintigraphy; and MRI. Orthop Clin North Am 1991;22:401–18.
[19] Schauwecker DS, Braunstein EM, Wheat LJ. Diagnostic imaging of osteomyelitis. Infect Dis Clin North Am 1990;4:441–63.
[20] Creutzig H. Bone imaging after total replacement arthroplasty. Eur J Nucl Med 1976;1:177–80.
[21] Gayle JM, Redding WR, Vacek JR, et al. Diagnosis and surgical treatment of periapical infection of the third mandibular molar in five horses. J Am Vet Med Assoc 1999;215: 829–32.
[22] Oyen WJ, Corstens FH. Scintigraphic techniques for delineation of infection and inflammation. Br J Hosp Med 1995;54:75–80.
[23] Ruther W, Hotze A, Moller F, et al. Diagnosis of bone and joint infection by leucocyte scintigraphy. A comparative study with 99mTc-HMPAO-labelled leucocytes, 99mTc-labelled antigranulocyte antibodies and 99mTc-labelled nanocolloid. Arch Orthop Trauma Surg 1990;110:26–32.
[24] Southwood LL, Kawcak CE, McIlwraith CW, et al. Use of scintigraphy for assessment of fracture healing and early diagnosis of osteomyelitis following fracture repair in rabbits. Am J Vet Res 2003;64:736–45.
[25] Cleveland KB. General principles of infection. In: Canale ST, editor. Operative orthopaedics. Philadelphia: Mosby; 2005. p. 643–59.
[26] Reef V, Reimer J, Reid CF. Ultrasonographic findings in horses with osteomyelitis. In: Blake-Caddel L, editor. Proceedings of the 37th Annual Convention of the American Association of Equine Practitioners. San Francisco (CA); 1991. p. 381–91.
[27] Nguyen TM, Gauthier DW, Myles TD, et al. Detection of group B streptococcus: comparison of an optical immunoassay with direct plating and broth-enhanced culture methods. J Matern Fetal Med 1998;7:172–6.
[28] del Rio ML, Gutierrez B, Gutierrez CB, et al. Evaluation of survival of Actinobacillus pleuropneumoniae and Haemophilus parasuis in four liquid media and two swab specimen transport systems. Am J Vet Res 2003;64:1176–80.
[29] Elsayed S, Gregson DB, Church DL. Comparison of direct selective versus nonselective agar media plus LIM broth enrichment for determination of group B streptococcus colonization status in pregnant women. Arch Pathol Lab Med 2003;127:718–20.
[30] Bertone AL. Update on infectious arthritis in horses. Equine Vet Educ 1999;11:143–52.
[31] Meijer MC, van Weeren PR, Rijkenhuizen AB. Clinical experiences of treating septic arthritis in the equine by repeated joint lavage: a series of 39 cases. J Vet Med A Physiol Pathol Clin Med 2000;47:351–65.
[32] Southwood LL, Frisbie DD, Kawcak CE, et al. Evaluation of serum biochemical markers of bone metabolism for early diagnosis of nonunion and infected nonunion fractures in rabbits. Am J Vet Res 2003;64:727–35.
[33] Ohishi T, Takahashi M, Kushida K, et al. Changes of biochemical markers during fracture healing. Arch Orthop Trauma Surg 1998;118:126–30.

[34] Ingle BM, Hay SM, Bottjer HM, et al. Changes in bone mass and bone turnover following distal forearm fracture. Osteoporos Int 1999;10:399–407.
[35] Raekallio J, Makinen PL. Alkaline and acid phosphatase activity in the initial phase of fracture healing. Acta Pathol Microbiol Scand 1969;75:415–22.
[36] Volpin G, Rees JA, Ali SY, et al. Distribution of alkaline phosphatase activity in experimentally produced callus in rats. J Bone Joint Surg Br 1986;68:629–34.
[37] Mariani BD, Martin DS, Levine MJ, et al. The Coventry Award. Polymerase chain reaction detection of bacterial infection in total knee arthroplasty. Clin Orthop 1996;331:11–22.
[38] Trampuz A, Osmon DR, Hanssen AD, et al. Molecular and antibiofilm approaches to prosthetic joint infection. Clin Orthop 2003;414:69–88.
[39] Dernell WS. Treatment of severe orthopedic infections. Vet Clin North Am Small Anim Pract 1999;29:1261–74.
[40] Godber LM, Walker RD, Stein GE, et al. Pharmacokinetics, nephrotoxicosis, and in vitro antibacterial activity associated with single versus multiple (three times) daily gentamicin treatments in horses. Am J Vet Res 1995;56:613–8.
[41] Ross MW, Orsini JA, Richardson DW, et al. Closed suction drainage in the treatment of infectious arthritis of the equine tarsocrural joint. Vet Surg 1991;20:21–9.
[42] Bertone AL, Davis M, Cox HU, et al. Arthrotomy versus arthroscopy and partial synovectomy for treatment of experimentally induced infectious arthritis in horses. Am J Vet Res 1992;53:585–91.
[43] Klemm KW. Antibiotic bead chains. Clin Orthop 1993;295:63–76.
[44] Dipiro JT, Bivins BA, Record KE, et al. The prophylactic use of antimicrobials in surgery. Curr Probl Surg 1983;20:69–132.
[45] Kahn DS, Pritzker KP. The pathophysiology of bone infection. Clin Orthop 1973;96:12–9.
[46] Bassett CA. Clinical implications of cell function in bone grafting. Clin Orthop 1972;87:49–59.
[47] Bonfiglio M, Jeter WS. Immunological responses to bone. Clin Orthop 1972;87:19–27.
[48] Gray JC, Elves MW. Early osteogenesis in compact bone isografts: a quantitative study of contributions of the different graft cells. Calcif Tissue Int 1979;29:225–37.
[49] Goldberg VM, Stevenson S. Bone transplantation. In: Evarts CM, editor. Surgery of the musculoskeletal system. New York: Churchhill Livingstone; 1989. p. 54–81.
[50] Urist MR. Bone: formation by autoinduction. Science 1965;150:893–9.
[51] Markel MD. Bone grafts and bone substitutes. In: Nixon A, editor. Equine fracture repair. Philadelphia: WB Saunders; 1996. p. 87–92.
[52] McDuffee LA, Anderson GI. In vitro comparison of equine cancellous bone graft donor sites and tibial periosteum as sources of viable osteoprogenitors. Vet Surg 2003;32:455–63.
[53] Harriss FK, Galuppo LD, Decock HE, et al. Evaluation of a technique for collection of cancellous bone graft from the proximal humerus in horses. Vet Surg 2004;33:293–300.
[54] Tobias KM, Schneider RK, Besser TE. Use of antimicrobial-impregnated polymethyl methacrylate. J Am Vet Med Assoc 1996;208:841–5.
[55] Holcombe SJ, Schneider RK, Bramlage LR, et al. Lag screw fixation of noncomminuted sagittal fractures of the proximal phalanx in racehorses: 59 cases(1973–1991). J Am Vet Med Assoc 1995;206:1195–9.
[56] Swinebroad EL, Dabareiner RM, Swor TM, et al. Osteomyelitis secondary to trauma involving the proximal end of the radius in horses: five cases(1987–2001). J Am Vet Med Assoc 2003;223:486–91.
[57] Schneider RK, Andrea R, Barnes HG. Use of antibiotic-impregnated polymethyl methacrylate for treatment of an open radial fracture in a horse. J Am Vet Med Assoc 1995;207:1454–7.
[58] Olmstead ML, Hohn RB, Turner TM. A five-year study of 221 total hip replacements in the dog. J Am Vet Med Assoc 1983;183:191–4.
[59] Trippel SB. Antibiotic-impregnated cement in total joint arthroplasty. J Bone Joint Surg Am 1986;68:1297–302.

[60] Calhoun JH, Mader JT. Antibiotic beads in the management of surgical infections. Am J Surg 1989;157:443–9.
[61] Buchholz HW, Elson RA, Heinert K. Antibiotic-loaded acrylic cement: current concepts. Clin Orthop 1984;190:96–108.
[62] Eckman JBJ, Henry SL, Mangino PD, et al. Wound and serum levels of tobramycin with the prophylactic use of tobramycin-impregnated polymethylmethacrylate beads in compound fractures. Clin Orthop 1988;237:213–5.
[63] Wahlig H, Dingeldein E, Bergmann R, et al. The release of gentamicin from polymethylmethacrylate beads. An experimental and pharmacokinetic study. J Bone Joint Surg Br 1978;60:270–5.
[64] Wininger DA, Fass RJ. Antibiotic-impregnated cement and beads for orthopedic infections. Antimicrob Agents Chemother 1996;40:2675–9.
[65] Henry SL, Seligson D, Mangino P, et al. Antibiotic-impregnated beads. Part I: bead implantation versus systemic therapy. Orthop Rev 1991;20:242–7.
[66] Adams K, Couch L, Cierny G, et al. In vitro and in vivo evaluation of antibiotic diffusion from antibiotic-impregnated polymethylmethacrylate beads. Clin Orthop 1992;278:244–52.
[67] Fish DN, Hoffman HM, Danziger LH. Antibiotic-impregnated cement use in US hospitals. Am J Hosp Pharm 1992;49:2469–74.
[68] Popham GJ, Mangino P, Seligson D, et al. Antibiotic-impregnated beads. Part II: factors in antibiotic selection. Orthop Rev 1991;20:331–7.
[69] DiMaio FR, O'Halloran JJ, Quale JM. In vitro elution of ciprofloxacin from polymethylmethacrylate cement beads. J Orthop Res 1994;12:79–82.
[70] Bowyer GW, Cumberland N. Antibiotic release from impregnated pellets and beads. J Trauma 1994;36:331–5.
[71] Wininger DA, Fass RJ. Antibiotic-impregnated cement and beads for orthopedic infections. Antimicrob Agents Chemother 1996;40:2675–9.
[72] Downes S. Methods for improving drug release from poly(methyl)methacrylate bone cement. Clin Mater 1991;7:227–31.
[73] Wilson KJ, Cierny G, Adams KR, et al. Comparative evaluation of the diffusion of tobramycin and cefotaxime out of antibiotic-impregnated polymethylmethacrylate beads. J Orthop Res 1988;6:279–86.
[74] Flick AB, Herbert JC, Goodell J, et al. Noncommercial fabrication of antibiotic-impregnated polymethylmethacrylate beads. Technical note. Clin Orthop 1987;223:282–6.
[75] Farnsworth KD, White NA, Robertson J. The effect of implanting gentamicin-impregnated polymethylmethacrylate beads in the tarsocrural joint of the horse. Vet Surg 2001;30:126–31.
[76] Turner TM, Urban RM, Gitelis S, et al. Radiographic and histologic assessment of calcium sulfate in experimental animal models and clinical use as a resorbable bone-graft substitute, a bone-graft expander, and a method for local antibiotic delivery. One institution's experience. J Bone Joint Surg Am 1903;83:8–18.
[77] Santschi EM, McGarvey L. In vitro elution of gentamicin from plaster of Paris beads. Vet Surg 2003;32:128–33.
[78] Mackey D, Varlet A, Debeaumont D. Antibiotic loaded plaster of Paris pellets: an in vitro study of a possible method of local antibiotic therapy in bone infection. Clin Orthop 1982;167:263–8.
[79] Dahners LE, Funderburk CH. Gentamicin-loaded plaster of Paris as a treatment of experimental osteomyelitis in rabbits. Clin Orthop 1987;219:278–82.
[80] Dacquet V, Varlet A, Tandogan RN, et al. Antibiotic-impregnated plaster of Paris beads. Trials with teicoplanin. Clin Orthop 1992;282:241–9.
[81] Cook VL, Bertone AL, Kowalski JJ, et al. Biodegradable drug delivery systems for gentamicin release and treatment of synovial membrane infection. Vet Surg 1999;28:233–41.
[82] Artzi Z, Givol N, Rohrer MD, et al. Qualitative and quantitative expression of bovine bone mineral in experimental bone defects. Part 2: morphometric analysis. J Periodontol 2003;74:1153–60.

[83] Poynton AR, Zheng F, Tomin E, et al. Resorbable posterolateral graft containment in a rabbit spinal fusion model. J Neurosurg 2002;97:460 3.
[84] Houser BE, Mellonig JT, Brunsvold MA, et al. Clinical evaluation of anorganic bovine bone xenograft with a bioabsorbable collagen barrier in the treatment of molar furcation defects. Int J Periodontics Restorative Dent 2001;21:161–9.
[85] da Costa F, Taga R, Taga EM. Rabbit bone marrow response to bovine osteoinductive proteins and anorganic bovine bone. Int J Oral Maxillofac Implants 2001;16:799–808.
[86] Ethell MT, Bennett RA, Brown MP, et al. In vitro elution of gentamicin, amikacin, and ceftiofur from polymethylmethacrylate and hydroxyapatite cement. Vet Surg 2000;29:375–82.
[87] Sanchez E, Baro M, Soriano I, et al. In vivo-in vitro study of biodegradable and osteointegrable gentamicin bone implants. Eur J Pharm Biopharm 2001;52:151–8.
[88] Whitehair KJ, Bowersock TL, Fessler JF, et al. Regional limb perfusion for antibiotic treatment of experimentally induced septic arthritis. Vet Surg 1992;21:367–73.
[89] Whitehair KJ, Adams SB, Parker JE, et al. Regional limb perfusion with antibiotics in three horses. Vet Surg 1992;21:286–92.
[90] Whitehair KJ, Blevins WE, Fessler JF, et al. Regional perfusion of the equine carpus for antibiotic delivery. Vet Surg 1992;21:279–85.
[91] Palmer SE, Hogan PM. How to perform regional limb perfusion in the standing horse. In: Proceedings of the 45th Annual American Association of Equine Practitioners Convention, Albuquerque, NM. American Association of Equine Practitioners; 1999. p. 124–7.
[92] Santschi EM, Adams SB, Murphey ED. How to perform equine intravenous digital perfusion. In: Proceedings of the 44th Annual American Association of Equine Practitioners Convention, Baltimore (MD): American Association of Equine Practitioners; 1998. p. 198–201.
[93] Murphey ED, Santschi EM, Papich MG. Regional intravenous perfusion of the distal limb of horses with amikacin sulfate. J Vet Pharmacol Ther 1999;22:68–71.
[94] Schaadt J, Crowley R, Miller D, et al. Isolated limb perfusion: a literature review. J Extra Corpor Technol 2002;34:130–43.
[95] Scheuch BC, Van Hoogmoed LM, Wilson WD, et al. Comparison of intraosseous or intravenous infusion for delivery of amikacin sulfate to the tibiotarsal joint of horses. Am J Vet Res 2002;63:374–80.
[96] Olson ME, Ceri H, Morck DW, et al. Biofilm bacteria: formation and comparative susceptibility to antibiotics. Can J Vet Res 2002;66:86–92.
[97] Anwar H, Strap JL, Costerton JW. Kinetic interaction of biofilm cells of Staphylococcus aureus with cephalexin and tobramycin in a chemostat system. Antimicrob Agents Chemother 1992;36:890–3.
[98] Mattson SE, Pearce SG, Boure LP, et al. Comparison of intraosseous and intravenous infusion of technetium Tc 99m pertechnate in the distal portion of forelimbs in standing horses by use of scintigraphic imaging. Am J Vet Res 2005;66:1267–72.
[99] Butt TD, Bailey JV, Dowling PM, et al. Comparison of 2 techniques for regional antibiotic delivery to the equine forelimb: intraosseous perfusion vs. intravenous perfusion. Can Vet J 2001;42:617–22.
[100] Parra A, Lugo J, Boothe D, et al. Pharmacokinetics of enrofloxacin and amikacin after intravenous regional perfusion of the distal limb. In: Proceedings of the American College of Veterinary Surgeons; 2005 [available as CDROM].
[101] Gagnon H, Ferguson JG, Papich MG, et al. Single-dose pharmacokinetics of cefazolin in bovine synovial fluid after intravenous regional injection. J Vet Pharmacol Ther 1994;17:31–7.
[102] Werner LA, Hardy J, Bertone AL. Bone gentamicin concentration after intra-articular injection or regional intravenous perfusion in the horse. Vet Surg 2003;32:559–65.

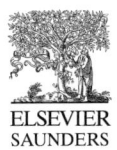

VETERINARY
CLINICS
Equine Practice

Infections in the Equine Abdomen and Pelvis: Perirectal Abscesses, Umbilical Infections, and Peritonitis

Yvonne A. Elce, DVM

College of Veterinary Medicine, North Carolina State University, 4700 Hillsborough Street, Raleigh, NC 27606, USA

Infections of the abdomen and pelvis can pose a diagnostic and therapeutic challenge to equine clinicians. Often, treatment is expensive and prolonged. The continued development of diagnostic and therapeutic modalities as well as indices to predict prognosis accurately is important in the overall management of these cases. The purpose of this article is to outline briefly the latest diagnostics and treatments available for several common infections in the abdomen. Perirectal abscesses, umbilical infections, and peritonitis, particularly focal peritonitis, are discussed [1]. These conditions are not uncommon, and their management has not been addressed in detail in the recent literature. As with many infections, surgical drainage or removal and appropriate medical therapy are crucial to successful resolution. In the current climate of antimicrobial resistance, early detection and local treatment are becoming more important and appropriate for many local infections.

Perirectal abscesses

Perirectal abscesses have been reported in all types of equids: horses and miniature horses, male and female horses, and horses of various ages [2–6].

Pathophysiology

The etiology of perirectal abscesses is often unknown. Some etiologies are obvious, such as after repair of rectal tears or rectovaginal fistulas, postfoaling trauma, lymph node abscessation, or gravitation of an abscess from the gluteal muscles after an intramuscular injection [2,3,7]. Other causes are

E-mail address: yvonne_elce@ncsu.edu

more speculative. Perirectal abscess formation after presumed migration of an abscess after an intramuscular injection was reported in two horses and in one horse after mucosal trauma incurred during dystocia [2]. There are two reports of a perirectal abscess occurring after a rectal tear repair [6,7]. Anorectal lymphadenopathy leading to abscess formation occurred in three young horses [3]. These three horses were all less than 15 months of age, and the authors speculated that the young age correlated to a naive immune system [3]. This was presumed to render the horses susceptible to common pyogenic bacteria forming abscesses in lymph nodes from local or hematogenous spread [3]. The cause is unknown in many cases, with no history of trauma, intramuscular injection, or rectal palpation [4,5]. Theories for the formation of perirectal abscesses in these horses include mounting or trauma from other horses, rectal inflammation (subsequent to diarrhea), or iatrogenic trauma from thermometers or rectal punctures seeding the perirectal tissues with bacteria [4].

Perirectal abscessation is common in people and is described as one of the most commonly encountered conditions in general surgery [8]. In human patients, perirectal abscesses are reported after impaction of colonic diverticula that become inflamed [5]. There is usually an underlying cause in people, such as neoplasia, immune deficiency, diabetes, surgery, trauma, or steroid therapy [9].

Diagnosis

Horses with perirectal abscesses are often presented with signs of abdominal pain. Other common presenting signs include pyrexia, anorexia, depression, dyschezia, reduced fecal output or rectal impaction, and tenesmus. Two horses presented with visible swelling dorsal to the anus (Fig. 1) [4,5], and one horse had dysuria, presumably from neuritis associated with regional inflammation [3]. Diagnosis is confirmed with physical examination, rectal palpation, ultrasound, and fine needle aspiration. Rectal palpation confirms the presence and location of a mass causing an extraluminal obstruction. The masses tend to be firm and oval with occasional soft areas, and they can be located a variable distance from the rectum. The mass was located dorsal to the rectum in nine horses and lateral in three horses [2–5]. The presence of mucopurulent material on the feces or rectal sleeve of the clinician indicates a communication with the rectum [3].

The differential diagnoses for a perirectal mass include neoplasia, lymphadenopathy, hematoma, and abscess. Ultrasound is indicated to aid in determining the extent of the abscess and to monitor progress during treatment. A fine needle aspirate obtained percutaneously or transrectally should be performed to determine the cause of the mass. The risk of introducing bacteria into the mass is greater when aspiration is performed transrectally [3]. A percutaneous approach is recommended because this decreases the risk of iatrogenic infection and obtains a more reliable sample for culture [3].

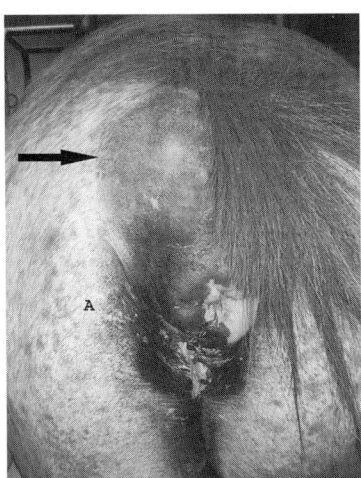

Fig. 1. Large perirectal mass (*arrow*) with visible swelling dorsal to the rectum externally. A, external anal sphincter.

A percutaneous approach can be performed after sterile preparation of the perineal region and insertion of a needle of appropriate length. Larger gauge needles (14–18 gauge) may aid in aspiration of thick purulent material. If a percutaneous approach is not practical, inserting a 14- to 18-gauge needle guarded in the palm of the hand into the rectum and then into the abscess can be readily performed. Attaching the needle to an extension set and syringe facilitates aspiration. Use of ultrasound to guide needle aspiration is recommended for deep masses to ensure penetration of the needle into the mass. The fine needle aspirate obtained this way should be submitted for cytologic examination as well as culture and sensitivity testing. Bacteria that have been isolated from perirectal abscesses include *Streptococcus zooepidemicus* and *Escherichia coli* [2,3]. In human patients, polymicrobial infections of aerobic and anaerobic bacteria are common, with anaerobic bacteria being isolated more often [9]. The most frequently isolated organisms in human patients are those originating from the skin (*Staphylococcus aureus* and *Streptococcus* spp) or gastrointestinal tract (*Bacteroides fragilis* and *E coli*) [9]. With increasing bacterial resistance, obtaining and submitting fluid for culture and sensitivity testing of aerobic and anaerobic bacteria is important for optimal treatment and prevention of unnecessary antimicrobial use.

If ultrasound and palpation are indicative of extension into the abdomen, an abdominocentesis is indicated to determine the presence and degree of any abdominal inflammation and infection [2,10]. Most cases are caudal to the peritoneal reflection at the pelvic inlet, and involvement of the peritoneal cavity is uncommon. The results of hematology and serum biochemistry may be normal or may reflect the presence of infection with leukocytosis and hyperfibrinogenemia [3].

Treatment

Treatment includes management of the abscess and facilitating defecation and urination. Feeding a fecal softening diet of feeds with high water content, fresh grass, or pellets and administration of mineral oil via a nasogastric tube can be used to help the passage of fecal material through the partially occluded rectum [3]. Initially, feces may need to be manually evacuated; in some instances, gentle gravity-flow lubricant enemas may be required to relieve the rectal impaction oral to the abscess. The administration of analgesics and anti-inflammatory drugs is recommended to control discomfort and reduce the inflammation associated with the abscess. Administration of intravenous balanced electrolyte solutions may be required if the horse is not maintaining adequate hydration.

Guidelines for systemic antimicrobial use have not been established for equine perirectal abscesses. The abscess environment impairs the function of many antimicrobial drugs. The abscess capsule prevents antimicrobial penetration, the acidic pH alters some antimicrobial function, and protein binding or enzymes can inactivate antimicrobials [9]. Adequate local treatment of the abscess when there is no peritoneal involvement may negate the need for systemic antimicrobials [2]. The administration of systemic antimicrobials may be indicated in select cases, such as anorectal lymphadenopathy, if the horse is febrile so as to combat the presumed bacterial stimulus and bacteremia, as well as for those cases in which the abscess is close to or involving the peritoneum [2,3]. Most horses in the reported literature were treated with antimicrobials consisting of various combinations of trimethoprim-sulfa, ampicillin, penicillin, and rifampin [2–5]. Antimicrobial therapy should be based on culture and sensitivity test results when this information is available and on the most commonly isolated bacteria when test results are unavailable (*Streptococcus* spp and *E coli*).

The definitive treatment for perirectal abscessation is surgical drainage [8–11]. Abscess drainage is the treatment of choice for human patients and is commonly performed using ultrasound guidance [8–11]. Medical management alone, however, has been used successfully in foals with lymphadenopathy [3]. Inadequate drainage is the leading cause of abscess recurrence and treatment failure in human patients [8]. Perirectal abscesses can be drained in a variety of ways depending on their location. The abscess is drained into the rectum for dorsally located abscesses, into the vagina in mares with ventral abscesses, or ventral to the anus in male horses with ventral abscesses (Fig. 2). Abscesses located lateral to the rectum may be drained into the rectum or lateral to the anus [2,11]. Surgical drainage can be readily accomplished in the standing horse using sedation and combinations of local and epidural anesthesia. Topical lidocaine can be used on the rectal mucosa if the abscess is being drained into the rectum. A guarded number 10 blade can then be introduced into the rectum in the hand of a surgeon and used to create a drainage hole from the abscess into the rectum. If

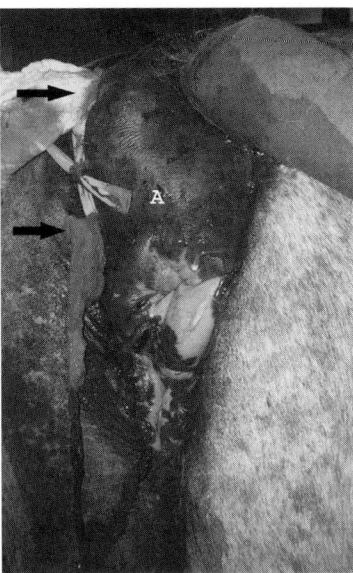

Fig. 2. Drainage of the perirectal abscess through the perineum rather than into the rectum. Gauze packing (*arrows*) and a Penrose drain (A) exit the mass at the most ventral aspect to ensure complete drainage.

the abscess is being drained perineally, a local line block using 2% lidocaine or epidural anesthesia can be used. Again, a number 10 scalpel blade can be used to create one or multiple drainage holes through the skin, subcutaneous tissues, and abscess capsule (depending on the size of the abscess). Creating a drainage hole at the most ventral aspect of the abscess is recommended for complete drainage (see Fig. 2). There are several large vessels lateral to the rectum, and ultrasound guidance is recommended when operating in this area. If the abscess involves the peritoneal cavity, general anesthesia with lavage and exploration of the abdomen are warranted as well as drainage of the abscess. A Foley catheter may be placed within the abscess rectally or perineally to facilitate drainage and lavage of deep abscesses.

The drainage site is then managed to prevent early apposition of the skin or mucosal edges before abscess resolution with daily lavage of the abscess and cleaning of the surrounding skin or mucosa. Petrolatum jelly may be placed on the skin ventral to the drainage to prevent scalding in cases that have been drained percutaneously.

Prognosis and complications

The prognosis for horses with perirectal abscesses has been excellent with adequate surgical drainage. Surgical drainage and medical treatment have been successful in 12 (92%) of 13 reported cases [2–5]. The prognosis is reportedly poor (1 [50%] of 2 cases) for successful resolution when the abscess involves the peritoneum; however, this has only been reported in 2 horses [2]. The most common complication is recurrence of the abscess because of inadequate surgical drainage [8]. Other complications include rectal stricture if the submucosa of the rectum is damaged, hemorrhage, extension into the abdomen, and complications associated with bacteremia (eg, laminitis, endocarditis).

Umbilical remnant infections

Umbilical remnant infections in foals are commonly encountered in equine practice. The umbilical cord divides at birth. It is composed of the amniotic sheath, the umbilical vein, two umbilical arteries, and the urachus (Fig. 3). It is not uncommon for more than one structure to become infected, with the arteries and urachus affected most frequently (omphaloarteritis) [12]. Infection of the umbilical remnants can be successfully diagnosed and treated. If left undiagnosed or treated inappropriately, however, an infected umbilicus can lead to potentially fatal complications by seeding bacteria to other parts of the body. Umbilical remnant infection has been linked to the development of infected joints, hernias, patent urachus, sepsis, meningitis, liver abscesses, peritonitis, and intra-abdominal adhesions [12–14].

Pathophysiology

The division of the cord at birth and subsequent time until complete atrophy and loss of the external remnant create an avenue for bacteria to enter the foal. Care of the umbilical remnant and the environment in

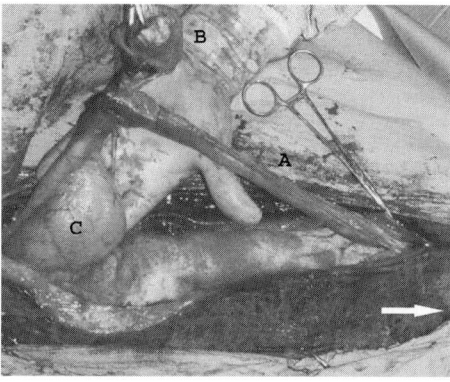

Fig. 3. Umbilical remnant structures. The arrow points toward the head of the foal. A, umbilical vein; B, external remnant; C, bladder with urachal attachment to B and the two umbilical arteries.

which the foal lives are important in reducing the risk of infection. Other important factors in the development of infection include adequate passive transfer of immunity postpartum and intrauterine infection prepartum [12]. There is extensive literature on the appropriate care of the umbilical cord of human infants and the relation of that care to the development of umbilical remnant infection and associated septic complications. In developed countries, where standards of hygiene are good, there is little advantage of topical antimicrobial or disinfectant application over simple daily cleaning and drying of the cord [15–19]. There are a few reports, however, of reduced colonization of the cord by bacteria when topical antiseptics or antimicrobials are used [18,19]. In developing countries, umbilical cord infections constitute a major cause of neonatal morbidity and mortality, and this may be related to a decreased ability to keep the cord clean compared with that in developed countries [15,17]. By extrapolation from human infant care, improving the daily cleaning of the remnant and the environment of the foal would result in a decreased rate of clinically significant umbilical infections. Recommendations include daily cleaning and inspection of the umbilical remnant and avoiding harsh cauterants, such as 7% iodine, because these may be detrimental to healthy tissue [12]. Dilute povidone-iodine solutions or dilute 4% chlorhexidine solutions can be used for daily cleaning [12,19]. The use of gloves when handling and cleaning the umbilicus reduces the transfer and colonization of the umbilicus by common skin organisms, such as *Staphylococcus* spp and *Streptococcus* spp.

Umbilical remnant infection predisposes a foal to a variety of diseases. Umbilical remnant infection should always be considered in a foal with a patent urachus. Localized inflammation and necrosis in the arteries or veins can result in the urachus losing its seal, and infection within the urachus itself can result in an acquired patent urachus [12]. A congenital patent urachus can act as an opening for bacterial invasion. Inflammation and necrosis of the umbilical remnant have been shown in calves to increase the risk of hernia formation by 82%. It is thought that infection and inflammation weaken the body wall and delay closure of the umbilical ring [20]. Localized inflammation around the umbilical remnant inside the abdomen in foals has been linked to the development of abdominal adhesions [21]. Infection in the umbilical vein can lead to hepatic abscessation, and hematogenous spread of bacteria accounts for the other complications seen with infected umbilical remnants (eg, septic arthritis, meningitis) [12]. Suspicion of umbilical remnant infection should exist in any foal with signs of bacteremia or sepsis from an unknown source. It is important to remember that umbilical infection can be present without obvious abnormalities of the external remnant (Fig. 4). Bacteria that have been cultured from umbilical remnant infections include *E coli*, *Streptococcus* spp, *Salmonella* spp, *Staphylococcus* spp, *Klebsiella* spp, *Actinobacillus* spp, and *Clostridium perfringens* [12–14, 22,23].

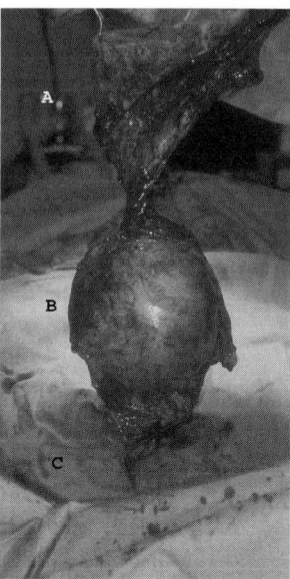

Fig. 4. Normal umbilical remnant externally (A) with a large internal abdominal abscess (B). The abscess originated from the umbilicus, but the original source of the infection (urachus versus umbilical arteries) was no longer evident at the time of surgery. C, abdominal wall.

Diagnosis

There is a large body of human literature devoted to early detection of infection in the neonate through sampling of umbilical cord blood and examination of the placenta [24–30]. These tests may prove most useful in foals that are at high risk (preterm), have failure of passive transfer of immunity, or are born to high-risk mares in a hospital environment. Early diagnosis and treatment of bacterial invasion before the onset of clinical signs has improved patient outcome in human infants. Tests that have shown promise in predicting neonatal umbilical remnant infection and sepsis are leukocyte invasion of the placenta, high concentrations of cytokines (interleukin-6, interleukin-8, C-reactive protein, and procalcitonin), and an abnormal complete blood cell count in umbilical cord blood [24–30]. Umbilical cord blood is easy to sample, and the previously mentioned tests have strong associations with the development of umbilical remnant infection and sepsis [24–30]. Interleukin-6, interleukin-8, and C-reactive protein concentrations in umbilical cord blood have all been shown to be strongly predictive of early neonatal sepsis and are increased before the development of clinical signs [25,28,29]. The interleukins have a shorter half-life, and their concentration decreases, giving false-negative results if sampled 12 to 24 hours after the onset of inflammation [29]. Obtaining a positive blood culture from umbilical cord blood is also predictive of sepsis [29]. The value of these tests should be investigated to aid early diagnosis and treatment of sepsis and infection, particularly in high-risk foals.

Early diagnosis and early aggressive treatment are crucial to avoiding complications. Physical examination and palpation of the external remnant are important. Ultrasound of the internal structures of the umbilicus is necessary to detect infection that may not be palpable externally (see Fig. 4). Any foal with fever, septic joints, or evidence of bacteremia or sepsis should have a careful ultrasound examination of the umbilicus. Ultrasound parameters of normal and abnormal umbilical remnants have been established [31,32]. The results of hematology and serum biochemistry may reflect the presence of infection with leukocytosis and hyperfibrinogenemia. Blood cultures should be performed. CT or MRI techniques are other modalities that could be used in the future if ultrasound findings are equivocal. The drawbacks would be the necessity for general anesthesia and the expense.

Treatment

There are two approaches for treatment of umbilical remnant infections: systemic antimicrobial therapy and surgical excision. Systemic broad-spectrum antimicrobial therapy is recommended to treat the infection and also to prevent the development of complications. Culture and sensitivity test results are obtained if possible. It has been the experience of many clinicians that mild infections can be successfully treated with antimicrobials alone and that the development of complications while on intravenous broad-spectrum antimicrobial therapy is low. Surgery is recommended if antimicrobial therapy alone has failed to resolve the infection [22]. Other clinicians, however, have reported improved survival rates after surgical excision compared with antimicrobial therapy alone (66.6% survival with excision, 42.9% survival without excision) [12]. Surgical excision of the infected umbilical remnant reduces the length of time that the foal requires treatment with antimicrobials. Surgery is indicated to remove the source of infection if complications are present, such as evidence of septicemia or joint infection [12]. If ultrasound evaluation reveals a discrete abscess in the umbilicus, surgery is also recommended because of the decreased ability of antimicrobials to penetrate abscesses effectively [9]. If the foal is otherwise healthy and ultrasound examination does not reveal a discrete abscess, medical management can be attempted with serial ultrasound, physical, hematologic, and serum biochemical assessments.

Surgical removal of umbilical remnants has been well described using a routine celiotomy and a laparoscopic approach [22,23,33,34]. Laparoscopy greatly reduces the length of the abdominal incision needed to remove infected remnants and is less invasive [22]. Laparoscopy reduces the risk of leaving inaccessible areas of the infected umbilical remnant in the abdomen [22]. Removal of deep infected remnants can be limited because of poor exposure with the routine celiotomy approach. The decreased invasiveness of laparoscopy compared with a celiotomy approach should reduce the risk of abdominal adhesion formation [32]. Laparoscopy is technically more demanding, however, and may initially take longer to perform. Marsupialization of the umbilical vein has been described for foals and calves when infection within the vein extends to and involves the liver so as to provide drainage for the hepatic infection [35]. Incomplete removal of an infected umbilical vein and not providing drainage for hepatic abscesses have been associated with a high (50%) mortality rate in affected foals [32].

Prognosis and complications

The prognosis for foals with umbilical infections depends on the number and type of complications caused by the infected umbilicus [12,13,32]. Antimicrobial resolution of mild infection carries a good prognosis. Surgical removal of an uncomplicated infected umbilical remnant carries a small risk of anesthetic and incisional complications. Combining the results from four reports in the literature, 10 (91%) of 11 (laparoscopy) and 45 (86.5%) of 52 (routine celiotomy) foals undergoing surgical removal of the umbilical remnant survived, and 10 (59%) of 17 foals treated with medical therapy only survived [12,22,32,33]. It is worth noting that 2 of 4 foals died after surgical excision of an umbilical remnant, with extensive infection of the umbilical vein extending into the hepatic parenchyma on ultrasound [32]. These umbilical veins were not marsupialized or removed laparoscopically; thus, complete removal or drainage of the infection was likely not accomplished [32]. The prognosis for simple infections is thus good with surgical removal, and the prognosis declines with the type and severity of complications associated with umbilical remnant infection, such as septic joints, meningitis, and intra-abdominal adhesions or peritonitis.

Peritonitis

Peritonitis, or inflammation of the peritoneum, can occur in horses of any age or breed. There are many known causes, most of which are secondary to gastrointestinal disease, hematogenous spread from an upper respiratory tract bacterial infection in younger horses (*Streptococcus* spp and *Rhodococcus* spp), or idiopathic in origin, such as many infections caused by *Actinobacillus* spp.

Abdominal abscesses

Pathophysiology

Abdominal abscesses in horses and foals have been found in a variety of locations with a variety of causes. Ulceration or compromised viability of the gastrointestinal tract, perforation of the gastrointestinal tract by worms or foreign bodies, and hematogenous spread to mesenteric lymphatics from respiratory pathogens, particularly *Streptococcus equi* subsp *equi*, are well-known causes [36–41]. In many cases, however, the originating cause of the abscess is unknown [42–44]. It is hypothesized that abscesses form as a result of a failure by the individual animal to develop adequate immunity to an organism to which it has been exposed, such as *S equi*, *S zooepidemicus*, or *Corynebacterium pseudotuberculosis* [43]. In one study of 25 horses with abdominal abscesses, all but 5 horses had a history of respiratory catarrh in the recent past and 3 had a history of subcutaneous abscesses [43]. Abscesses have been reported in association with the mesenteric lymph nodes, liver, kidney, spleen, uterus, bladder, gastrointestinal tract, and abdominal wall as well as with or without adhesions to multiple structures [36,42]. Bacteria that have been cultured include *Streptococcus* spp, *Rhodococcus* spp, *Corynebacterium* spp, *Clostridium* spp, *Bacteroides* spp, and *E coli*.

Diagnosis

Diagnosis of intra-abdominal abscesses in the horse can be challenging. Horses are often presented with a history of colic, fever, weight loss, depression, and anorexia and may have a history of a cough or subcutaneous abscesses. A history of *S equi* infection or *Rhodococcus equi* exposure in younger horses should heighten suspicion of an intra-abdominal abscess, and appropriate ELISAs and titers can be performed [40]. In one study, 63.3% of horses with internal *C pseudotuberculosis* abscesses had a history or presence of external abscesses [36]. Serum synergistic hemolysin inhibition titers were greater than 1:512 in 96.4% of horses with internal *C pseudotuberculosis* abscesses [36]. Horses with neoplasia may have a similar history and clinical signs and present a diagnostic dilemma of some importance [42]. Hematology and serum biochemistry results can be nonspecific in cases of neoplasia with indications of infection, such as leukocytosis, neutrophilia, or hyperfibrinogenemia. Peritoneal fluid analysis was useful in identifying neoplasia on cytology in 11 of 25 horses. In comparing abscesses and neoplasia, however, peritoneal fluid cytology was only diagnostic of an abscess in 3 of 15 horses [42,43]. Peritoneal fluid from horses with abdominal neoplasia is also often classified as an exudate. Peritoneal lavage greatly enhances the diagnostic accuracy of peritoneal fluid analysis in human and canine patients (from 47% to 96%); however, this may not be practical in the horse [42]. Investigations into the use of small volumes of peritoneal lavage and the subsequent enhanced diagnostic accuracy are warranted in the horse. Serial abdominocentesis may improve the chance of obtaining a diagnosis. Intracellular or free bacteria in the abdominal fluid would be indicative of an internal abscess; however, culture of peritoneal fluid is rarely productive (0 of 14 cases had a positive culture in one report) but should be performed [43]. Rectal palpation may be used to confirm the presence of a mass but not the type of mass. Ultrasound examination, externally and rectally, of the abdomen can detect those abscesses close to the body wall or rectum.

Nuclear scintigraphy is used in people to search for the cause of fever of unknown origin and to track the progression of an infection in a patient undergoing treatment. Radiolabeled autologous leukocytes have been used in horses to locate sites of infections [45]. This technique has limitations, however. The labeling process is labor-intensive and not always available. Leukocytes are fragile and may be destroyed during labeling or can disassociate from the radionuclide [46]. The most common radionuclides used for labeling leukocytes are ^{111}In-oxine and ^{99m}Tc-hexamethylpropyleneamine oxime (HMPAO). Most leukocytes labeled are neutrophils. Each radionuclide has a distinct normal distribution that must be taken into account during image interpretation [46]. ^{111}In is normally distributed to the liver, spleen, and bone marrow, and ^{99m}Tc is normally distributed to the urinary and gastrointestinal tract, making it an unattractive option for imaging abdominal abscesses in the horse. Clinical experience with use of ^{99m}Tc-HMPAO labeled leukocytes in horses has been positive when infections involve the musculoskeletal system but disappointing when used for investigation of nonorthopedic inflammation, with low numbers of positive scans [47]. ^{111}In-labeled leukocytes are imaged 24 hours after injection in people; in the horse, images can be seen starting at 22 hours after injection [45,46]. ^{99m}Tc-labeled leukocytes are imaged 2 to 4 hours after injection [46]. Because of the labor-intensive and problem-prone extracting, labeling, and injecting procedures associated with radiolabeled autologous leukocytes, alternatives are being developed involving a radiolabeled protein or molecule that binds to leukocytes in vivo. These include peptides and antigranulocytic/antibody fragments, which have been developed and are being used successfully in clinical trials in human patients [46]. Fanolesomab, for example, is an antigranulocytic antibody that is labeled with ^{99m}Tc-pertechnetate and binds to CD15 receptors on neutrophils after intravenous injection. This agent has a normal distribution limited to the vasculature and seems to be safe and nontoxic [46].

Another possibility that has great potential for veterinary medicine is that of radiolabeled antimicrobials. The advantage of radiolabeled antimicrobials is that they bind specifically to the bacteria, thus distinguishing between sterile and infected inflammation, which radiolabeled leukocytes do not. The use of radiolabeled ciprofloxacin for diagnosing and localizing infection has been reported in the literature [48,49]. Use of ^{99m}Tc-ciprofloxacin for detection of gastrointestinal and abdominal infections in human patients has a positive predictive value of 92%, negative predictive value of 77%, sensitivity of 79%, specificity of 91%, and accuracy of 84% [48]. This technique has also been used in people to monitor the progression of infection and to determine response to treatment [49]. Nuclear scintigraphy is a noninvasive technique that does not require anesthesia and is already used in many institutions and private equine practices. The main drawbacks include the necessity for handling radioactive material and special licensing. In addition to its use as a diagnostic tool, the use of scintigraphy to monitor the response to therapy is attractive to aid in accurate assessment of complete resolution.

A standing abdominal laparoscopy is increasingly popular as another more invasive technique that does not require general anesthesia and may be useful for finding abdominal abscesses, obtaining a culture or biopsy of a mass, and helping to determine the method of treatment. A standing laparoscopic examination of the dorsal abdomen, including the liver, spleen, and intestines, can be readily accomplished. Laparoscopic guidance can be used to aid in obtaining accurate samples for histopathologic examination or culture from intra-abdominal masses.

Treatment

Abdominal abscesses in the horse can be treated with long-term antimicrobials or surgery. Depending on the location and involvement of various abdominal structures, complete surgical excision, surgical drainage and lavage, marsupialization, or bypass of adhered or involved intestines is indicated [50–52]. In the case of intestinal adhesions, it is recommended that an intestinal bypass procedure be performed to limit complications [51]. Surgical resolution of an abscess results in a greatly shortened period of antimicrobial administration [53]. A short duration of antimicrobial use is desirable to limit deleterious side effects, such as diarrhea and the development of resistance. If drainage and lavage are performed or surgery is not an option, long-term antimicrobial therapy is required. Broad-spectrum antimicrobials should be used until a culture of the abscess can be obtained. An antimicrobial with activity against anaerobic bacteria should be considered, because anaerobic bacteria were isolated from 8 of 35 horses with peritonitis and abdominal abscesses [44]. Antimicrobial therapy should be discontinued only after serum fibrinogen concentration, blood leukocyte counts, ultrasound, nuclear scintigraphy, or laparoscopy has confirmed resolution of the infection.

Prognosis and complications

There are various case reports and retrospective studies in the literature that have reported on prognosis [36–44,51–53]. The severity of hyperfibrinogenemia was associated with outcome [43]. In horses with a fibrinogen concentration of greater than 800 mg/dL, 9 (60%) of 15 horses survived, and 8 (80%) of 10 horses with a fibrinogen concentration of less than 800 mg/dL survived [43]. Eight (32%) of 25 horses with intra-abdominal abscesses died or were euthanized [43]. The presence of anaerobic bacteria worsened the prognosis, with 4 (50%) of 8 horses with anaerobic bacteria surviving and

9 (60%) of 15 horses without anaerobic bacteria surviving [44]. The prognosis for complicated abdominal abscesses that involve multiple organs and intestinal adhesions is obviously less favorable than the prognosis for a simple abscess. The prognosis and potential for complications need to be determined on an individual level after diagnosis and assessment of the abscess and the inciting cause. In a retrospective study of horses with internal *C pseudotuberculosis* abscesses, 17 (71%) of 24 horses survived with long-term antimicrobials.

Diffuse peritonitis

New information from the human literature may be worth considering in cases of equine peritonitis. In the human literature, extensive ongoing research is looking at the peritoneal and blood concentrations of inflammatory cytokines and markers, such as activated protein C or procalcitonin, for use in prognosis and monitoring the response to treatment [54–56]. The most promising tests are those measuring procalcitonin and activated protein C because these tests are commercially available assays and procalcitonin can be measured bedside using a dipstick test [54]. Procalcitonin is the 116–amino acid propeptide of the hormone calcitonin. The source of procalcitonin is extrathyroidal and does not seem to be consistently related to calcium concentration but rather is involved in the inflammatory response to infection [54]. The pathophysiology of this response is not yet understood, but calcitonin concentrations have repeatedly been shown to increase significantly in patients with infection or sepsis [54]. Activated protein C plays a role in the control of microvascular coagulation (possessing antithrombotic activities) and is anti-inflammatory. It has also been shown in many studies to increase in the presence of inflammation and infection [55].

The concentration of blood procalcitonin in human patients with abdominal sepsis and inflammation has been shown to be an early and reliable indicator of prognosis and is also used to monitor patients after elective abdominal procedures to predict the development of complications [54]. Persistent high concentrations of procalcitonin have been shown to be a sensitive predictor of septic complications and can also reflect the effectiveness of therapy, such as surgical lavage [54]. Serum procalcitonin concentration had a sensitivity of 84% and a specificity of 91% in distinguishing between survivors and nonsurvivors in the first 4 days after abdominal lavage for treatment of septic peritonitis [54]. Activated protein C is less related to infection and more to inflammation [55]. It has been shown to be significantly and persistently lower in patients who died after developing septic shock with peritonitis versus those who survived [55]. Other cytokines that have been studied include peritoneal concentrations of interleukin-6, interleukin-1β, and tumor necrosis factor-α. These cytokines were higher in the peritoneal fluid of patients with peritoneal sepsis, with a higher potential for the development of septic complications [56]. Determining normal and abnormal levels of these cytokines in various clinical diseases in the horse may aid in therapeutic monitoring and assessing prognosis.

In a retrospective study of horses with diffuse peritonitis, horses were less likely to survive if they showed signs of abdominal pain or had distended small intestine on rectal examination, nasogastric reflux, serosanguineous peritoneal fluid, or higher total solids than those horses that did not show these signs. Overall, 43 (78%) of 55 horses with primary diffuse peritonitis survived to discharge, with 36 (65%) of 55 horses surviving without surgical treatment. Showing signs of abdominal pain on presentation reduced the chance of survival to less than 50%. Surgical treatment is recommended in those horses showing signs of abdominal pain, distended small intestine on rectal examination, nasogastric reflux, or serosanguineous peritoneal fluid (L.L. Southwood, BVSc, PhD, unpublished data, 2005).

Summary

Abdominal or pelvic infections in the neonate or adult horse can be diagnosed and treated successfully. Increasing the use of more advanced diagnostic and prognostic tests should improve our early recognition and enable us to monitor the effectiveness of our treatment on an improved level. The use of radionuclide-labeled antimicrobials has the potential to improve the diagnosis of abscesses in the pelvic region or abdomen using a noninvasive method. This technique may also aid in the decision to discontinue therapy. Serum procalcitonin or other inflammatory markers could be used for the prognosis and assessment of horses with diffuse or local intra-abdominal infection. Tests such as these may help veterinarians to assess the effectiveness of the treatment being used through a simple blood assay. Similar tests using umbilical cord blood can also aid in early detection of neonatal infections and enable aggressive early treatment. The standard tenants of maintaining a clean healthy environment to prevent infection and the establishment of drainage or removal of the source of infection as the best treatment still hold true. Surgical drainage or lavage is the recommended therapy for infection and shortens the duration of antibiotic therapy required, which is crucial in this age of antibiotic resistance.

References

[1] Davis JL. Treatment of peritonitis. Vet Clin North Am Equine Pract 2003;19:7765–78.
[2] Sanders-Shamis M. Perirectal abscesses in six horses. J Am Vet Med Assoc 1985;187(5): 499–500.
[3] Magee AA, Ragle CA, Hines MT, et al. Anorectal lymphadenopathy causing colic, perirectal abscesses, or both in five young horses. J Am Vet Med Assoc 1997;210(6):804–7.
[4] Torkelson J. Perirectal abscess, colic, and dyschezia in a horse. Can Vet J 2002;43:127–8.
[5] Ayres SL, Wagner P. Perirectal abscess in an American Miniature Horse. Equine Pract 1994; 16(9):33–5.

[6] Wilson DG, Stone WC. Antimesenteric enterotomy for repair of a dorsal rectal tear in a mare. Can Vet J 1990;31:705–7.
[7] Freeman DE, Richardson DW, Tulleners EP, et al. Loop colostomy for management of rectal tears and small-colon injures in horses: 10 cases (1976–1989). J Am Vet Med Assoc 1992;9: 1365–71.
[8] Onaca N, Hirshberg A, Adar R. Early reoperation for perirectal abscess, a preventable complication. Dis Colon Rectum 2001;44(10):1469–73.
[9] Brook I, Frazier EH. The aerobic and anaerobic bacteriology of perirectal abscesses. J Clin Microbiol 1997;35(11):2974–6.
[10] Neilsen MB, Torp-Pedersen S. Sonographically guided transrectal or transvaginal one-step catheter placement in deep pelvic and perirectal abscesses. AJR Am J Roentgenol 2004;183: 1035–6.
[11] Freeman DE. Rectum and anus. In: Auer JA, Stick JA, editors. Equine surgery. Philadelphia: WB Saunders; 1999. p. 286–93.
[12] Adams SB, Fessler JF. Umbilical cord remnant infections in foals: 16 cases (1975–1985). J Am Vet Med Assoc 1987;190:316–8.
[13] Patterson-Kane JC, Bain FT, Donahue JM, et al. Meningoencephalomyelitis in a foal due to Salmonella agona infection. NZ Vet J 2001;49:159–61.
[14] Ndung'u FK, Ndegwa MW, deMaar TWJ. Patent urachus with subsequent joint infection in a free-living Grevy's zebra foal. J Wildl Dis 2003;39(1):244–5.
[15] Zupan J, Garner P, Omari AA. Topical umbilical cord care at birth. Cochrane Database Syst Rev 2004;3:CD001057.
[16] Evens K, George J, Ansgt D, et al. Does umbilical cord care in preterm infants influence bacterial colonization or detachment? J Perinatol 2004;24(2):100–4.
[17] Mullany LC, Darmstadt GL, Tielsch JM. Role of antimicrobial applications to the umbilical cord in neonates to prevent bacterial colonization and infection: a review of the evidence. Pediatr Infect Dis J 2003;22(11):996–1002.
[18] Janssen PA, Selwood BL, Dobson SR, et al. To dye or not to dye: a randomized, clinical trial of a triple dye/alcohol regime versus dry cord care. Pediatrics 2003;111(1):15–20.
[19] Meberg A, Schoyen R. Bacterial colonization and neonatal infections. Effect of skin and umbilical disinfection in the nursery. Acta Paediatr Scand 1985;74:366–71.
[20] Steenholdt C, Hernandez J. Risk factors for umbilical hernia in Holstein heifers during the first two months after birth. J Am Vet Med Assoc 2004;224(9):1487–90.
[21] Freeman DE, Orsini JA, Harrison IW, et al. Complications of umbilical hernias in horses: 13 cases (1972–1986). J Am Vet Med Assoc 1988;192(6):804–7.
[22] Fischer AT Jr. Laparoscopically assisted resection of umbilical structures in foals. J Am Vet Med Assoc 1998;214(12):1813–6.
[23] Lillich JD, DeBowes RM. Bladder. In: Auer JA, Stick JA, editors. Equine surgery. Philadelphia: WB Saunders; 1999. p. 596–610.
[24] Korbage de Araujo MC, Schultz R, Latorre MO, et al. A risk factor for early onset infection in premature newborns: invasion of chorioamniotic tissues by leukocytes. Early Hum Dev 1999;54:1–15.
[25] Hatzidaki E, Gourgiotis D, Manoura A, et al. Interleukin-6 in preterm premature rupture of membranes as an indicator of neonatal outcome. Acta Obstet Gynecol Scand 2005;84(7): 632–8.
[26] Yoon BH, Romero R, Shim JY, et al. C-reactive protein in umbilical cord blood: a simple and widely available clinical method to assess the risk of amniotic fluid infection and funisitis. J Matern Fetal Neonatal Med 2003;14:85–90.
[27] Kordek A, Giedrys-Kalemba S, Pawlus B, et al. Umbilical cord blood serum procalcitonin concentration in the diagnosis of early neonatal infection. J Perinatol 2003;23(2):148–53.
[28] Santana C, Guindeo MC, Gonzalez G, et al. Cord levels of cytokines as predictors of early neonatal sepsis. Acta Paediatr 2001;90(10):1176–81.

[29] Volante E, Moretti S, Pisani F, et al. Early diagnosis of bacterial infection in the neonate. J Matern Fetal Neonatal Med 2004;16:13–6.
[30] Dollner H, Vatten L, Halgunset J, et al. Histologic chorioamnionitis and umbilical cord serum levels of pro-inflammatory cytokines and cytokine inhibitors. BJOG 2002;109(5):534–9.
[31] Reef VB, Collatos C. Ultrasonography of umbilical structures in clinically normal foals. Am J Vet Res 1987;49:2143–6.
[32] Reef VB, Collatos C, Spencer PA, et al. Clinical, ultrasonographic and surgical findings in foals with umbilical remnant infections. J Am Vet Med Assoc 1989;195:69–72.
[33] Robertson JT, Embertson RM. Surgical management of congenital and perinatal abnormalities of the urogenital tract. Vet Clin North Am Equine Pract 1988;4:359–77.
[34] Boure L, Marcoux M, Laverty S. Laparoscopic abdominal anatomy of foals positioned in dorsal recumbency. Vet Surg 1997;26:1–6.
[35] Edwards RD III, Fubini SL. A one-stage marsupialization procedure for management of infected umbilical vein remnants in calves and foals. Vet Surg 1995;24:32–5.
[36] Pratt SM, Spier SJ, Carroll SP, et al. Evaluation of clinical characteristics, diagnostic test results, and outcome in horses with internal infection caused by Corynebacterium pseudotuberculosis: 30 cases (1995–2003). J Am Vet Med Assoc 2005;227:441–8.
[37] DiPietro JA, Boero M, Ely RW. Abdominal abscess associated with Parascaris equorum infection. J Am Vet Med Assoc 1983;182:991–2.
[38] Hanselaer JR, Nyland TG. Chyloabdomen and ultrasonographic detection of an intraabdominal abscess in a foal. J Am Vet Med Assoc 1983;183(12):1465–7.
[39] Aleman M, Watson JL, Jang SS. Clostridium novyi type A intra-abdominal abscess in a horse. J Vet Intern Med 2003;17:934–6.
[40] Higuchi T, Hashikura S, Gojo C, et al. Clinical evaluation of the serodiagnostic value of enzyme-linked immunosorbent assay for Rhodococcus equi infection in foals. Equine Vet J 1997;29:274–8.
[41] Sweeney CR, Whitlock RH, Meirs DA, et al. Complications associated with Streptococcus equi infection on a horse farm. J Am Vet Med Assoc 1987;191:1446–8.
[42] Zicjer SC, Wilson D, Medearis I. Differentiation between intra-abdominal neoplasms and abscesses in horses, using clinical and laboratory data: 40 cases (1973–1988). J Am Vet Med Assoc 1990;196:1130–4.
[43] Rumbaugh GE, Smith BP, Carlson GP. Internal abdominal abscesses in the horse: a study of 25 cases. J Am Vet Med Assoc 1978;172:304–9.
[44] Sweeney RW, Sweeney CR, Weiher J. Clinical use of metronidazole in horses: 200 cases (1984–1989). J Am Vet Med Assoc 1991;198:1045–8.
[45] Koblik PD, Lofstedt J, Jakowski RM, et al. Use of ^{111}In-labelled autologous leukocytes to image an abdominal abscess in a horse. J Am Vet Med Assoc 1985;186:1319–22.
[46] Love C, Palestro CJ. Radionuclide imaging of infection. J Nucl Med Technol 2004;32:47–57.
[47] Ramzan PHL, Malton RJ, McGladdery AJ. Use of ^{99m}technetium hexamethylpropyleneamine oxime labeled leucocyte scintigraphy in equine medical investigations: 8 cases. Equine Veterinary Education 2004;16:122–7.
[48] Artiko V, Davidovic B, Nikolic N, et al. Detection of gastrointestinal and abdominal infections by 99mTc-ciprofloxacin. Hepatogastroenterology 2005;52(62):491–5.
[49] Singh B, Mittal BR, Battacharya A, et al. Technetium-99m ciprofloxacin imaging in the diagnosis of post-surgical bony infection and evaluation of response to antibiotic therapy: a case report. J Orthop Surg (Hong Kong) 2005;13:190–4.
[50] Rigg DL, Gatlin SJ, Reinertson EL. Marsupialization of an abdominal abscess caused by Serratia marcescens in a mare. J Am Vet Med Assoc 1987;191:222–4.
[51] Prades M, Peyton L, Pattio N, et al. Surgical treatment of an abdominal abscess by marsupialisation in the horse: a report of two cases. Equine Vet J 1989;21:459–61.
[52] Skidell J. Resection of an intra-abdominal abscess in a horse using stapling technique. Equine Vet J 1996;8:140–2.

[53] Blot S, De Waele JJ. Critical issues in the clinical management of complicated intra-abdominal infections. Drugs 2005;65:1611–20.
[54] Rau B, Kruger CM, Schilling MK. Procalcitonin: improved biochemical severity stratification and postoperative monitoring in severe abdominal inflammation and sepsis. Langenbecks Arch Surg 2004;389:134–44.
[55] Karamarkovic A, Radenkovic D, Milic N, et al. Protein C as an early marker of severe septic complications in diffuse secondary peritonitis. World J Surg 2005;29:759–65.
[56] Yamamoto T, Umegae S, Kitagawa T, et al. Intraperitoneal cytokine productions and their relationship to peritoneal sepsis and systemic inflammatory markers in patients with inflammatory bowel disease. Dis Colon Rectum 2005;48:1005–15.

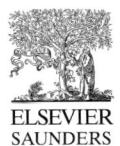

Enteritis and Colitis in Horses

Darien J. Feary, BVSc, MS[a],
Diana M. Hassel, DVM, PhD[b],*

[a]*Department of Medicine and Epidemiology, School of Veterinary Medicine,
University of California, Davis, CA 95616, USA*
[b]*Department of Clinical Sciences, College of Veterinary Medicine and Biological Sciences,
Colorado State University, Fort Collins, CO 80526, USA*

Inflammatory diseases of the equine gastrointestinal tract include a wide variety of disorders that, despite many recent advances in monitoring and therapy, remain an important cause of morbidity and mortality in horses. Some of the more common known infectious and noninfectious causes of enteritis and colitis in adults and foals are listed in Table 1. This article begins with a review of the diagnosis and treatment of specific disease entities known to cause enterocolitis, including salmonellosis, Potomac horse fever (PHF), clostridiosis, parasitic enteritis, proliferative enteropathy (*Lawsonia intracellularis*), and duodenitis–proximal jejunitis (DPJ). Recent advances in the diagnosis, treatment, and monitoring of horses with acute enterocolitis are then described.

Classic treatment of infectious enterocolitis in horses consists primarily of replacement of fluid and electrolyte losses, control of enteric inflammation and reduction of fluid secretion, control of endotoxemia and sepsis, and re-establishment of normal flora. These are accomplished through the administration of intravenous crystalloids and colloids, antidiarrheal agents (eg, bismuth subsalicylate solutions), nonsteroidal anti-inflammatory drugs (NSAIDs), therapeutic agents to combat endotoxemia (eg, J-5 hyperimmune plasma, polymyxin B sulfate), antimicrobial therapy, probiotics or transfaunation, and feeding to re-establish short-chain fatty acid colonic content. Standard additional monitoring includes hematologic and serum biochemical analysis, which is often characterized by moderate to severe leukopenia, a mild to moderate left shift, toxic changes in the neutrophils [1], azotemia, high serum sorbitol dehydrogenase and γ-glutamine aminotransferase

---

* Corresponding author.
E-mail address: dhassel@colostate.edu (D.M. Hassel).

Table 1
Causes of infectious and noninfectious enteritis and colitis in adults and foals

Adult		Foals (<8 months old)	
Infectious	Noninfectious	Infectious	Noninfectious
Salmonellosis	Carbohydrate overload	Salmonellosis	Gastroduodenal ulceration
Antimicrobial-associated colitis	Antimicrobial-associated colitis	*Lawsonia intracellularis* (proliferative enteropathy)	Peritonitis
Clostridial enterocolitis (*Clostridium difficile*, *Clostridium perfringens*)	Right dorsal ulcerative colitis (nonsteroidal anti-inflammatory drug toxicity)	*C difficile*	Sepsis
Neorickettsia risticii (Potomac horse fever)	Intoxications: cantharidin (blister beetle), hoary alyssum, arsenic, caster oil	*C perfringens*	Nutritional Dietary indiscretion Overfeeding
Cyathostomiasis/strongylosis Duodenitis–proximal jejunitis	Peritonitis Sand enteropathy Infiltrative or inflammatory bowel disease: eosinophilic, granulomatous, lymphocytic or plasmacytic enteritis, alimentary lymphosarcoma, Duodenitis–proximal jejunitis	Rotavirus *Rhodococcus equi* *Strongyloides westeri*	Lactose intolerance

activity, and hyperlactatemia [2]. Advances in monitoring and treatment beyond standard supportive care measures have improved our abilities to treat horses with acute severe enterocolitis of any origin successfully.

Salmonellosis

Diagnosis

Equine colitis caused by *Salmonella* spp infection is clinically indistinguishable from colitis caused by other infectious and noninfectious causes. Severe cases may exhibit peracute enterocolitis with or without diarrhea that is rapidly fatal despite aggressive therapy. Other recognized syndromes of *Salmonella* spp infection include a latent subclinical carrier state that may revert to active fecal shedding with or without clinically apparent infection and bacteremia or septicemia in neonatal foals. Established risk factors associated with progression of latent infection to active shedding, nosocomial infection, and clinical disease include "stressors," such as transportation [3], gastrointestinal tract disorders [4,5], change in or withholding of feed [5,6], abdominal surgery [7,8], high ambient temperature [5,9], and antimicrobial therapy [5,7,8]. The prevalence of fecal shedding of *Salmonella* spp among the general horse population in the United States is estimated to be 0.8% [10], and it is estimated to be between 1.4% and 20% among horses admitted to veterinary teaching hospitals [11]. Within the hospitalized population of horses, those with gastrointestinal disease, notably impaction of the small colon [12], and foals [7,8] show an increased frequency of shedding *Salmonella* spp.

Bacterial culture and isolation of *Salmonella* spp from blood, tissues, or five or more sequential daily fecal samples is considered to be the "gold standard" for diagnosis of *Salmonella* spp infection in horses and remains the currently recommended protocol [13]. *Salmonella* spp are shed intermittently in feces, however, and cannot be consistently isolated from horses with salmonellosis [13,14], particularly those with profuse watery diarrhea [15]. Further, a positive fecal culture for *Salmonella* spp from a horse with compatible clinical signs does not necessarily confirm a diagnosis of salmonellosis. Rectal mucosal biopsies are more sensitive compared with fecal samples for isolation of *Salmonella* spp from infected horses but are less frequently used because the technique is invasive and carries more risk to the patient [14]. The disadvantages of bacterial culture of feces are the lag in time required to obtain test results (2–5 days), suboptimal sensitivity (55% for a single sample) [13], and cost of performing multiple cultures to improve sensitivity. Use of polymerase chain reaction (PCR) techniques has been developed and investigated as an alternative to or to be used in conjunction with bacterial culture for identification of *Salmonella* spp in fecal and environmental samples [16,17]. The advantages of a PCR assay over conventional bacterial culture are the short time (24 hours) required to obtain test results, the ability to detect *Salmonella* spp present in low numbers early in the course of disease that may be undetectable by bacterial culture, considerably greater sensitivity [16,17], the requirement for fewer samples, and the associated reduced cost [16]. Some studies report a discrepancy between results comparing PCR assay and bacterial culture of fecal and environmental samples, however, leading to the suggestion that a PCR assay for detection of *Salmonella* spp DNA in equine feces is less accurate than previously thought [16,18]. In addition, a PCR assay does not provide antimicrobial sensitivity results or permit serotyping or speciation of isolates, which are important for clinical and surveillance purposes.

Culture of peripheral blood is indicated in neonates if bacteremia or septicemia is suspected. *Salmonella* spp are rarely cultured from blood in infected adult horses [2]. The sensitivity of culture for microorganisms in peripheral blood may be enhanced by careful aseptic technique, collection of multiple samples (three or more samples) comprising 10 to 30 mL of blood from central and peripheral venipuncture sites during a period of high fever ($\geq 103°F$), and if the patient has not received antimicrobial agents for at least 24 hours before collection.

Salmonella spp culture requires selective techniques and multiple steps that are not performed during routine culture of feces for other microorganisms. Techniques for *Salmonella* spp isolation do not seem to be highly standardized among microbiology testing laboratories [19] and depend on cost, efficiency, and accuracy of the testing method used. A positive test result should not terminate ongoing testing for other causes of enterocolitis, nor should prior antimicrobial therapy prevent culturing of *Salmonella* spp from feces of infected horses, despite in vivo bacterial sensitivity to the antimicrobial agent [13]. For a detailed review of sample and laboratory techniques for *Salmonella* spp culture, the reader is referred to a previous review [19].

Use of a PCR assay in conjunction with bacterial culture of feces may be beneficial for the detection of infected horses early in the course of disease, and PCR assay seems to have the greatest agreement (70%) with bacterial culture when two or more positive PCR results are used to define a horse as actively shedding *Salmonella* spp [20].

Determining the most practical and accurate method(s) for the detection of *Salmonella* spp from equine patients is an area of active research, accelerated by an apparent increase in the number of equine hospital outbreaks, the emergence of multidrug resistance in equine *Salmonella* spp isolates, the associated cost (financial and mortality), and a negative public perception.

Treatment

The use of antimicrobial therapy for the treatment of salmonellosis in horses is controversial. The apparent association between administration of antimicrobials and increased risk of fecal shedding of *Salmonella* spp [4,5,20] suggests that antimicrobials can cause salmonellosis. They may act by inhibiting normal competitive gastrointestinal flora, by reducing the infective dose required to produce disease, or by allowing proliferation and active shedding of salmonellae from previously latently infected horses.

Antimicrobial treatment does not reduce fecal shedding of *Salmonella* spp, even if the strain is sensitive to the antimicrobial agent used [13]. There is no evidence that antimicrobial therapy is beneficial in altering the course of salmonellosis in adult horses [2,21], and antimicrobial administration negatively affects gastrointestinal immunity, suggesting that antimicrobial treatment is more likely to be detrimental to hospitalized horses with salmonellosis. Situations in which antimicrobial therapy may be indicated include septicemia or immunocompromised horses, as indicated by severe neutropenia. In these cases, selection of a narrow-spectrum agent with bactericidal activity, intracellular penetration, and minimal effect on commensal flora should be considered.

The emergence of multidrug-resistant (MDR) *Salmonella* spp in documented nosocomial outbreaks of equine patients complicates the selection of antimicrobials when they are indicated. Choice of an appropriate antimicrobial agent should also take results of an antibiogram into consideration when one is available. A review of MDR *Salmonella* spp and nosocomial infection in equine veterinary hospitals has been published [20].

Systemic fluoroquinolone (enrofloxacin) administration is currently recommended at a dose of 5 mg/kg administered intravenously once daily [22] because of its favorable pharmacokinetic properties. In addition, the MDR *Salmonella* spp involved in nosocomial outbreaks in hospitalized equine patients do not seem to have developed widespread resistance to enrofloxacin, based on reported antibiogram results [20]. Resistance of *Salmonella* spp to the aminoglycoside amikacin is also rare. Although enrofloxacin and, to a lesser extent, amikacin may be good choices for the treatment of salmonellosis in horses, these antimicrobials should be reserved for those cases in which they are indicated to avoid the emergence of further MDR isolates.

The authors advocate the administration of gentamicin (6.6 mg/kg administered intravenously or intramuscularly once daily) to horses with salmonellosis or acute enterocolitis of unknown etiology in which antimicrobial therapy is indicated. Narrow-spectrum antimicrobial agents directed against gram-negative bacteria, such as the aminoglycosides, pose minimal risk for disruption of colonic luminal microflora and should be effective against most isolates.

The use of antimicrobial agents in horses with enterocolitis suspected to be caused by *Salmonella* spp infection should always be judicious and based on antibiogram results, with the goal of preventing systemic dissemination while supporting the natural immune response to infection rather than eliminating fecal shedding or carrier states.

The use of probiotic agents for the treatment and prevention of enterocolitis in horses is discussed elsewhere in this article.

Potomac horse fever (*Neorickettsia risticii*)

Diagnosis

PHF, or equine monocytic ehrlichiosis, is an infectious but not contagious cause of fever and colitis in horses. The causative agent, *Neorickettsia risticii* (formerly *Ehrlichia risticii*), is a rickettsial organism that infects mononuclear cells, specifically blood monocytes and tissue macrophages, with a predilection for intestinal epithelial crypt cells and mast cells in the large and small intestines. PHF has been reported to exist throughout most of the United States and in parts of Canada, Europe, Venezuela, India, Italy, Uruguay, Brazil, and Australia [23–26].

Significant developments in our understanding of this disease have occurred in the past 15 years. Briefly, recent evidence suggests that under natural conditions, *N risticii* is transmitted via the oral route to horses through the accidental ingestion of infected digenetic trematodes (eg, *Acanthatrium* spp, *Lecithodendrium* spp) in the secretions of first (operculate freshwater snails) and second (aquatic insects, such as caddisflies, dragonflies, stoneflies, and mayflies) intermediate hosts [27]. A broad range of host genera have been implicated in each phase of the complex aquatic life cycle and vary depending on the particular endemic geographic region of the United States.

PHF has a distinct seasonal distribution, with a peak incidence of clinical cases occurring sporadically during the warmer months between June and September in horses grazing pastures bordering creeks or rivers and under certain circumstances, such as outbreaks on racetracks [28].

Identifying PHF as the cause for signs of enterocolitis in a horse is important, because specific treatment is effective if administered early in the course of disease and is contraindicated in other causes of infectious colitis, such as salmonellosis and clostridiosis. A provisional diagnosis of PHF can often be made based on recognition of typical clinical signs and the seasonal and geographic occurrence of the disease [29].

Clinical manifestations of PHF are similar to those of enterocolitis in adult horses attributable to other causes and include acute onset of dullness, anorexia, fever (102°F–107°F), and reduced to absent gastrointestinal motility, often followed by mild to severe diarrhea (10%–60% of cases) within 12 to 48 hours, with or without abdominal pain. Laminitis may develop as a serious complication in up to 40% of naturally infected horses [29]. Abortion or fetal reabsorption attributable to fetal infection with *N risticii* may occur several months after clinical disease in pregnant mares [29]. Abortion is accompanied by placentitis and retained fetal membranes in the mare [29]. The fetus is expelled in good condition, with enterocolitis, periportal hepatitis, myocarditis, and lymphoid hyperplasia of the mesenteric lymph nodes and spleen identified microscopically [30]. Infected foals may be born alive but are severely maladjusted [24].

Typical hematologic abnormalities in horses with PHF include an initial leukopenia (<5000 cells/μL) with a toxic left shift and a marked rebound leukocytosis (>14,000 cells/μL) [31]. Anemia, thrombocytopenia, and evidence for coagulopathy are variable findings, as are plasma protein, electrolyte, and acid-base abnormalities, depending on the severity of diarrhea. In contrast to the other rickettsia known to cause disease in horses (*Anaplasma phagocytophila*), visual examination of Romanowsky-stained blood smears is not useful for diagnosis of PHF, because only a small number of blood monocytes are infected with *N risticii*, even during acute bacteremia [24].

A definitive diagnosis of PHF should be based on isolation or detection of *N risticii* from the blood or feces of infected horses [29], but culture isolation is time-consuming ($\leq$3 weeks for a positive diagnosis) and impractical for most diagnostic laboratories and clinical situations [23]. Although serologic diagnosis using the indirect fluorescent antibody (IFA) test has had widespread use in the past, serologic diagnosis has limited value in clinical disease for a number of reasons: (1) the high incidence of seropositive horses without evidence of clinical disease in endemic areas [32], (2) the large number of false-positive test results in some laboratories [33], (3) difficulty in demonstrating a rise in antibody titer in affected horses given the close temporal association between onset of clinical signs and the rapid rise in serum antibody titer [34,35], and (4) inability to distinguish between active and previous infection or vaccination [33]. Indirect [35] and monoclonal competitive [36] ELISA tests are reported to be more sensitive than the IFA test; however, at this time, a rapid and reliable field serodiagnostic test has not yet become available [24].

Use of a PCR assay to detect *N risticii* DNA in whole blood and feces of infected horses is a rapid, sensitive, and accurate method of diagnosis of PHF [33,37]. In the future, conventional PCR methods are likely to be replaced by real-time PCR assays for routine diagnosis of PHF and epidemiologic investigations because of more rapid test results (within 2 hours), lower risk of contamination, less cost, and the ability to test larger sample numbers. The use of the TaqMan (Applied Biosystems, Foster City, California) PCR assay also allows quantitation of *N risticii* DNA and may be helpful in monitoring the course of infection and quantifying material for experimental infection or antigen production [38]. A PCR assay can detect *N risticii* DNA in feces or blood mononuclear cells at the time of clinical disease [27] and in formalin-fixed intestinal tissue when a postmortem diagnosis is required [25]. Submission of whole blood and fecal samples for PCR testing is recommended, because the presence of *N. risticii* in blood and feces may not necessarily coincide [23]. It is also noteworthy that fecal samples may be refrigerated at 4°C but not frozen (<-20°C), because freezing significantly reduces the sensitivity of a PCR assay [37].

The only distinguishing postmortem features in horses with PHF are a lack of severe invasive lesions, foul odor, or significant inflammatory infiltration of the intestine and the presence of significantly depleted inactive lymphoid tissue. *N risticii* may be identified in epithelial cells and macrophages of the small and large intestines and small colon in histopathologic sections by immunoperoxidase or modified silver stains, where they appear as densely packed morulae or as larger, individually, tightly enveloped forms within the cytoplasm of host cells [24].

Treatment

The treatment of choice for PHF is the intravenous administration of oxytetracycline (6.6 mg/kg twice daily) in addition to nonspecific supportive care, such as intravenously administered crystalloid and colloid therapy; anti-inflammatory, antiendotoxic, and antidiarrheal therapy; and management of abdominal pain and specific treatment of adverse sequelae, including laminitis and other complications of the systemic inflammatory response syndrome (SIRS). If administered early in the clinical course of the disease, treatment is reported to be effective in preventing progression of the disease and results in significant clinical improvement within 12 hours as well as resolution of clinical disease within 3 to 5 days in most cases [29].

N risticii is able to survive intracellularly because of its ability to inhibit phagosome-lysosome fusion, and thus to resist lysosomal digestion [39]. In small animal and human patients, doxycycline is the drug of choice for treatment of ehrlichial diseases [39]. Intravenous administration of doxycycline is reported to cause cardiotoxicity and sudden death in horses and should be avoided. Oral doxycycline (10 mg/kg administered orally twice daily) could be considered for the treatment of PHF, although minimizing the risk of adverse effects on gastrointestinal microflora in horses with enterocolitis may include avoiding an oral tetracycline. Alternatively, oral administration of the erythromycin and rifampin combination is reported to be effective in experimental studies in horses [40], despite poor in vitro activity against *N risticii* [24]. The use of macrolide antimicrobial agents in adult horses poses significant risk for development of colitis, and these would not be among the first drugs of choice for the treatment of PHF.

Despite having an effective antimicrobial treatment for the disease, the case fatality rate for horses with PHF can be as high as 30%, and there do not seem to be any recent advances reported with regard to specific therapy. Successful treatment relies on early recognition of disease and prompt instigation of antimicrobial therapy, supportive care, and prevention and management of adverse sequelae. Naturally and experimentally infected horses are most often euthanized because of severe abdominal pain, unresponsive severe diarrhea, endotoxemia, or laminitis [25].

Equine clinicians should be aware of the risk of inducing acute renal failure when administering systemic oxytetracycline to infected horses that may be hypovolemic and may also be receiving other potentially nephrotoxic drugs, such as NSAIDs, concurrently. This complication can be avoided with the prior administration of intravenous or oral fluids and monitoring of renal parameters via blood biochemical analysis.

Clostridial enterocolitis

Diagnosis

A variety of *Clostridium* spp have been associated with acute enterocolitis in mature horses and foals, but *Clostridium difficile* and *Clostridium perfringens* are the most commonly isolated species and are the focus of this review. *C perfringens* type C and, less commonly, type A as well as the more recently identified β_2-toxigenic *C perfringens* have been most frequently associated with enterocolitis in adult horses and foals. *C difficile* is the most common cause of antimicrobial-associated diarrhea in human patients. A dramatic increase in incidence over the past 20 years has been associated with the increased use of third-generation cephalosporins, and *C difficile* continues to be an important cause of nosocomial infection in human patients. Similar to the case in human patients, *C difficile* has emerged, and is being reported, with increasing frequency as a cause of nosocomial and antimicrobial-associated enterocolitis in equine patients [41].

Diagnosis of Clostridium difficile infection

The clinical signs of enterocolitis caused by *C difficile* are indistinguishable from other infectious and noninfectious causes of acute enterocolitis in mature horses. The association of certain predisposing factors, the most common of which is antimicrobial therapy, in combination with underlying stress factors, such as hospitalization, transport, surgery, and dietary changes, in a horse with signs of acute enterocolitis should alert the equine clinician to the likelihood of a *C difficile* infection.

C difficile is not considered part of the normal flora of the equine adult gastrointestinal tract and is uncommonly isolated from normal mature horses. The isolation rate may increase in asymptomatic horses being treated with antimicrobials [42], however, and up to 42% of horses that develop acute colitis during treatment with antimicrobials can have *C difficile* isolated [41,43,44]. These studies emphasize the need to include laboratory testing for *C difficile* as part of the routine workup in all horses with colitis, especially in combination with antimicrobial therapy.

The clinical importance of *C difficile* in foals seems to be different from that in mature horses. Although most information suggests that *C difficile* is uncommonly isolated from healthy foals (<3%) [43], one recent study reported an isolation rate of 29% in healthy foals less than 14 days old [41]. *C difficile* is being increasingly recognized as a cause of neonatal foal diarrhea, and disease is less frequently associated with administration of antimicrobials in foals compared with mature horses [45]. This evidence suggests that neonatal foals become colonized with *C difficile* during the first few weeks of life, as is observed in human infants and puppies, and that they can be asymptomatic carriers. It has been suggested that *C difficile* may be a primary pathogen in neonatal foals [45], and this was confirmed by Arroyo and colleagues [46], who demonstrated the primary pathogenic nature of *C difficile* in foals in a model that fulfilled Koch's postulates of disease.

The current understanding of *C difficile* infection is that the manifestation of clinically important disease depends on the production of two large protein exotoxins, toxin A (enterotoxin) and toxin B (cytotoxin), which act synergistically to cause intestinal tissue disruption and secondary inflammation with associated clinical signs. Some virulent strains may only produce toxin B [47]. A third known toxin has recently been identified as binary toxin (ADP-ribosyltransferase) in human isolates as well as a small number of equine isolates and is unrelated to either of the more prevalent toxins A and B [48]; however, its role in the pathogenesis of equine colitis is unclear.

The laboratory diagnosis of *C difficile* is based on two types of tests performed on fecal samples: bacterial culture and toxin detection. *C difficile* is a spore-forming, obligately anaerobic, gram-positive rod. Successful culture requires inoculation of approximately 25 g of feces collected directly from the rectum into a rectal sleeve or plastic bag with excess air evacuated or application of a rectal swab sample onto selective media (cycloserine-cefoxitin-fructose agar [CCFA]), anaerobic incubation for 36 to 48 hours at 37°C, and identification of bacterial colonies based on specific morphologic characteristics, Gram stain results, and results of biochemical testing. Culture is a sensitive test but lacks specificity because of the existence of nontoxigenic isolates. Approximately 25% of *C difficile* strains are reported to be nontoxigenic in horses, and thus not clinically important [49]. The slow turnaround time, low specificity, and discrepant results, depending on fecal sample handling and storage, make culture an insufficient test for diagnosis of *C difficile* enterocolitis on its own. In addition, unless fecal samples are processed within 2 hours, recovery of *C difficile* from aerobically stored and refrigerated (4°C) fecal samples significantly decreases from 76% after 24 hours to only 29% after 72 hours [49]. Therefore, samples should be stored refrigerated under anaerobic conditions (via anaerobic transport medium, such as BBL Port-A-Cul Tubes [Becton Dickinson, Franklin Lakes, New Jersey]) or frozen at $-20°C$ [50]. Fecal samples should also be collected on a daily basis to enhance the likelihood of *C difficile* detection. In contrast to culture, stability of toxin in equine feces is reportedly better than that of the organism and storage may be adequate with refrigeration only. The amount of feces available from a rectal swab sample is inadequate for toxin detection, however.

Definitive diagnosis of *C difficile* enterocolitis requires demonstration of production of toxin A or B or both in fecal samples from affected horses. The gold standard test for toxin detection involves demonstration of cytotoxicity (toxin B) in cell culture. This technique is sensitive and specific but requires specific laboratory facilities, is expensive, and necessitates a 6- to 48-hour incubation period. Several immunoassays detecting toxin A alone or toxins A and B directly in feces have been developed and are commercially available. These assays are rapid (<1 hour) and practical, and although they are less sensitive than cell culture and not validated for use in horses, their use in the clinical setting for diagnosis of *C difficile* in horses is becoming more common. The Triage *C difficile* Panel (Biosite Diagnostics, San Diego, California) is an enzyme immunoassay (EIA) for the simultaneous detection of the *C difficile* common antigen (glutamine dehydrogenase) and toxin A (Fig. 1). The combination of the antigen and the toxin immunoassay in one test increased the sensitivity and specificity in human patients [51]. Other combination immunoassays currently in development [52] may prove to be useful in horses. It is important to realize that because toxin A is more stable and more enterotoxic than toxin B, development of available immunoassays has focused on detection of toxin A alone. The prevalence of toxin A-negative/toxin B-positive strains of *C difficile* is unknown in horses but has been reported [45], emphasizing the need to perform further testing for detection of toxin B if clinical signs and culture results support toxigenic *C difficile* infection.

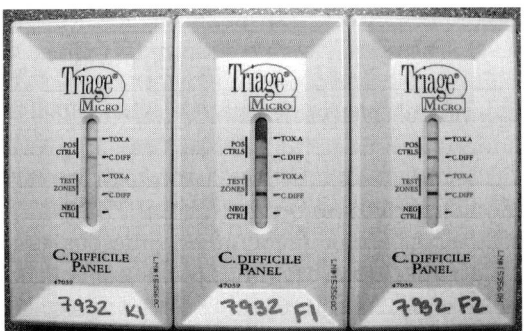

Fig. 1. Triage *C difficile* Panel (Biosite Diagnostics, San Diego, California) is an EIA for the simultaneous detection of the *C difficile* common antigen (glutamine dehydrogenase) and toxin A.

PCR methods for the detection of *C difficile* in equine feces have been employed but have not gained widespread use. A conventional PCR assay is used to detect the presence of the genes for toxins A and B (but not their expression), and its clinical use in equine isolates has produced discrepant results [45]. Novel real-time PCR techniques and methods detecting gene expression are likely to be increasingly used in laboratories with these facilities. An arbitrarily primed PCR assay and PCR ribotyping have been used in epidemiologic investigation of *C difficile* from human and animal sources [53] and have a role in the investigation of suspected nosocomial infection in equine facilities.

Although a consensus regarding definitive laboratory diagnostic criteria for *C difficile* colitis in horses has not been established, many authors support the view that the diagnosis of *C difficile* colitis requires isolation of the organism in combination with demonstration of toxin A or B or both directly in the feces [45,50]. In cases of culture-positive and toxin-negative results, especially early in disease, toxin assays should be repeated on subsequent fecal samples [46] or colonies should be tested for toxin production with a commercially available toxin immunoassay [47].

The most frequently reported method of antimicrobial susceptibility testing of *C difficile* isolates from horses is the Etest (AB Biodisk, Solna, Sweden). This test is a simple agar diffusion technique used to determine the minimal inhibitory concentration (MIC) of antimicrobials for *C difficile*. Recently, Båverud and coworkers [54] reported the use of broth microdilution as an alternative method of susceptibility testing of *C difficile* isolates from horses with reliable and reproducible results. The importance of susceptibility testing may increase in the future because of the existence of metronidazole-resistant strains of *C difficile* in horses [55].

Diagnosis of Clostridium perfringens infection

C perfringens is a bacterium that is widely distributed as spores and vegetative cells in the environment. *C perfringens* type A can be isolated in small numbers (<10^3 colony-forming units [CFUs]/g of feces) from normal horses. In horses, *C perfringens* is most commonly associated with enterocolitis in neonatal foals that develops within the first few days of life. Early colonization of the neonatal gastrointestinal tract with clostridial organisms seems to occur normally in neonatal foals, with a subsequent decline in numbers as other anaerobes and microflora become established. The development of infection and exotoxin production by *C perfringens* and the subsequent clinical signs of enterocolitis are believed to be associated with this early colonization and apparent tolerance to the organism, the presence of trypsin inhibitors in ingested mare's colostrum, and a variety of environmental factors that increase the risk of disease [56,57]. There also seems to be geographic and seasonal variation associated with neonatal clostridial enterocolitis [50]. In North America, enterocolitis in foals caused by *C perfringens* is most commonly associated with type C, which produces the cytotoxic β-toxin in addition to α-toxin and, occasionally, with certain subtypes of *C perfringens* type A [50].

Clinical signs of disease tend to occur in previously healthy vigorous foals that ingest an adequate to large amount of good-quality colostrum. At 24 to 72 hours of age, affected foals develop acute abdominal pain, fever, mild to severe hemorrhagic diarrhea, and hypovolemic and septic shock. Some foals die before the development of diarrhea. The disease is associated with a high case fatality rate (54%–68%) despite aggressive medical treatment [57].

Clinical signs of disease in adult horses are similar, although the disease seems to occur less commonly, or is less commonly diagnosed, in adult horses compared with neonatal foals. Factors associated with the development of disease in adult horses are also different and poorly understood.

C perfringens strains, predominantly type A, containing the novel $β_2$-toxin gene (*cpb2*) have been correlated with enterocolitis in adult horses, specifically typhlocolitis [58]. In addition, $β_2$-toxigenic *C perfringens* can be isolated from healthy as well as diseased animals and is widespread in nature, suggesting that predisposing factors are necessary for the development of disease associated with $β_2$-toxin [59].

Diagnosis of enterocolitis caused by *C perfringens* in adult horses and foals may be made based on the combination of isolation of large numbers of *C perfringens*, identification of the toxin gene, and associated clinical features of enterocolitis. In suspect cases, fresh feces should be shipped refrigerated or fecal swabs collected and placed in anaerobic transport medium. Samples should be processed as soon as possible or frozen if extended storage is required. Cultivation requires anaerobic media, and recovery may be optimized by employing more than one method and using enrichment media [60]. In foals, blood culture should also be performed if bacteremia is suspected.

Demonstration of toxin production requires detection of the genes that encode the toxin using a multiplex PCR assay applied directly to feces or isolated bacteria [61]. DNA testing can be used to identify genotypes of

C perfringens types A through E as well as all major toxin types, β_2-toxin, and enterotoxin. More recently, sophisticated techniques, including a multiplex PCR assay specific for *C perfringens* that does not require purified clostridial DNA [62] and microarray-based assays [63], have been developed.

Postmortem findings in cases of fatal enterocolitis are characterized by acute hemorrhagic enteritis as well as by colitis and villi necrosis. Features that may distinguish disease caused by *Clostridium* spp from other causes of enterocolitis include identification of large numbers of gram-positive rods in stained smears and sections of affected intestine obtained immediately after death and the presence of mural emphysema. Immunohistochemistry employing antitoxin antibodies has been used to detect β_2-toxin in intestinal sections and may be a useful diagnostic tool when bacterial culture and PCR methods are not feasible [64].

When interpreting results of diagnostic tests for *C perfringens* in suspect cases, it should be remembered that demonstration of the toxin gene does not necessarily imply clinically important toxin expression. In addition, at least in the western United States, *C perfringens* type A can be isolated from the environment as well as from most normal broodmares and foals and does not seem to be associated with disease on its own and β_2-toxigenic *C perfringens* can be isolated occasionally from normal mares and foals [65]. α-Toxin and enterotoxin are believed to have low pathogenicity in horses, and their role in disease is questionable [65]. *C perfringens* type C is rarely found in the environment or in the feces of normal horses or foals, however, and is more likely to be associated with disease [65].

It is undoubtedly challenging to establish a definitive diagnosis of enterocolitis caused by *C perfringens* in horses. It may also seem to be less important compared with other causes of colitis in horses because it does not seem to be directly infectious, result in outbreaks of disease, or exist as a carrier state. Nevertheless, in suspected cases, an effort should be made to identify the organism and interpret its significance so that specific treatment and preventative management practices may be instituted.

Treatment

Clostridium difficile

The treatment of *C difficile* enterocolitis in mature horses depends somewhat on the clinical presentation. Recommendations for the treatment of *C difficile*–associated diarrhea (CDAD) in human patients may provide reasonable guidelines for the treatment of horses, although there are some exceptions. The first step is to discontinue antimicrobial therapy, if possible, and to administer appropriate supportive care to normalize fluid, electrolyte, and colloid deficits. Interestingly, antidiarrheal medications and opiates are avoided in human patients because of toxin release and slowed clearance of *C difficile* secondary to reduced gastrointestinal motility [66]. In up to 25% of patients, conservative therapy is sufficient to resolve symptoms.

Specific pharmacotherapy with conventional antimicrobial treatment is reserved for patients that do not respond adequately to supportive care as well as for older patients, patients with comorbid conditions, and those in which continued antimicrobial treatment is necessary.

As is the case with human patients, metronidazole has been considered the first-line treatment for *C difficile* colitis in horses [43,45]. Resolution of diarrhea and inability to isolate *C difficile* or to detect toxin in feces of affected foals are reported within 18 to 72 hours of oral metronidazole therapy (15 mg/kg administered orally three times daily) [46]. The reported use of vancomycin in horses is variable. Because of the concern for emergence of resistant bacteria in human medicine, vancomycin is considered an inappropriate antimicrobial for use in horses with *C difficile* colitis. Metronidazole-resistant strains have been reported in up to 43% of isolates from horses [45,55] in certain geographic regions, however, as well as in human patients in whom isolates were previously considered to be predictably susceptible to metronidazole [67]. Therefore, some authors consider the judicious use of vancomycin to be indicated in horses with documented resistance to or poor clinical response to metronidazole and appropriate supportive care [45]. These studies emphasize the importance of culture and susceptibility testing of *C difficile* isolates from horses as part of the routine diagnostic procedure in horses with acute enterocolitis.

Although metronidazole is considered the initial drug of choice for equine *C difficile* colitis, it is noteworthy that empiric metronidazole use in the treatment of human patients with presumptive CDAD may not be justified in most (75%) patients and that empiric metronidazole use should be reserved for the patients at highest risk [68]. Although this may be a logical approach to enterocolitis in mature horses, it may not necessarily apply to equine neonates. Because of the potentially primary pathogenic nature of *C difficile* in foals, the apparent clinical effectiveness of metronidazole in affected foals [46], and the high-risk nature of equine neonates, it seems reasonable to initiate metronidazole therapy (10–15 mg/kg administered orally two or three times daily) in foals with diarrhea with or without a *C difficile* toxin-positive fecal sample, especially in certain geographic regions in which clostridial-associated diarrhea is frequently recognized. The importance of ongoing daily fecal sample submission for isolation and toxin detection for *C difficile*, followed by antimicrobial susceptibility testing, should be emphasized, however.

Metronidazole has been administered parenterally to adult horses and foals. Limited data from human patients suggest that intravenously administered metronidazole may also be useful in the treatment of *C difficile*–associated colitis, with intracolonic therapeutic concentrations achieved by excretion of the drug into bile and exudation across inflamed tissue [69].

Bacitracin for the treatment of acute enterocolitis in horses should no longer be considered appropriate based on recent studies documenting widespread resistance among *C difficile* isolates [41,55].

Adjunctive therapeutic options for the management of *C difficile* colitis in horses include oral administration of probiotics, such as *Saccharomyces* spp, *Lactobacillus* spp, di-tri-octahedral (DTO) smectite (Bio-sponge; Platinum Performance, Buellton, California), adsorbent and immune products, and fecal transfaunation. The use of these treatments in horses is based on evidence from studies in human medicine, and few prospective investigations exist in equine patients, although the use of these treatments seems to be a growing area of interest. These alternative therapies are discussed in further detail elsewhere in this article.

Clostridium perfringens

The treatment of diarrhea in foals has recently been reviewed [70]. Briefly, successful treatment of enterocolitis in neonatal foals caused by *C perfringens* requires early and aggressive intravenous fluid therapy with a combination of crystalloid and colloid fluids. In severe cases, acid-base abnormalities may not correct with replacement fluid therapy alone and require specific treatment with isotonic sodium bicarbonate. The use of inotropic or vasopressor support should also be considered when physical parameters and markers of tissue perfusion do not respond adequately to volume resuscitation. Broad-spectrum systemic antimicrobial therapy with good anaerobic coverage, such as intravenous penicillin in combination with an aminoglycoside, and orally or intravenously administered metronidazole (10–15 mg/kg administered twice daily) are indicated. There is some anecdotal evidence that oral administration of metronidazole may be more effective than intravenous administration as a means of inhibiting small intestinal bacterial proliferation locally. To the authors' knowledge, resistance of *C perfringens* to metronidazole has not been documented as it has with *C difficile*. Additional therapy includes complete withholding of milk feeding for 24 to 96 hours or longer, because villous necrosis leads to malabsorption and feeding contributes to the development of osmotic diarrhea and abdominal pain. There is also some suggestion that milk provides a favorable medium for ongoing bacterial proliferation and toxin production [71].

Advances in the management of *C perfringens* enterocolitis in neonates lie in early recognition of the disease, withholding feed, and immediate or early institution of partial or total parenteral nutrition. A practical, easy-to-administer, and cost-effective recipe for parenteral nutrition has been described [70,72]. Reintroduction to oral fluids should occur gradually, with the feeding of small frequent meals. Observing tolerance to oral electrolyte solutions may be attempted before milk feeding. Addition of oral lactase (Lactaid tablets; 6000 U per 50-kg foal administered orally every 3 to 8 hours) can aid in small intestinal absorption of milk. The suggested off-label use of *C perfringens* type C and D antitoxins orally (10–20 mL administered orally once daily) early in the course of the disease may be beneficial, although there is no scientific evidence for efficacy. Hyperimmune plasma specific for *C perfringens* is also available (MG Biologics, Ames, Iowa) and may be administered for its potential specific immune effects and nonspecific beneficial coagulation and oncotic effects. Antiulcer medication, including sucralfate, is a preventative therapy commonly used by the authors. Anti-inflammatory therapy in the form of intravenously administered ketoprofen (1.1 mg/kg twice daily or 2.2 mg/kg once daily) should be considered and used judiciously in neonates. Control of abdominal pain is usually adequately achieved with low doses of intravenously or intramuscularly administered butorphanol (0.04–0.1 mg/kg). In severe cases, the degree of intestinal blood loss requires whole blood transfusion. Adjunctive treatment with DTO-smectite, administered as a paste, and *Saccharomyces* spp may be beneficial.

Successful treatment of acute disease may be followed by the development of segmental infarction of intestine secondary to coagulopathy and vessel thrombosis, intestinal adhesions secondary to fibrinous peritonitis, or long-term ill-thrift [56].

Treatment of adult horses is generally the same as that in neonatal foals, except that the use of broad-spectrum antimicrobial therapy is less often indicated unless significant neutropenia is documented or there is suspicion of septicemia. Metronidazole therapy alone or in combination with penicillin is recommended, although the risk of antimicrobial-induced colitis is much greater in adult horses; thus, these drugs should be used cautiously. Interestingly, in some European countries, gentamicin has been shown to induce β_2-toxin production in vitro. In addition, horses clinically affected with typhlocolitis attributable to β_2-toxigenic *C perfringens* showed reduced disease after cessation of gentamicin therapy [73]. The significance of this finding in clinical cases requires further investigation.

Equine proliferative enteropathy (*Lawsonia intracellularis*)

Diagnosis

Equine proliferative enteropathy (EPE) is a well-described transmissible enteric disease caused by the bacterium *L intracellularis*. The disease has been reported in horses as sporadic isolated cases in various parts of the United States, Canada, and Australia. Proliferative enteropathy, or intestinal adenomatosis, is best described in swine, in which it is an endemic disease typically causing reduced growth rates and diarrhea in weanling age pigs. In addition to swine, proliferative enteropathy has been sporadically observed in a variety of other species [74].

Definitive antemortem diagnosis of proliferative enteropathy in horses involves a combination of recognition of characteristic clinical findings and laboratory confirmation by serologic testing for the presence of antibodies to *L intracellularis* and pathogen detection in feces using a PCR assay.

EPE primarily affects weanling foals between the ages of 3 and 6 months and is characterized by profound dullness, fever, weight loss, colic, diarrhea, and hypoproteinemia causing ventral edema. Typical clinicopathologic abnormalities include leukocytosis, mild anemia, mild to severe hypoproteinemia, and occasional hyperfibrinogenemia. Electrolyte and acid-base abnormalities reflect the degree of gastrointestinal losses secondary to diarrhea and may include hyponatremia, hypokalemia, hypocalcemia, and metabolic acidosis. Less consistent abnormalities include the presence of azotemia, a high creatine kinase level, and hypoglycemia. Abdominal ultrasound is a useful diagnostic aid and typically reveals loops of moderate to markedly thickened small intestine (Fig. 2). Peritoneal fluid analysis is often unremarkable.

Gross pathologic lesions in EPE are characteristic of the disease and are typified by segmental mucosal hypertrophy involving the ileum and terminal jejunum, although the entire small intestine may be involved in severe cases [74]. Histologic examination of intestinal tissue, coupled with Warthin-Starry silver staining or immunohistochemistry, is diagnostic for EPE and reveals the hallmark findings of small intestinal hyperplasia and the presence of curved intracellular bacteria in the apical cytoplasm of crypt cells [73]. Organisms can also be identified in mucosal smears of proliferative small intestine or in cell culture monolayers by the modified Ziehl-Neelsen stain with dilute carbol fuchsin [75]. Because of the obvious disadvantages of postmortem diagnostic testing for EPE, efforts over the past few years have led to some major advances in the development and improvement of antemortem diagnosis.

A diagnosis of EPE can be established in clinically affected animals using molecular diagnostic techniques, such as demonstrating *L intracellularis* in fecal samples or tissue specimens by PCR and serologic testing for the presence of antibody to *L intracellularis* (D.J. Feary, BVSc, MS, unpublished data, 2005). Because of the organism's obligatory intracellular nature, isolation of the bacterium requires cell culture medium and is not routinely performed.

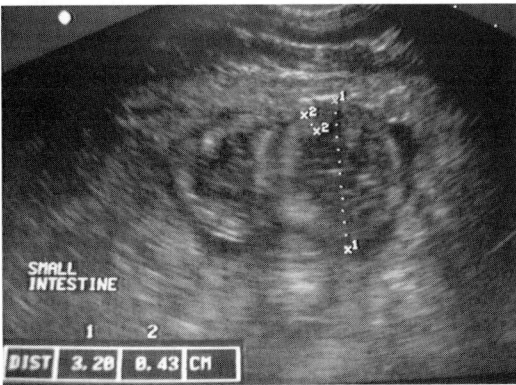

Fig. 2. Abdominal ultrasound image of moderately thickened loops of small intestine in a foal with EPE.

Nested [76] and multiplex PCR [77] techniques have been developed and are considered to have a high specificity in animals with active infection. Novel real-time PCR assays are available and may replace conventional methods for diagnosis of *L intracellularis* infection because of rapid test results, reduced risk of contamination, and the ability to test large sample numbers and to quantitate bacterial DNA. The sensitivity of PCR assays on fecal samples can be reduced, however, because of the presence of PCR-inhibitory factors that inactivate or interfere with components of the test [78] and by the time of sampling, as determined by the degree of bacterial shedding in feces, resulting in false-negative results.

The detection of *L intracellularis* in feces corresponds to the sloughing of infected intestinal epithelial cells in clinically affected animals [73]. The time of initial detection and duration of fecal shedding of *L intracellularis* in equids have not been determined, nor has the sensitivity of a PCR assay on equine feces. Results of a PCR assay on feces may remain positive for only a short time after initiation of specific antimicrobial therapy (D.J. Feary, BVSc, MS, unpublished data, 2005). Based on proliferative enteropathy in swine, reported cases in equids, and clinical observation of EPE, it seems likely that the sensitivity of detection of *L intracellularis* by PCR assay on fecal samples of horses with clinical disease would be improved by collection of samples before initiating specific antimicrobial therapy, or from environmental fecal samples retrospectively if this is not possible, followed by sequential daily fecal samples. *L intracellularis* DNA may be detected in environmental fecal samples after a few days (D.J. Feary, BVSc, MS, personal observation, 2005). Ideally, fecal samples should be refrigerated if transportation to the testing laboratory for analysis is required.

Serologic analysis for the presence of antibodies to *L intracellularis* using a serum IFA test or an immunoperoxidase monolayer assay (IPMA) is another means of diagnosis. Positive serum titers for naturally infected horses are commonly reported between 1:30 and 1:120 [79] but have been detected as high as 1:960 in one foal [80]. Because studies reporting experimental infection of horses with *L intracellularis* are not yet available, the time of detection and duration of serologic responses in horses are unknown. Antibodies to *L intracellularis* have been detected approximately 14 days after infection, however, and 7 to 14 days after the appearance of clinical signs in experimentally infected swine [73]. Negative serologic results at the time of presentation reflect acute infection and inadequate time to mount a detectable specific immune response. In addition, serologically positive foals and adult horses without clinical signs have been detected on the premises where a clinically affected foal was housed (D.J. Feary, BVSc, MS, unpublished data, 2005) and in the dam of an affected foal [81]. These findings suggest that the presence or magnitude of the serologic response alone may not be a sensitive test for definitive diagnosis of EPE.

Submission of serum and multiple fecal samples for PCR testing is recommended to enhance the chance of obtaining a diagnosis of EPE, because the presence of antibodies to *L intracellularis* in serum and fecal shedding of the organism may not necessarily coincide.

Treatment

L intracellularis proliferative enteropathy in foals, unlike the case in swine, is a debilitating and invariably fatal disease if left untreated. The prognosis is excellent with accurate diagnosis and prompt initiation of supportive care and specific antimicrobial therapy directed against intracellular bacteria, however.

Most cases successfully treated involved the use of erythromycin alone (15–25 mg/kg administered orally three or four times daily) or in combination with rifampin (5–10 mg/kg administered orally twice daily) for a period of 21 days [79,81]. Other effective antimicrobial agents used for the treatment of EPE include penicillin, ampicillin, chloramphenicol, and doxycycline [82]. The authors have successfully treated EPE with azithromycin at a dose of 10 mg/kg administered orally once daily for 5 days, followed 10 mg/kg administered orally every other day, in combination with rifampin (5 mg/kg administered orally twice daily). The use of azithromycin alone or in combination with rifampin may be an effective alternative, because azithromycin has been shown to be more effective in the treatment of *Rhodococcus equi* in foals and has fewer side effects and reduced frequency of administration compared with erythromycin [83].

Supportive care for the management of foals with EPE may include correction of fluid and electrolyte deficits with a combination of crystalloid and colloid therapy; anti-inflammatory, antidiarrheal, and antiulcer therapy; and pain management. The early parenteral administration of colloids in the form of plasma or hetastarch should be emphasized, because affected foals can be profoundly hypoproteinemic. Hypoproteinemia and subsequent peripheral edema may be exacerbated by administration of crystalloid fluids; thus, close patient monitoring may be necessary. Normalization of the plasma protein concentration in response to therapy may be slow compared with improvement in clinical signs and other measurements [79]. Nutritional support in the form of enteral or parenteral nutrition should also be addressed. Foals that tolerate enteral feeding may be fed small frequent meals consisting of low-bulk and easily digestible complete pelleted feeds as well as good-quality alfalfa hay. In severe cases, foals that continue to show signs of abdominal pain, are anorexic, or are in poor body condition may require additional support in the form of parenteral nutrition.

Parasitic enteritis

Diagnosis

The most commonly implicated parasites that may result in acute or chronic enterocolitis in horses are strongyles. Strongyle infections are caused by two groups of nematodes: large (strongylosis) and small (cyathostomiasis) strongyles. Although large strongyle infections were identified as an important cause of colic, and occasionally chronic diarrhea, in horses before the development of modern anthelmintics, the small strongyles have emerged in more recent years as a major cause of acute and chronic diarrhea as well as being implicated as a cause of colic. Advances in the diagnosis and treatment of larval cyathostomiasis are thus the focus of this section.

With the widespread use of interval treatment with broad-spectrum anthelmintics in recent decades, such as the benzimidazoles, pyrantel, and ivermectin, cyathostomes have become ubiquitous parasites and virtually all grazing horses from temperate regions are assumed to be infected with them. Interval treatment with these drugs is highly effective at reducing the prevalence of large strongyles, such as *Strongylus vulgaris*, but it is relatively ineffective at controlling the cyathostomes [84]. Cyathostomes are currently believed to be the most commonly identified cause of chronic diarrhea in the horse and also may be associated with acute and potentially fatal colitis [2]. Paradoxically, one risk factor associated with the development of acute larval cyathostomiasis is recent treatment with adulticidal anthelmintics. Other risk factors for clinical cyathostomiasis are the age of the horse, with horses aged 1 to 6 years most commonly affected, and seasonal occurrence [85]. In temperate zones, most cases classically occur in association with emergence of larvae from a hypobiotic state in the mucosa of the large intestine in the late winter and spring months [2]. In the southeastern United States and subtropical regions, emergence occurs in late fall and winter [2].

Definitive diagnosis of cyathostomiasis can be difficult, but in cases of clinical cyathostomiasis, diagnosis typically consists of evaluation of signalment, history, and epidemiologic risk factors as described previously as well as fecal examination, hematologic examination, serum biochemistry, and histologic examination of cecal or large colon biopsies if surgical exploration has been performed [84]. Cyathostome larvae may be visible with the naked eye in the feces or on a glove after rectal examination. Larvae vary in size and appearance depending on the species of cyathostome and may be red or white in color. Fecal worm egg counts are of little help diagnostically, because disease is caused by larval stages of the parasite. Routine hematologic examination may reveal leukocytosis with neutrophilia and, occasionally, anemia or mild eosinophilia. Profound hypoalbuminemia is usually present, but hyperglobulinemia may mask this when evaluating total protein (TP) concentration. Histologic examination of rectal biopsies is often nondiagnostic; however, if biopsies of the cecum or large colon are possible, they are likely to show characteristic pathologic changes, including edema and eosinophilic inflammation, with or without identification of mucosal larvae [84].

The identification of prepatent infection with cyathostomes remains difficult, because life-threatening burdens of larval stages of the parasite may exist in a subclinical state. These inhibited (hypobiotic) larvae are also relatively resistant to several of the currently available anthelmintics [84].

Current research efforts are focused on investigating the host immune responses that the mucosal larvae invoke, and molecular tools have been developed to help facilitate identification of larval and egg stages of cyathostomes [86]. Research is also in progress to develop an immunodiagnostic test that allows numbers of mucosal larvae to be estimated. This test uses antigen-specific IgG(T) serum antibody responses as markers of infection [86]. Additionally, studies are underway to develop molecular methods for the early detection of anthelmintic-resistant genotypes [86].

Treatment

There are currently three chemical classes of anthelmintics with a broad spectrum of activity in common use in horses. Each has a discrete mode of action, and they include the macrocyclic lactones (eg, ivermectin, moxidectin), benzimidazoles (eg, fenbendazole), and pyrimidines (eg, pyrantel pamoate). The selection pressure of frequent administration of deworming doses for parasite control programs has been associated with the development of resistance of small strongyles to the effects of benzimidazoles, with up to 97.7% of farms in the southern United States reported to have fenbendazole-resistant cyathostomes [87]. Resistance to ivermectin has not been recognized to date [88]; however, repeated dosing is necessary, because efficacy is primarily directed toward the maturing larvae as they begin development from an arrested state [84]. Specifics regarding anthelmintic treatment of parasite-associated disease have been reviewed [89].

In acute colitis secondary to larval cyathostomiasis, death rates may be as high as 60% in severe cases [84]. In addition to the standard supportive care for colitis consisting of fluids, electrolytes, colloids, antidiarrheal agents, and nutritional support, treatment of horses with colitis secondary to cyathostomiasis may include anthelmintic and corticosteroid therapy. A suggested corticosteroid protocol consists of dexamethasone (50 µg/kg administered intravenously or intramuscularly) for 1 to 5 days, followed by oral prednisolone (1 mg/kg administered orally) until the diarrhea has resolved [84].

Duodenitis–proximal jejunitis

Diagnosis

Equine DPJ is an inflammatory condition characterized by functional ileus of the small intestine and resulting in distention, abdominal pain, and gastric reflux [90]. Clinically, horses with this condition may have signs of severe endotoxemia and dehydration but relatively mild pain [91]. Horses may show abdominal pain initially; after gastric decompression, volume replacement, and analgesic therapy, the colic signs subside but signs of lethargy and depression predominate [90]. Differentiating DPJ from a strangulating or nonstrangulating mechanical obstruction of the small intestine can be a diagnostic challenge. Differentiating characteristics may include persistent abdominal pain until surgical repair or visceral rupture has occurred in horses with mechanical obstructions and large volumes of nasogastric reflux with each decompressive effort that are often malodorous and orange brown or red brown in color in horses with DPJ. Horses with DPJ also commonly have a low-grade fever, endotoxemia and dull mentation, and high liver enzyme activity [92] and typically exhibit high peritoneal fluid protein concentrations (as with strangulating obstructions) without concurrent increases in nucleated cell count [90]. Although horses with strangulating obstructions may have low peritoneal fluid nucleated cell counts initially, the cell count tends to increase over time as necrosis of the affected segment of bowel progresses.

Abdominal ultrasound examination is a useful aid in diagnosis of DPJ and for evaluating the efficacy of therapy or the development of small intestinal ileus. Differentiation of strangulated small intestine from generalized ileus caused by DPJ may be difficult via ultrasound examination; both may be associated with thickening of the intestinal wall and loss of intestinal motility, but identification of duodenal involvement or progressive peritoneal fluid accumulation associated with peritonitis from ischemic bowel may provide a clue as to the disease etiology.

Although the initiating cause of DPJ is unknown, several studies have suggested several etiologic agents, including *Clostridium* spp [93,94], *Salmonella* spp, and mycotoxins [95]. The most recent work suggests *C difficile* as an agent likely involved in the pathogenesis of DPJ [94]. Toxigenic strains of *C difficile* were successfully cultured from a small population of horses with DPJ, and similar histopathologic changes were identified in horses with fatal *C difficile*–associated enterocolitis and in nonsurvivors with DPJ [94]. Additional recent work demonstrated that feeding larger quantities of concentrate in the diet and pasture grazing are risk factors for DPJ [96].

Treatment

Treatment for DPJ typically entails the following therapeutic objectives: alleviation of gastric and small intestinal distention, replenishing fluid and electrolyte losses, combating endotoxemia, and restoring normal gastrointestinal motility. This is accomplished primarily via supportive care, such as intravenous fluid, electrolyte, and colloid supplementation; NSAIDs; and gastric decompression. Advanced monitoring techniques, including the use of arterial blood pressure monitoring, central venous pressure (CVP), and serial abdominal ultrasonography, to assess efficacy of treatment and progression of ileus may be advantageous. The use of antimicrobial agents remains controversial, but surgical exploration, followed by oral metronidazole administration after gastric decompression, has been advocated by some authors based on evidence of a clostridial etiology for the disease [91].

Prokinetic medications are routinely used with variable efficacy in the hope of shortening the course of the disease. Current theory suggests that ileus occurs primarily as a consequence of extensive local inflammation within the intestinal wall, resulting in the release of mediators that disrupt motility. The most commonly used prokinetic medications used in horses include lidocaine, erythromycin, metoclopramide, and cisapride. Lidocaine is the preferred first-choice prokinetic agent based on a recent survey of American College of Veterinary Surgeons (ACVS) diplomates who perform intestinal surgery [97]. Its efficacy likely results from its anti-inflammatory effects rather than from blockade of sympathetic inhibitory reflexes [98]. It is known to decrease neutrophil recruitment and activation [98]. Added benefits of lidocaine include analgesia and reduction of inhalant anesthetic requirements while under general anesthesia. The dose most frequently used is a 1.3-mg/kg intravenously administered loading dose, followed by a 0.05-mg/kg/min constant rate infusion (CRI).

Erythromycin is thought to initiate the migrating motor complex via motilin receptors. Even when using the low doses administered for prokinetic effects, a potentially serious side effect is fatal colitis. Metoclopramide is a dopamine receptor antagonist and also promotes acetylcholine release from cholinergic neurons via 5-hydroxytryptamine $(HT)_4$ receptors. The most commonly used dose is a 0.04-mg/kg/h CRI. A new prokinetic agent (Tegaserod, Novartis Pharmaceuticals Corp., East Hanover, New Jersey), a gastrointestinal-specific $5\text{-}HT_4$ receptor agonist that increases borborygmi and defecation in normal horses without the side effects of other $5\text{-}HT_4$ receptor agonists [99], has recently been investigated.

The authors have had good success with the use of a lidocaine CRI (0.05 mg/kg/min) in combination with a metoclopramide CRI (0.03–0.04 mg/kg/h) in horses with ileus secondary to DPJ. Anecdotally, the use of these agents concurrently seems to be more effective than either drug alone.

Advances in monitoring

Adult horses and foals with enterocolitis often have life-threatening hemodynamic abnormalities that require intensive therapy. It is these most critical patients in which the use of advanced monitoring techniques can potentially improve patient management and survival. Regular repeated or continuous monitoring in equine patients with enterocolitis facilitates the early detection of correctable abnormalities and directed therapeutic intervention. A complete and detailed review of routine and advanced monitoring in critically ill equine patients is available [99]. In this article, the authors provide a brief overview of the application of monitoring techniques that may be relevant to mature horses and foals with enterocolitis.

The major hemodynamic abnormality in equine patients with enterocolitis is volume depletion because of large fluid deficits and ongoing losses related to gastric reflux or diarrhea. Hypovolemia and subsequent hypoperfusion of vital organ systems and tissue microcirculation eventually lead to multiple organ dysfunction. This can be complicated by sepsis in the neonate and endotoxemia in the mature horse. Thus, the mainstay of treatment of horses and foals with enterocolitis is fluid therapy using a combination of crystalloids and colloids.

Some or all of the following monitoring aids can provide important information about the metabolic and circulatory status of the equine patient and response to fluid therapy. Detecting trends in monitored variables provides more valuable information than the result of a single test, emphasizing the need for monitoring at regular intervals.

Clinical assessment

Although seemingly obvious, a thorough physical examination provides the easiest and least expensive means of detecting deficits in volume and perfusion, remembering that clinical abnormalities are generally undetectable until the degree of dehydration reaches greater than 5%. Physically detectable indicators of hypovolemia include the following: (1) tachycardia, (2) pale mucous membranes, (3) prolonged capillary refill time, (4) dull mentation, (5) cool extremities, (6) poor peripheral pulse quality, (7) prolonged jugular refill, and (8) reduced urine output. Physically detectable indicators of hypoperfusion include the following: (1) dry mucous membranes, (2) sunken eyes (especially foals), (3) reduced tear film production, and (4) decreased skin turgor compared with normal [100].

Additional information obtained from hematology and serum biochemistry that support these findings includes elevated packed cell volume (PCV), TP plasma concentration, and prerenal azotemia (elevated creatinine or blood urea nitrogen [BUN] level). Unfortunately, PCV and TP are not sensitive markers of circulatory status in horses or foals with enterocolitis, because splenic contraction and individual variation can greatly influence PCV and gastrointestinal protein loss resulting in hypoproteinemia is common. Critically ill neonatal foals have been observed to mount an appropriate physiologic response to hypotension and hypoperfusion [101] inconsistently, making heart rate and PCV unpredictable indicators of circulatory status in foals [102].

The creatinine concentration at presentation rarely exceeds 4 mg/dL if azotemia is prerenal in origin. Serial monitoring of PCV and TP, at least at 12-hour intervals, and of creatinine plus or minus BUN levels, every 12 to 24 hours initially, provides more useful information and is indicated for monitoring the response to intravenous fluid therapy. Failure of the creatinine concentration to return to normal values within 24 hours suggests ongoing volume deficits or underlying renal disease.

Electrolytes

Electrolyte and acid-base abnormalities are common in horses and foals with gastrointestinal disease. Hypocalcemia and hypomagnesemia are also commonly detected in equine patients with various gastrointestinal diseases, endotoxemia, and sepsis [103–105]. Calcium and magnesium levels should be frequently evaluated in horses with gastrointestinal disease because of their important role in maintaining normal visceral and vascular smooth muscle function, and deficits should be promptly corrected so as to reduce their contribution to gastrointestinal ileus. Serum ionized calcium and magnesium concentrations are more sensitive than total values, and the magnitude of ionized hypocalcemia and hypomagnesemia tends to increase with the severity of disease [103,106]. Ionized hypocalcemia has been detected in 80% of horses with enterocolitis [104]. A recent report has shown that ionized hypocalcemia in horses with gastrointestinal disease is significantly associated with the development of paralytic ileus and the probability of reduced short-term survival [106]. The need for repeated calcium supplementation in these patients correlated with decreased overall survival, although this finding was not statistically significant [106].

Results of these studies emphasize the importance of measuring ionized calcium and magnesium in adult horses and foals with enterocolitis. Sodium and chloride deficits are common in patients with enterocolitis secondary to gastrointestinal and potentially concurrent renal loss. These abnormalities are generally rapidly and easily corrected with isotonic intravenous fluid therapy. Particular attention should be paid to serum potassium concentrations, which can be significantly decreased in patients with colitis because of reduced dietary intake. Hypokalemia may contribute to ileus and dull mentation. Hypokalemia may be refractory to supplementation, especially in the face of concurrent hypomagnesemia. Prompt recognition of hypokalemia and supplementation with potassium aimed at restoring serum concentrations to within the normal range are recommended to support gastrointestinal and cardiovascular function.

Arterial blood pressure

Blood pressure, as an estimate of blood flow, is determined by cardiac output (heart rate × stroke volume) and systemic vascular resistance (vasomotor tone). Mean arterial pressure (MAP) rather than systolic or diastolic pressure is more important for perfusion and is more practically measured via indirect techniques in clinically ill horses and foals [99,107,108]. Serial monitoring of MAP in equine patients with enterocolitis can be used to assess the adequacy of fluid therapy or the need for additional support using inotropic or pressor agents. Because MAP poorly reflects blood flow when systemic vascular resistance is altered, such as during sepsis and endotoxemia, MAP should be used in conjunction with other markers of oxygen delivery, such as venous oxygen saturation (Svo_2) and blood lactate [99,109].

Indirect blood pressure in normal adult horses is approximately 90 to 120 mm Hg and ranges between 60 and 120 mm Hg for normal neonatal foals [99]. Lower values for MAP may be observed in premature foals and in the immediate postpartum period (K.G. Magdesian, DVM, personal communication, 2005). Ideally, measurements should be repeated three times, with the average value for MAP recorded. The exact blood pressure at which therapeutic intervention in the form of volume, inotropic, or pressor support is indicated is unknown for unanesthetized equine patients with gastrointestinal disease. Some authors support the recommendation that tissue perfusion in neonatal foals is inadequate when MAP is less than 60 mm Hg, however [109,110]. At values less than 60 mm Hg in other mammalian species, pressure autoregulation of vital organs fails and flow becomes pressure dependent. Organ perfusion may be adequate at a MAP considerably lower than this in premature foals, as is the case in preterm human infants [111]. A recent study demonstrated a poor correlation between blood pressure and cardiac output, at least in anesthetized foals [112]. Measurement of cardiac output in critical adult horses and foals may become a practical method of assessing circulatory status of clinical cases in the future, with promising developments in noninvasive volumetric echocardiography techniques [112].

Central venous pressure

CVP is an invasive but valuable monitoring tool used to direct fluid therapy in hypovolemic patients. CVP provides an estimate of venous return to the heart, reflecting the balance between central venous blood volume, venous capacitance, and right-sided cardiac function [100]. It has been suggested that CVP may be a better indicator of intravascular volume status than arterial blood pressure, because there is less influence of vascular resistance and autoregulation [113]. CVP can be particularly useful in equine patients with enterocolitis because their frequently hypoproteinemic state or the presence of acute renal failure predisposes them to iatrogenic fluid overload and secondary edema formation.

A low CVP ($<7-12$ cm H_2O) in adult horses and ponies and $<2.8-12$ cm H_2O in foals) is consistent with hypovolemia (or venodilation) [99]. A rise in CVP to within the normal range indicates adequate fluid resuscitation, and a persistent increase in CVP indicates overzealous fluid administration or right-sided heart failure. Monitoring of CVP requires placement of a catheter into the central venous compartment via the jugular vein and has been described [99]. Monitoring trends in CVP as a means of directing fluid therapy is more useful than a single measurement, remembering that CVP may also be increased by pleural or pericardial effusion, vasoconstriction, patient positioning, and technical factors (eg, air within the lines, catheter occlusion) [99].

Colloid osmotic (oncotic) pressure

Plasma osmotic pressure refers to the force created by large solute molecules (mainly albumin) that are not freely movable across the vascular membrane, and are thus important for retention of fluid within the vascular compartment. The balance between the colloid osmotic pressure (COP;

favoring retention) and the opposing force exerted by hydrostatic pressure (favoring filtration) is often unbalanced in equine patients with acute enterocolitis. Inflammation of the intestinal wall attributable to a variety of causes leads to endothelial damage and consequent increased capillary permeability. Leakage of protein (mainly albumin) into the interstitium results in decreased plasma oncotic pressure, increased interstitial oncotic pressure, and net efflux of fluid from the capillary into the interstitium (edema). This imbalance may be compensated for early in disease by increased lymph flow that serves to reduce the interstitial protein concentration. The administration of crystalloid fluids exacerbates the disruption in Starling's forces by diluting plasma proteins, increasing hydrostatic pressure, and promoting net fluid efflux from the capillary into the interstitium, resulting in overt edema.

Hypoproteinemia is of concern because it can lead to hypovolemia and because interstitial edema occurs in all body tissues, in addition to the subcutaneous tissues, potentially resulting in organ dysfunction. Measurement of total plasma solids using refractometry proves a rough estimation of colloid oncotic pressure, with values less than 4.0 to 4.2 g/dL in horses generally associated with overt edema. COP can be estimated indirectly by calculation from plasma albumin and globulin measurements (eg, Landis-Pappenheimer equation), but these are not as predictive of COP in sick adult horses and foals [114] compared with healthy patients. COP can be measured directly with the use of commercial analyzers (Wescor 4420 colloid osmometer; Wescor, Logan, Utah). Normal COP in adult horses is similar to that in other animals (approximately 20–25 mm Hg) and is lower in foals (15–22 mm Hg) [99,114]. Monitoring the response to synthetic colloid administration also requires direct osmometry, because indirect measurements do not reflect the contribution of synthetic colloids to COP.

Lactate

Lactate is produced as the end product of anaerobic glycolysis. Hyperlactatemia most commonly reflects inadequate tissue perfusion and oxygen delivery associated with hypovolemia and dehydration; thus, it is a useful monitoring and prognostic tool in horses and foals with enterocolitis. Other pathophysiologic causes of lactate accumulation should always be considered when interpreting hyperlactatemia, however. These include other reasons for reduced tissue perfusion, such as hypotension and hypoxemia; impaired lactate clearance by the liver in liver disease; and hypermetabolic states, such as sepsis, vigorous exercise, and seizures [115]. High concentrations of circulating endogenous and exogenous catecholamines can also increase blood lactate, as can exogenous glucose administration and severe alkalosis [115]. Endotoxemia is frequently associated with the pathophysiology of enterocolitis in adult horses and can cause hyperlactatemia without inadequate tissue oxygenation. This can be explained by endotoxin-mediated inhibition of the enzyme pyruvate dehydrogenase, which is necessary for the oxidation of pyruvate in the mitochondria [115]. Thiamine is a cofactor for pyruvate dehydrogenase, and although rarely recognized in horses, thiamine deficiency also increases blood lactate via a similar mechanism to endotoxin [115]. Blood lactate in normal adult horses is less than 2 mmol/L and less than 2.5 mmol/L in normal 24-hour-old neonatal foals [99], and it can increase to 30 mmol/L in critically ill equine patients (D.J. Feary, BVSc, MS, personal observation, 2005). The degree of hyperlactatemia and lactic acidosis is fairly well correlated with the severity of tissue hypoperfusion and has prognostic value in horses with acute abdominal disease [116]. Recently, Corley and colleagues [102] showed a significant association between admission lactate level, severity of illness, and hospital survival in critically ill neonatal foals. Interestingly, foals with a diagnosis of colitis in this study were found to have the lowest average admission lactate levels of the groups of foals examined [102]. In one study, the mean plasma lactate concentration at admission for horses with acute colitis and subclinical disseminated intravascular coagulopathy (DIC) was 6.5 mmol/L [117].

As with other monitoring tools, serial blood lactate measurement provides much more useful information than a single measurement. A rapid decrease in lactate concentration in response to specific treatment of hypoperfusion is a favorable prognostic indicator and likely has a predictive value equal to if not better than the lactate concentration before therapy. Lactate is a sensitive indicator of tissue hypoperfusion and can be used to detect occult hypovolemic or hypotensive states before measurable changes in clinical parameters; therefore, evaluation of lactate concentration may be useful when tailoring specific therapy, particularly inotropic or vasopressor support.

Measurement of lactate in body fluids in addition to blood is a useful tool in the evaluation of sepsis and ischemia. Peritoneal fluid lactate has been shown to be a useful predictor of intestinal ischemia attributable to strangulating obstruction in horses with colic [118,119], and future studies may reveal the potential prognostic value of peritoneal fluid lactate in equine patients with severe enterocolitis.

Advances in treatment

Di-tri-octahedral smectite

DTO-smectite is a natural hydrated aluminomagnesium silicate that is commercially available for use in horses (Bio-sponge). DTO-smectite has been shown to adsorb substances, such as endotoxins and exotoxins, in the human gastrointestinal tract effectively and, more recently, to bind equine-origin *C difficile* toxins A and B as well as *C perfringens* enterotoxin in vitro without any effect on bacterial growth or the action of metronidazole [120]. In vivo studies on the treatment of enterocolitis have not been published, but at this time, the authors use DTO-smectite at an initial dose of 1 to 2 lb mixed with water and delivered via a nasogastric tube, followed by 0.5 to 1 lb every 6 to 12 hours in mature horses with acute colitis. Results of a recent randomized clinical trial evaluating the use of DTO-smectite in postoperative colic patients revealed a marked reduction in the prevalence of postoperative diarrhea and improved clinical and hematologic parameters in treated horses compared with controls [121]. Treatment with DTO-smectite seems to have few if any adverse effects in mature horses and foals, and anecdotal reports suggest that it is effective at reducing the volume and duration of acute diarrhea in horses. Although its specific beneficial effect in clinical equine enterocolitis caused by *C difficile* is yet to be determined, the authors advocate its use in clinical cases. Treatment early in the course of disease seems to be most effective.

Probiotics

The role of biotherapy (therapy involving probiotics) in human medicine is evolving as a means to control CDAD. The theoretic beneficial effect of probiotic use as a means of preventing and treating CDAD is to provide naturally occurring bacteria to restore "colonization resistance" in the gastrointestinal tract attributable to disturbances caused by antimicrobial use, for example. Probiotics that have been proposed for this use in human beings include various bacteria (*Bifidobacterium* spp, *Lactobacillus* GG, *Lactobacillus rhamnosus*, *Lactobacillus casei*, *Lactobacillus plantarum* 299v, and *Enterococcus faecium*) and yeasts (*Saccharomyces boulardii* and *Saccharomyces cerevisiae*) [122,123]. Although showing early promising beneficial effects, a systematic review of randomized controlled trials of probiotic therapy for the prevention and treatment of CDAD in adult human patients found a paucity of eligible studies that did not provide convincing evidence to support a clinical benefit of probiotics [123].

Several studies have reviewed commercially available probiotic products for use in people and horses and have found that label descriptions of most products were inaccurate [124,125]. Products did not specifically list their contents, did not contain the organisms stated, contained lower concentrations of viable organisms than stated, contained additional species, or contained organisms that had no probiotic effect or were even potentially pathogenic [124,125]. Veterinary products performed particularly poorly [125]. These studies emphasize the fact that probiotic preparations are considered nutritional supplements rather than pharmacologic agents; as a result regulatory control does not require scientific evidence for efficacy or safety [126]. In addition, even if probiotic preparations contained the labeled concentration of viable organisms at the time of use, the dose required to be efficacious is not reported for horses. Based on extrapolation from human dosing regimens, it is highly unlikely that the amount required would be achievable in adult horses.

Weese and Rousseau [126] recently demonstrated the urgent need for safety and efficacy testing of all potential equine products with a randomized controlled clinical trial evaluating the efficacy of *Lactobacillus pentosus* WE7 for prevention of equine neonatal diarrhea. Although this organism demonstrated potentially beneficial properties in vitro, these were not evident in vivo, and administration was actually associated with the development of diarrhea and other significant clinical abnormalities.

In summary, although the use of probiotic preparations in horses is not generally associated with adverse effects, equine practitioners should educate clients regarding the lack of evidence supporting their use. Until scientific data become available through randomized controlled clinical trials conducted in horses, the administration of commercially available probiotics for treatment or prevention of equine acute enterocolitis seems to be the least supported of all available adjunctive therapies, and labeled claims should be cautiously evaluated. The use of probiotics in neonatal foals less than 24 hours of age should not be recommended because of the potential for reducing absorption of colostral immunoglobulin or nonselective absorption of potentially pathogenic organisms in the probiotic preparation.

S boulardii and *S cerevisiae* are yeasts that are commercially available in purified lyophilized capsules or granules that may be found in commercial horse feeds and as human and equine supplements [127]. Randomized controlled clinical trials evaluating the effectiveness of orally administered *S boulardii* for the prevention of antimicrobial-associated diarrhea in adults and children have established efficacy [128,129]. A recent report established efficacy of *S boulardii* for decreasing the duration and severity of clinical signs in horses with enterocolitis [130]. Further, the presence of viable yeast in feces of clinically normal horses after oral administration of the organism at a dosage of 25 g administered orally twice daily for 14 days was established [130]. Proposed mechanisms by which *S boulardii* exerts its beneficial effect are based on studies in laboratory animals and include inactivation of *C difficile* toxin A receptor, enhanced immunologic function in the gastrointestinal tract, competition for attachment sites, and its ability to block *C difficile* adherence to cells in vitro [131–133].

These studies support the use of *S boulardii* as an adjunctive treatment in people and horses undergoing antimicrobial therapy for certain diseases. In addition, yeasts are an excellent source of dietary fiber, chromium, and B-vitamins (with the exception of vitamin B_{12}) and are likely to be beneficial for resident microflora and colonocyte health [127]. Adverse effects, such as the development of *S boulardii* fungemia in severely ill or immunocompromised patients, have been reported, however [134].

The authors have experienced an apparent clinical response to the administration of *S cerevisiae* and *Lactobacillus* spp as a commercial equine supplement (Forco Feed Supplement; Forco Products, Flagler, Colorado) in horses with watery diarrhea (20 g administered orally four times daily), although response is unpredictable and patient-dependent.

Several prebiotic agents, such as psyllium and germinated barley foodstuff, have potential for the management of enterocolitis in horses, increasing fecal bulk by water absorption in the large colon and promoting bacterial growth, proliferation, and short-chain fatty acid production, an important energy source for supporting colonocyte function [127].

Fecal transfaunation

Administration of fecal enemas prepared from stool samples from healthy individuals has been reported to be effective in recurrent and refractory cases of *C difficile*–associated colitis in human patients [69]. The administration of donor stool via nasogastric tube has also been reported to be effective in preventing further diarrhea in recurrent *C difficile* infection [135]. Although stool transplantation may be associated with some risk of transmission of infectious disease, this can be avoided by performing prior laboratory testing. An important factor in performing fecal transfaunation is the administration of oral antacids, such as omeprazole, before the procedure so as to minimize microbial inhibition by the acid gastric environment. All antimicrobials should also be discontinued. Anecdotal reports of successful fecal transfaunation in horses via nasogastric tube as therapy for chronic diarrhea warrant further investigation. Equine veterinarians may obtain cecal contents from a horse that has died recently or may obtain fresh feces via rectal evacuation from an available healthy horse.

Adsorbents and immune products

Recurrent *C difficile*–associated colitis has been treated with varied success with intravenous human immunoglobulin, but further investigation is required before these products are recommended in human patients. Hyperimmune plasma specific for *C difficile* (MG Biologics, Ames, Iowa) is available for use in horses and has been used clinically as therapy for neonatal foal diarrhea [70].

An immune whey protein concentrate derived from the milk of immunized cows contains high concentrations of specific IgA antibodies against *C difficile* toxins and whole bacterial cells. Given orally to human patients with recurrent CDAD, this therapy has shown promise in preliminary studies [136], and randomized clinical trials are underway.

A number of killed and live-attenuated vaccines are undergoing investigation for human patients with recurrent CDAD [69]. A *C difficile* toxoid vaccine has been shown to induce an immune response to toxins A and B and an associated favorable clinical response in affected human patients, supporting further investigation [137]. Surgery is rarely indicated in human patients with enterocolitis and only for recurrent severe *C difficile* colitis associated with serious complications [138]. In horses, persistent signs of colic in association with rapidly deteriorating clinical parameters, progressive abdominal distention, and generalized ileus may necessitate exploratory celiotomy. Unfortunately, most of these cases do not respond to surgical treatment; however, if surgery is performed, a large colon enterotomy with colonic evacuation and infusion of DTO-smectite (1 lb) intraluminally in water (1–2 L) is recommended by the authors (Fig. 3).

Colloids

Hypoalbuminemia has been associated with increased morbidity and mortality in human and animal patients and is a frequent consequence of colitis and enteritis in adult horses and foals. Equine clinicians have a variety of options for specifically treating hypoproteinemia in critically ill patients, including biologic solutions, such as plasma, and synthetic colloids. These solutions differ with respect to the type and size of component molecules, COP, cost, and side effects [139–141]. These solutions may also be used in combination with crystalloids as part of optimal fluid resuscitation and management of many diseases resulting in hypovolemia, systemic inflammatory response syndrome (SIRS), and sepsis.

Recently, there has been renewed interest in the use of human albumin in critically ill small animal patients and anecdotal use in critically ill horses. Albumin constitutes 75% to 80% of the plasma COP, with 40% of total body albumin within the intravascular space and 60% in the interstitial space. The plasma albumin concentration decreases in critical illness because of reduced production (secondary to hypergammaglobulinemia), increased use (catabolism), and increased loss (eg, enteritis or colitis, SIRS, vasculitis). Albumin synthesis is also reduced in response to administration of artificial colloids. In addition to its significant contribution to COP, albumin has important functions in hemostasis as a carrier protein for certain drugs, endogenous hormones, metals, and enzymes and as a free radical

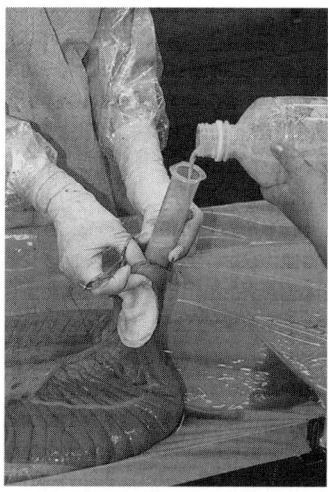

Fig. 3. Intraoperative administration of DTO-smectite (Platinum Performance, Buellton, California) in saline into the large colon through a pelvic flexure enterotomy.

scavenger in inflammatory states [142,143]. Human albumin is available as a 5% or concentrated (25%) solution and has an average COP of 200 mm Hg [142].

Nonsteroidal anti-inflammatory drugs

NSAID therapy has long been an integral component of therapy in horses with acute colitis to help negate the effects of endotoxin, subsequent cytotoxin release, and SIRS. These drugs are often used in combination with polymyxin B sulfate (3000 IU/kg in saline [1 L] administered intravenously twice daily) in an effort to bind circulating endotoxin to minimize the subsequent inflammatory response. The most commonly used NSAID in equine medicine is flunixin meglumine (0.25 mg/kg administered intravenously three times daily). Recent research has suggested that nonspecific inhibitors of the cyclooxygenase (COX) enzyme, such as flunixin meglumine, may have detrimental effects on the ability of the mucosa to repair itself after injury, however, thus potentially allowing further absorption of endotoxin from a damaged intestinal wall [144]. Prostaglandins play critical roles in the recovery process of injured gastrointestinal tissue, and traditional NSAIDs inhibit COX-1 and COX-2 in equine gastrointestinal tissue [145]. The COX-1 and COX-2 enzymes have recently been demonstrated to become markedly upregulated in response to ischemic injury of the large colon [145]. This suggests that COX-2 selective inhibitors may play an important role in the separation of proinflammatory and proreparative functions of COX-elaborated prostanoids, thus potentially optimizing treatment of horses with acute colitis.

Disseminated intravascular coagulopathy and heparin

DIC is a hot topic in human medicine that continues to evolve as our understanding of the pathophysiology of DIC changes. A unifying explanation of the pathophysiology of DIC is that it is a syndrome of dysregulated coagulation and inflammation that is associated with a diverse variety of clinical syndromes. In human patients, DIC is most commonly associated with sepsis. This is probably also true for foals; however, in adult horses, it seems to be most commonly associated with severe endotoxemia secondary to acute gastrointestinal disease. Widespread systemic activation of the coagulation, fibrinolytic, and antithrombotic systems creates a paradoxic disorder of microvascular thrombosis, hemorrhage, or both. Progression leads to multiple organ failure and death.

DIC remains a challenging syndrome to manage in equine patients with acute enterocolitis, which is probably the most common underlying disease associated with DIC in horses. In one study, the 1-year incidence of subclinical DIC in horses with acute colitis was 32% [146]. Thrombophlebitis, renal failure, and laminitis are all serious complications of acute enterocolitis in horses and are involved in the clinical progression of DIC in some cases, although this has not been demonstrated in clinical studies. Aortoiliac and digital artery thrombosis have been reported as serious and fatal complications of sepsis and enterocolitis in foals and adult horses [147,148]. Any means of preventing these complications would reduce morbidity, mortality, and cost of treatment.

The traditional definition of a diagnosis of DIC has revolved around the following criteria: three of six abnormal coagulation test results (platelet count, fibrinogen, prothrombin time [PT], activated partial thromboplastin time [PTT], antithrombin [AT], and fibrinogen degradation) combined with clinical signs of thrombosis or hemorrhage. Deficient AT is more likely to be detected in horses with enterocolitis because they have a greater risk for gastrointestinal and renal loss of AT as well as consumption in hypercoagulable states. In one study, horses with colitis and subclinical DIC were more likely to have AT deficiency and prolonged activated PTT than those without detectable DIC [146]. In a summary of findings across a group of studies comparing several coagulation tests and their correlation with outcome in equine patients, the PT was most consistently reported to correlate with survival [149]. The one routine test that has the least sensitivity for the diagnosis of DIC in horses is the fibrinogen concentration [150]. This is because horses seem to be quite efficient in their production of this acute-phase protein in response to inflammation. A lack of expected increase in fibrinogen concentration in response to inflammatory disease warrants further investigation in a horse that is likely to have DIC. The D-dimer assay is becoming a more widely used test of hemostasis in veterinary medicine. It is similar to fibrinogen degradation products (FDPs) in that it is a marker of fibrinolysis, but it is specific for the degradation of cross-linked fibrin. D-dimer measurement may be a useful indicator of a hypercoagulable state in horses with gastrointestinal disease and could potentially be useful in directing specific therapy for DIC.

Specific therapy for the prevention and treatment of DIC in high-risk patients includes providing stable clotting factors (II, VII, IX, and X), albumin, fibronectin, and AT in the form of fresh-frozen plasma as well as anticoagulants, such as aspirin and heparin. Thrombolytic agents, such as tissue plasminogen activator, streptokinase, and urokinase, are used for the treatment of macrovascular thrombosis in human and small animal patients and have been applied unsuccessfully in a small number of reported cases of thromboembolism in septic foals [148,151]. The most effective and important therapy for the DIC in any species is the identification and aggressive treatment of the underlying disease.

Current recommendations in critically ill small animal patients for the treatment of DIC are as follows. Prolongation of clotting times by 25% to 50% of the midrange of the reference interval (reference intervals vary considerably depending on the methodology used) indicates a significant defect in coagulation and warrants treatment with fresh-frozen plasma [152]. AT activity measured at less than 50% constitutes a significant risk for thrombosis or significant consumption. Therapy remains controversial, although AT administration (plasma or highly concentrated forms) seems the most promising method. Interestingly, quantities of AT in fresh-frozen plasma may be insufficient to alter hypercoagulable tendencies in small animals [153] and human beings [154]. Available evidence in these species suggests that supplementation of fresh-frozen plasma in patients with DIC syndromes characterized by hemorrhagic tendencies may be beneficial; however, for patients without significant risk for bleeding, administration of plasma is expensive and does not seem to improve survival rates [155]. In equine patients, it is important to consider carefully the risks of plasma therapy when making decisions regarding treatment. Although uncommon, the development of Theiler's disease (equine serum sickness) is being increasingly recognized as a highly fatal complication of plasma therapy in equine patients [156].

Heparin therapy for DIC in human patients has become controversial in recent years. There are positive and negative effects of heparin administration in animals and people with DIC. Positive effects include increased production of prostacyclin I_2, profound reduction of leukocyte activation and chemotaxis, and reduced transcription of inflammatory pathways through decreased nuclear factor (NF)-κB production [157]. Exogenous heparin has therapeutic effects in hypercoagulable thrombotic syndromes of DIC by augmentation of AT activity and inactivation of factors IIa (thrombin) and Xa (Stuart factor) of the clotting cascade. Administration of exogenous heparin inhibits the beneficial anti-inflammatory effects of AT, however [158]. This may have profound effects in patients with severe inflammatory diseases, such as enterocolitis.

Important advances with regard to heparin therapy in equine patients include the favorable pharmacokinetic properties of the low-molecular-weight heparins (LMWHs; dalteparin and enoxeparin) compared with conventional unfractionated heparin (UFH) therapy in horses [20,159]. LMWH is more expensive but has some important advantages over UFH that relate to its greater and more selective factor Xa inhibitory capacity and dose-dependent predictable pharmacokinetic properties. LMWH has a more rapid onset of action, higher bioavailability, and longer duration of action and does not have the cumulative individually variable side effects on red blood cells and platelets characteristic of UFH [160,161]. The reduced side effects of LMWH (dalteparin, 50 IU/kg administered subcutaneously once daily) compared with UFH in horses with colic have been reported in a clinical study, but effects on survival have not been reported [160]. It should be emphasized that LMWH does not affect clotting times as does UFH; therefore, the PTT should not used to predict plasma concentrations of heparin in treated animals.

References

[1] Smith BP. *Salmonella* infection in horses. Compend Contin Educ Pract Vet 1981;3(Suppl): S4–17.

[2] Jones SL. Inflammatory diseases of the gastrointestinal tract causing diarrhea. In: Reed SM, Bayly WM, Sellon DC, editors. Equine internal medicine. 2nd edition. St. Louis (MO): Elsevier; 2004. p. 884–913.
[3] Owen RR, Fullerton J, Barnum DA. Effects of transportation, surgery, and antibiotic therapy in ponies infected with Salmonella. Am J Vet Res 1983;44:46–50.
[4] Hird DW, Casebolt DB, Carter JD, et al. Risk factors for salmonellosis in hospitalized horses. J Am Vet Med Assoc 1986;188:173–7.
[5] House JK, Mainar-Jaime RC, Smith BP, et al. Risk factors for nosocomial Salmonella infection among hospitalized horses. J Am Vet Med Assoc 1999;214:1511–6.
[6] Traub-Dargatz JL, Salman MD, Jones RL. Epidemiologic study of salmonellae shedding in the feces of horses and potential risk factors for development of the infection in hospitalized horses. J Am Vet Med Assoc 1990;196:1617–22.
[7] Ernst NS, Hernandez JA, MacKay RJ, et al. Risk factors associated with fecal Salmonella shedding among hospitalized horses with signs of gastrointestinal tract disease. J Am Vet Med Assoc 2004;225:275–81.
[8] Schott HC, Ewart SL, Walker RD, et al. An outbreak of salmonellosis among horses at a veterinary teaching hospital. J Am Vet Med Assoc 2001;218:1152–9.
[9] Carter JD, Hird DW, Farver TB, et al. Salmonellosis in hospitalized horses: seasonality and case fatality rates. J Am Vet Med Assoc 1986;188:163–7.
[10] Traub-Dargatz JL, Garber LP, Fedorka-Cray PJ, et al. Fecal shedding of Salmonella spp by horses in the United States during 1998 and 1999 and detection of Salmonella spp in grain and concentrate sources on equine operations. J Am Vet Med Assoc 2000;217:226–30.
[11] Murray MJ. Salmonellosis in horses. J Am Vet Med Assoc 1996;209:558–60.
[12] Rhoads WS, Barton MH, Parks AH. Comparison of medical and surgical treatment for impaction of the small colon in horses: 84 cases (1986–1996). J Am Vet Med Assoc 1999;214: 1042–7.
[13] van Duijkeren E, Flemming C, Sloet van Oldruitenborgh-Oosterbaan M, et al. Diagnosing salmonellosis in horses: culturing of multiple versus single faecal samples. Vet Q 1995;17: 63–6.
[14] Palmer E, Whitlock RH, Benson CE, et al. Comparison of rectal mucosal cultures and fecal cultures in detecting Salmonella infection in horses and cattle. Am J Vet Res 1985;46:697–8.
[15] Cohen ND, Divers TL. Acute colitis in horses. Part I. Assessment. Compend Contin Educ Pract Vet 1998;20:92–8.
[16] Cohen ND, Martin LJ, Simpson RB, et al. Comparison of polymerase chain reaction and microbiological culture for detection of salmonellae in equine feces and environmental samples. Am J Vet Res 1996;57:780–6.
[17] Kurowski PB, Traub-Dargatz JL, Morley PS, et al. Detection of Salmonella spp in fecal specimens by use of real-time polymerase chain reaction assay. Am J Vet Res 2002;63: 1265–8.
[18] Alinovi CA, Ward MP, Couetil LL, et al. Detection of Salmonella organisms and assessment of a protocol for removal of contamination in horse stalls at a veterinary teaching hospital. J Am Vet Med Assoc 2004;223:1640–4.
[19] Hyatt DR, Weese JS. Salmonella culture: sampling procedures and laboratory techniques. Vet Clin North Am Equine Pract 2004;20:577–85.
[20] Dargatz DA, Traub-Dargatz JL. Multidrug-resistant Salmonella and nosocomial infections. Vet Clin North Am Equine Pract 2004;20:587–600.
[21] Divers TJ, Ball M. Medical treatment of acute enterocolitis in the mature horse. Equine Vet Educ 1996;8:204–7.
[22] Papich MG. Antimicrobial therapy for gastrointestinal diseases. Vet Clin North Am Equine Pract 2003;19:645–63.
[23] Madigan JE, Pusterla N. Neorickettsia risticii: Potomac horse fever. In: Proceedings of the 10th International Veterinary Emergency Critical Care Symposium. San Diego (CA): IVECCS; 2004. p. 197–201.

[24] Rikihisa Y. Rickettsial diseases. In: Reed SM, Bayly WM, Sellon DC, editors. Equine internal medicine. 2nd edition. St. Louis (MO): Elsevier; 2004. p. 96–109.
[25] Heller MC, McClure J, Pusterla N, et al. Two cases of Neorickettsia (Ehrlichia) risticii infection in horses from Nova Scotia. Can Vet J 2004;45:421–3.
[26] Dutra F, Schuch LF, Delucchi E, et al. Equine monocytic ehrlichiosis (Potomac horse fever) in horses in Uruguay and southern Brazil. J Vet Diagn Invest 2001;13:433–7.
[27] Madigan JE, Pusterla N, Johnson E, et al. Transmission of Ehrlichia risticii, the agent of Potomac horse fever, using naturally infected aquatic insects and helminth vectors: preliminary report. Equine Vet J 2000;32:275–9.
[28] Rikihisa Y, Reed SM, Sama RA, et al. Serosurvey of horses with evidence of equine monocytic ehrlichiosis. J Am Vet Med Assoc 1990;197:1327–32.
[29] Madigan JE, Pusterla N. Ehrlichial diseases. Vet Clin North Am Equine Pract 2000;16: 487–99.
[30] Long MT, Goetz TE, Kakoma I, et al. Evaluation of fetal infection and abortion in pregnant ponies experimentally infected with Ehrlichia risticii. Am J Vet Res 1995;10:1307–26.
[31] Dutta K, Penney BE, Myrup AC, et al. Disease features in horses with induced equine monocytic ehrlichiosis (Potomac horse fever). Am J Vet Res 1988;49:1747–51.
[32] Goetz TE, Holland CJ, Dawson JE, et al. Monthly prevalence (in 1986) of antibody titers against equine monocytic ehrlichiosis in apparently healthy horses in Illinois. Am J Vet Res 1989;50:1936–9.
[33] Mott J, Rikihisa Y, Zhang Y, et al. Comparison of PCR and culture to the indirect fluorescent-antibody test for diagnosis of Potomac horse fever. J Clin Microbiol 1997;35:2215–9.
[34] Palmer JE, Benson CE, Lotz GW. Serological response of experimental ponies orally infected with Ehrlichia risticii. Equine Vet J Suppl 1989;7:19–20.
[35] Pretzman CI, Rikihisa Y, Ralph D, et al. Enzyme-linked immunosorbent assay for Potomac horse fever disease. J Clin Microbiol 1987;25:31–6.
[36] Shankarappa B, Dutta SK, Sanusi J, et al. Monoclonal antibody mediated, immunodiagnostic competitive enzyme-linked immunosorbent assay for equine monocytic ehrlichiosis. J Clin Microbiol 1989;27:24–8.
[37] Biswas B, Dutta SK, Mukherjee D, et al. Diagnostic application of polymerase chain reaction for detection of Ehrlichia risticii in equine monocytic ehrlichiosis (Potomac horse fever). J Clin Microbiol 1991;29:2228–33.
[38] Pusterla N, Leuntenegger CM, Sigrist B, et al. Detection and quantitation of Ehrlichia risticii genomic DNA in infected horses and snails by real-time PCR. Vet Parasitol 2000;90: 129–35.
[39] Papich MG. Antimicrobial therapy for gastrointestinal diseases. Vet Clin North Am Equine Pract 2003;19:645–63.
[40] Palmer JE, Benson CE. Effect of treatment with erythromycin and rifampin during the acute stages of experimentally induced equine ehrlichial colitis in ponies. Am J Vet Res 1992;53:2071–6.
[41] Båverud V, Gustafsson A, Franklin A, et al. Clostridium difficile: prevalence in horses and environment, and antimicrobial susceptibility. Equine Vet J 2003;35:465–71.
[42] Gustafsson A, Båverud V, Gunnarsson A, et al. Study of faecal shedding of Clostridium difficile in horses treated with penicillin. Equine Vet J 2004;36:180–2.
[43] Weese JS, Staempfli HR, Prescott JF. A prospective study of the roles of Clostridium difficile and enterotoxigenic Clostridium perfringens in equine diarrhea. Equine Vet J 2001;33: 403–9.
[44] Magdesian KG, Madigan JE, Jang SS, et al. Colitis associated with Clostridium difficile in horses. J Vet Intern Med 1997;11:110.
[45] Magdesian KG, Hirsh DC, Jang SS, et al. Characterization of Clostridium difficile isolates from foals with diarrhea: 28 cases (1993–1997). J Am Vet Med Assoc 2002;220:67–73.
[46] Arroyo LG, Weese JS, Staempfli HR. Experimental Clostridium difficile enterocolitis in foals. J Vet Intern Med 2004;18:734–8.

[47] Delmée M, Van Broeck J, Simon A, et al. Laboratory diagnosis of Clostridium difficile-associated diarrhea: a plea for culture. J Med Microbiol 2005;54:187–91.
[48] Rupnik M, Dupuy B, Fairweather NF, et al. Revised nomenclature of Clostridium difficile toxins and associated genes. J Med Microbiol 2005;54:113–7.
[49] Weese JS, Staempfli HR, Prescott JF. Survival of Clostridium difficile and its toxins in equine feces: implications for diagnostic test selection and interpretation. J Vet Diagn Invest 2000;12:332–6.
[50] Jones RL. Clostridial enterocolitis. Vet Clin North Am Equine Pract 2000;16:471–85.
[51] Vanpoucke H, De Baere T, Claeys G, et al. Evaluation of six commercial assays for the rapid detection of Clostridium difficile toxin and/or antigen in stool specimens. Eur Soc Clin Microbiol Infect Dis CMI 2001;7:55–64.
[52] Massay V, Gregson DB, Chagla AH, et al. Clinical usefulness of components of the triage immunoassay, enzyme immunoassay for toxins A and B, and cytotoxin B tissue culture assay for the diagnosis of Clostridium difficile diarrhea. Am J Clin Pathol 2003;119:45–9.
[53] Arroyo LG, Kruth SA, Willey BM, et al. PCR ribotyping of Clostridium difficile isolates originating from human and animal sources. J Med Microbiol 2005;54:163–6.
[54] Båverud V, Gunnarsson A, Karlsson M, et al. Antimicrobial susceptibility of equine and environmental isolates of Clostridium difficile. Microbiol Drug Resist 2004;10:57–63.
[55] Jang SS, Hansen LM, Breher JE, et al. Antimicrobial susceptibilities of equine isolates of Clostridium difficile and molecular characterization of metronidazole-resistant strains. Clin Infect Dis 1997;25(Suppl):S266–7.
[56] MacKay RJ. Equine neonatal clostridiosis: treatment and prevention. Compend Contin Educ Pract Vet 2001;23:280–5.
[57] East LM, Dargatz DA, Traub-Dargatz JL, et al. Foaling-management practices associated with the occurrence of enterocolitis attributed to Clostridium perfringens infection in the equine neonate. Prev Vet Med 2000;46:61–74.
[58] Herholz C, Miserez R, Nicolet J, et al. Prevalence of β2-toxigenic Clostridium perfringens in horses with intestinal disorders. J Clin Microbiol 1999;37:358–61.
[59] Schotte U, Truyen U, Neubauer H. Significance of β2-toxigenic Clostridium perfringens infections in animals and their predisposing factors—a review. J Vet Med B Infect Dis Vet Public Health 2004;51:423–6.
[60] Netherwood T, Chanter N, Mumford JA. Improved isolation of Clostridium perfringens from foal feces. Res Vet Sci 1996;61:147–51.
[61] Garmory HS, Chanter N, Franch NP, et al. Occurrence of Clostridium perfringens β2-toxin amongst animals, determined using genotyping and subtyping PCR assays. Epidemiol Infect 2000;124:61–7.
[62] Baums CG, Schotte U, Amtsberg G, et al. Diagnostic multiplex PCR for toxin genotyping of Clostridium perfringens isolates. Vet Microbiol 2004;100:11–6.
[63] Al-Khaldi SF, Myers KM, Rasooly A, et al. Genotyping of Clostridium perfringens toxins using multiple oligonucleotide microarray hybridization. Mol Cell Probes 2004;18:359–67.
[64] Bacciarini LN, Boerlin P, Straub R, et al. Immunohistochemical localization of Clostridium perfringens β2-toxin in the gastrointestinal tract of horses. Vet Pathol 2004;40:376–81.
[65] Tillotson K, Traub-Dargatz JL, Dickinson CE, et al. Population-based study of fecal shedding of Clostridium perfringens in broodmares and foals. J Am Vet Med Assoc 2002;220:342–7.
[66] McFarland LV. Alternative treatments for Clostridium difficile disease: what really works? J Med Microbiol 2005;54:101–11.
[67] Kelly CP, Pothoulakis C, LaMont JT. Clostridium difficile colitis. N Engl J Med 1994;330:257–62.
[68] Vasa CV, Glatt AE. Effectiveness and appropriateness of empiric metronidazole for Clostridium difficile-associated diarrhea. Am J Gastroenterol 2003;98:354–8.
[69] Aslam S, Hamill RJ, Musher DM. Treatment of Clostridium difficile-associated disease: old therapies and new strategies. Lancet Infect Dis 2005;5:549–57.

[70] Magdesian KG. Neonatal foal diarrhea. Vet Clin North Am Equine Pract 2005;21: 295–312.
[71] Vilei EM, Schlatter Y, Perreten V, et al. Antibiotic-induced expression of a cryptic cpb2 gene in equine β2-toxigenic Clostridium perfringens. Mol Microbiol 2005;57: 1570–81.
[72] Tillotson K, Traub-Dargatz JL, Morgan PK. Partial parenteral nutrition in equine neonatal clostridial enterocolitis. Compend Contin Educ Vet Pract 2002;24:964–9.
[73] Lawson GHK, Gebhart CJ. Proliferative enteropathy. J Comp Pathol 2000;122:77–100.
[74] Cooper DM, Gebhart CJ. Comparative aspects of proliferative enteritis. J Am Vet Med Assoc 1998;212:1446–51.
[75] Lawson GHK, McOrist S. The enigma of the proliferative enteropathies: a review. J Comp Pathol 1993;108:41–6.
[76] Jones GF, Ward GE, Murtaugh MP, et al. Enhanced detection of intracellular organism of swine proliferative enteritis, ileal symbiont intracellularis, in feces by polymerase chain reaction. J Clin Microbiol 1993;31:2611–5.
[77] Cooper DM, Swanson DL, Gebhart CJ. Diagnosis of proliferative enteritis in frozen and formalin-fixed, paraffin-embedded tissues from a hamster, horse, deer and ostrich using a Lawsonia intracellularis-specific multiplex PCR assay. Vet Microbiol 1997;54:47–62.
[78] Jacobson M, Aspan A, Heldtander Königsson M, et al. Routine diagnostics of Lawsonia intracellularis performed by PCR, serological and post-mortem examination, with special emphasis on sample preparation methods for PCR. Vet Microbiol 2004;102:189–201.
[79] Lavoie JP, Drolet R, Parsons D, et al. Equine proliferative enteropathy: a cause of weight loss, colic, diarrhea and hypoproteinemia in foals on three breeding farms in Canada. Equine Vet J 2000;32:418–25.
[80] McClintock SA, Collins AM. Lawsonia intracellularis proliferative enteropathy in a weanling foal in Australia. Aust Vet J 2004;82:750–2.
[81] Schumacher J, Schumacher J, Rolsma M, et al. Surgical and medical treatment of an Arabian filly with proliferative enteropathy caused by Lawsonia intracellularis. J Vet Intern Med 2000;14:630–2.
[82] McOrist S, Mackie RA, Lawson GHK. Antimicrobial susceptibility of ileal symbiont intracellularis isolated from pigs with proliferative enteropathy. J Clin Microbiol 1995;33: 1314–7.
[83] Giguere S, Jacks S, Roberts GD, et al. Retrospective comparison of azithromycin, clarithromycin, and erythromycin for the treatment of foals with Rhodococcus equi pneumonia. J Vet Intern Med 2004;18:568–73.
[84] Mair T. Chronic diarrhea. In: Mair T, Divers T, Ducharme N, editors. Manual of equine gastroenterology. London: WB Saunders; 2002. p. 427–48.
[85] Reid SW, Mair TS, Hillyer MH, et al. Epidemiological risk factors associated with a diagnosis of clinical cyathostomiasis in the horse. Equine Vet J 1995;27:127–30.
[86] Matthews JB, Hodgkinson JE, Dowdall SM, et al. Recent developments in research into the Cyathostominae and Anoplocephala perfoliata. Vet Res 2004;35:371–81.
[87] Kaplan RM, Klei TR, Lyons ET, et al. Prevalence of anthelmintic resistant cyathostomes on horse farms. J Am Vet Med Assoc 2004;225:903–10.
[88] Meier A, Hertzberg H. Equine strongyles I. Development of anthelmintic resistance. Schweiz Arch Tierheilkd 2005;147:381–8.
[89] Love S. Treatment and prevention of intestinal parasite-associated disease. Vet Clin North Am Equine Pract 2003;19:791–806.
[90] McConnico RS. Duodenitis-proximal jejunitis (anterior enteritis, proximal enteritis). In: Reed SM, Bayly WM, Sellon DC, editors. Equine internal medicine. 2nd edition. St. Louis (MO): Elsevier; 2004. p. 884–913.
[91] Edwards GB, Proudman CJ. Diseases of the small intestine resulting in colic. In: Mair T, Divers T, Ducharme N, editors. Manual of equine gastroenterology. London: WB Saunders; 2002. p. 240–65.

[92] Davis JL, Blikslager AT, Catto K, et al. A retrospective analysis of hepatic injury in horses with proximal enteritis. J Vet Intern Med 2003;17:896–901.
[93] Griffiths NJ, Walton JR, Edwards GB, et al. The prevalence of Clostridium perfringens in the horse. Rev Med Microbiol 1997;8(Suppl):S52–4.
[94] Arroyo LG, Staempfli H, Rousseau JD, et al. Culture evaluation of *Clostridium* spp. in the nasogastric reflux of horses with duodenitis proximal jejunitis. In: Proceedings of the Eighth International Equine Colic Research Symposium. Lexington (KY): AAEP Foundation; 2005. p. 51–2.
[95] Schumacher J, Mullen J, Shelby R, et al. An investigation of the role of Fusarium moniliforme in duodenitis/proximal jejunitis of horses. Vet Hum Toxicol 1995;37:39–45.
[96] Cohen N, Murphy E, Roussel A, et al. Is duodenitis-proximal jejunitis associated with high concentrate diets? In: Proceedings of the Eighth International Equine Colic Research Symposium. Lexington (KY): AAEP Foundation; 2005. p. 49.
[97] Van Hoogmoed LM, Nieto JE, Snyder JR, et al. Survey of prokinetic use in horses with gastrointestinal injury. Vet Surg 2004;33:279–85.
[98] Cook VL. Update on postoperative ileus. In: Mazzaferro EM, editor. Proceedings of the 11th International Veterinary Emergency and Critical Care Symposium. Atlanta (GA): VECCS; 2005. p. 341–4.
[99] Magdesian KG. Monitoring the critically ill equine patient. Vet Clin North Am Equine Pract 2004;20:11–39.
[100] Macintire DK, Drobatz KJ, Haskins SC, et al. Manual of small animal emergency and critical care. Baltimore (MD): Lippincott Williams & Wilkins; 2005. 71–88.
[101] Corley KTT. Monitoring and treating hemodynamic disturbances in critically ill neonatal foals. Part I: hemodynamic monitoring. Equine Vet Educ 2002;14:270–9.
[102] Corley KTT, Donaldson LL, Furr MO. Arterial lactate concentration, hospital survival, sepsis and SIRS in critically ill neonatal foals. Equine Vet J 2005;37:53–9.
[103] Garcia-Lopez JM, Provost PJ, Rush JF, et al. Prevalence and prognostic importance of hypomagnesemia and hypocalcemia in horses that have colic surgery. Am J Vet Res 2001; 62:7–12.
[104] Toribio RE, Kohn CW, Chew DJ, et al. Comparison of serum parathyroid hormone and ionized calcium and magnesium concentrations and fractional urinary clearance of calcium and phosphorus in healthy horses and horses with enterocolitis. Am J Vet Res 2001;62: 938–47.
[105] Toribio RE, Kohn CW, Hardy J, et al. Alterations in serum parathyroid hormone and electrolyte concentrations and urinary excretion of electrolytes in horses with induced endotoxemia. J Vet Intern Med 2005;19:223–31.
[106] Delesalle C, Dewulf J, Schuurkes JAJ, et al. Ionized calcium as a prognostic parameter in colic horses. In: Proceedings of the Eighth Equine Colic Research Symposium. Lexington (KY): AAEP Foundation; 2005. p. 181–2.
[107] Corley KTT. Monitoring and treating the cardiovascular system in neonatal foals. Clin Tech Equine Pract 2003;2:42–55.
[108] Nout YS, Corley KTT, Donaldson LL, et al. Indirect oscillometric and direct blood pressure measurements in anesthetized and conscious neonatal foals. J Vet Emerg Crit Care 2002;12:75–80.
[109] Giguère S, Knowles HA, Valverde A, et al. Accuracy of indirect measurement of blood pressure in neonatal foals. J Vet Intern Med 2005;19:571–6.
[110] Corley KTT. Monitoring and treating hemodynamic disturbances in critically ill neonatal foals. Part II: assessment and treatment. Equine Vet Educ 2002;14:328–36.
[111] Seri I, Evans J. Controversies in the diagnosis and management of hypotension in the newborn infant. Curr Opin Pediatr 2001;13:116–23.
[112] Giguère S, Bucki E, Adin DB, et al. Cardiac output measurement by partial carbon dioxide rebreathing, 2-dimensional echocardiography, and lithium-dilution method in anesthetized neonatal foals. J Vet Intern Med 2005;19:737–43.

[113] Marino PL. Central venous pressure and wedge pressure. In: The ICU book. 2nd edition. Baltimore (MD): Lippincott Williams & Wilkins; 1998. p. 166–8.
[114] Magdesian KG, Fielding CL, Madigan JE. Measurement of plasma colloid osmotic pressure in neonatal foals under intensive care: comparison of direct and indirect methods and the association of COP with selected clinical and clinicopathological variables. J Vet Emerg Crit Care 2004;14:108–14.
[115] Marino PL. Tissue oxygenation. In: The ICU book. 2nd edition. Baltimore (MD): Lippincott Williams & Wilkins; 1998. p. 187–203.
[116] Furr MO, Lessard P, White NA. Development of a colic severity score for predicting the outcome of equine colic. Vet Surg 1995;24:97–101.
[117] Dolente BA, Wilkins PA, Boston RC. Clinicopathological evidence of disseminated intravascular coagulation in horses with acute colitis. J Am Vet Med Assoc 2002;220: 1034–8.
[118] Latson KM, Nieto JE, Beldomenico PM, et al. Evaluation of peritoneal fluid lactate as a marker of intestinal ischaemia in equine colic. Equine Vet J 2005;37:342–6.
[119] Grosche A, Schrodl W, Schusser GF. Specific parameters of blood and peritoneal fluid of colic horses to indicate intestinal ischemia. In: Proceedings of the Eighth Equine Colic Research Symposium. Lexington (KY): AAEP Foundation; 2005. p. 102–3.
[120] Weese JS, Cote NM, DeGannes RVG. Evaluation of in vitro properties of di-tri-octahedral smectite on clostridial toxins and growth. Equine Vet J 2003;35:638–41.
[121] Hassel DM, Smith PA, Nieto JE, et al. Di-tri-octahedral smectite for the prevention of postoperative diarrhea in equine colic patients: results of a randomized clinical trial [abstract]. Vet Surg 2004;33:E11.
[122] Plummer S, Weaver MA, Harris JC, et al. Clostridium difficile pilot study: effects of probiotic supplementation on the incidence of C. difficile diarrhea. Int Microbiol 2004;7: 59–62.
[123] Dendukuri N, Costa V, McGregor M, et al. Probiotic therapy for the prevention and treatment of Clostridium difficile-associated diarrhea: a systematic review. CMAJ 2005;173: 167–70.
[124] Canganella F, Paganini S, Ovidi M, et al. A microbiological investigation on probiotic pharmaceutical products used for human health. Microbiol Res 1997;152:171–9.
[125] Weese JS. Microbiological evaluation of commercial probiotics. J Am Vet Med Assoc 2002; 220:794–7.
[126] Weese JS, Rousseau J. Evaluation of Lactobacillus pentosus WE7 for prevention of diarrhea in neonatal foals. J Am Vet Med Assoc 2005;226:2031–4.
[127] Tillotson K, Traub-Dargatz JL. Gastrointestinal protectants and cathartics. Vet Clin North Am Equine Pract 2003;19:599–615.
[128] Surawicz CM, Elmer GW, Speelman P, et al. Prevention of antibiotic-associated diarrhea by Saccharomyces boulardii. Gastroenterology 1989;96:981–8.
[129] Kotowska M, Albrecht P, Szajewska H. Saccharomyces boulardii in the prevention of antibiotic-associated diarrhea in children: a randomized double-blind placebo-controlled trial. Aliment Pharmacol Ther 2005;21:583–90.
[130] Desrochers AM, Dolente BA, Roy MF, et al. Efficacy of *Saccharomyces boulardii* for treatment of horses with acute enterocolitis. J Am Vet Med Assoc 2005;227:954–9.
[131] Quamar A, Aboudola A, Warny M, et al. Saccharomyces boulardii stimulates intestinal immunoglobulin A immune response to Clostridium difficile toxin A in mice. Infect Immun 2001;69:2762–5.
[132] Tasteyre A, Barc MC, Karjalainen T, et al. Inhibition of in vitro call adherence of Clostridium difficile by Saccharomyces boulardii. Microb Pathog 2002;32:219–25.
[133] Wilson KH, Perini I. Role of competition for nutrients in suppression of Clostridium difficile by the colonic microflora. Infect Immun 1988;56:2610–4.
[134] Lherm T, Monet C, Nougiere B, et al. Seven cases of fungemia with S. boulardii in critically ill patients. Intensive Care Med 2002;28:797–801.

[135] Aas J, Gessert CE, Bakken JS. Recurrent Clostridium difficile colitis: case series involving 18 patients treated with donor stool administered via nasogastric tube. Clin Infect Dis 2003; 36:580–5.
[136] van Dissel JT, de Groot N, Hensgens CMH, et al. Bovine antibody-enriched whey to aid in the prevention of a relapse of Clostridium difficile-associated diarrhea: preclinical and preliminary clinical data. J Med Microbiol 2005;54:197–205.
[137] Sougioultzis S, Kyne L, Drudy D, et al. Clostridium difficile toxoid vaccine in recurrent C. difficile-associated diarrhea. Gastroenterology 2005;128:764–70.
[138] Stroehlein JR. Treatment of Clostridium difficile infection. Curr Treat Options Gastroenterol 2004;3:235–9.
[139] Southwood LL. Post-operative management of the large colon volvulus patient. Vet Clin North Am Equine Pract 2004;20:167–97.
[140] Magdesian KG, Madigan JE. Volume replacement in the neonatal ICU: crystalloids and colloids. Clin Tech Equine Pract 2003;2:20–30.
[141] Seahorn JL, Seahorn TL. Fluid therapy in horses with gastrointestinal disease. Vet Clin North Am Equine Pract 2003;19:665–79.
[142] Macintire DK, Drobatz KJ, Haskins SC, et al. Manual of small animal emergency and critical care. Baltimore (MD): Lippincott Williams & Wilkins; 2005. 55–70.
[143] Mazzaferro EM, Rudloff E, Kirby R. The role of albumin replacement in the critically ill veterinary patient. J Vet Emerg Crit Care 2002;12:113–24.
[144] Tomlinson JE, Blikslager AT. Effects of ischemia and the cyclooxygenase inhibitor flunixin on in vitro passage of lipopolysaccharide across equine jejunum. Am J Vet Res 2004;65: 1377–83.
[145] Morton AJ, Rotting AK, Freeman DE, et al. Characterization of cyclooxygenase 1 and cyclooxygenase 2 expression in normal and ischemic-injured equine left dorsal colon. In: Scientific Abstracts of the 2005 American College of Veterinary Surgeon Veterinary Symposium. Rockville (MD): ACVS; 2005. p. 18.
[146] Dolente BA, Wilkins PA, Boston RC. Clinicopathological evidence of disseminated intravascular coagulation in horses with acute colitis. J Am Vet Med Assoc 2002;220: 1034–8.
[147] Brianceau P, Divers TJ. Acute thrombosis of limb arteries in horses with sepsis: five cases (1988–1998). Equine Vet J 2001;33:105–9.
[148] Duggan VE, Holbrook TC, Dechant JE, et al. Diagnosis of aorto-iliac thrombosis in a Quarter Horse foal using Doppler ultrasound and nuclear scintigraphy. J Vet Intern Med 2004;18:753–65.
[149] Henry-Barton M. Dyshemostasis in equine sepsis. In: Proceedings of the 11th Veterinary Emergency Critical Care Symposium. Atlanta (GA): IVECCS; 2005. p. 267–72.
[150] Dallap BL. Coagulopathy in the equine critical care patient. Vet Clin North Am Equine Pract 2004;20:231–51.
[151] Forrest LJ, Cooley JA, Darien BJ. Digital artery thrombosis in a septicemic foal. J Vet Intern Med 1999;13:382–5.
[152] Bateman S. Coagulation defects: when is therapy required? In: Proceedings of the 11th Veterinary Emergency Critical Care Symposium. Atlanta (GA): IVECCS; 2005. p. 191–3.
[153] Rozanski E, Hughes D, Scotti M, et al. The effect of heparin and fresh frozen plasma on plasma antithrombin III activity, prothrombin time and activated partial thromboplastin time in critically ill dogs. J Vet Emerg Crit Care 2001;11:15–21.
[154] Leese T, Holliday M, Watkins M, et al. A multicentre controlled clinical trial of high-volume fresh frozen plasma therapy in prognostically severe acute pancreatitis. Ann R Coll Surg Engl 1991;73:207–14.
[155] Bateman S. DIC and heparin. In: Proceedings of the 11th Veterinary Emergency Critical Care Symposium. Atlanta (GA): IVECCS; 2005. p. 195–8.
[156] Aleman M, Nieto JE, Carr EA, et al. Serum hepatitis associated with commercial plasma transfusion in horses. J Vet Intern Med 2005;19:120–2.

[157] Oelschlager C, Romisch J, Staubitz A, et al. Antithrombin III inhibits nuclear factor kappa B activation in human monocytes and vascular endothelial cells. Blood 2002;99:4015–20.
[158] Hoffmann JN, Vollmar B, Laschke MW, et al. Adverse effect of heparin on antithrombin action during endotoxemia: microhemodynamic and cellular mechanisms. Thromb Haemost 2002;88:242–52.
[159] Ward MP, Brady TH, Couetil LL, et al. Investigation and control of an outbreak of salmonellosis caused by multidrug-resistant Salmonella typhimurium in a population of hospitalized horses. Vet Microbiol 2005;107:233–40.
[160] Feige K, Schwarzwald CC, Bombeli T. Comparison of unfractioned and low molecular weight heparin for prophylaxis of coagulopathies in 52 horses with colic: a randomised double-blind clinical trial. Equine Vet J 2003;35:506–13.
[161] Monreal L, Villatoro AJ, Monreal M, et al. Comparison of the effects of low-molecular-weight and unfractioned heparin in horses. Am J Vet Res 1995;56:1281–5.

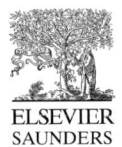

Septicemia and Cardiovascular Infections in Horses

Sophy A. Jesty, DVM[a],*, Virginia B. Reef, DVM[b]

[a]*Cornell University Hospital for Animals, PO Box 34, Ithaca, NY 14853, USA*
[b]*New Bolton Center, University of Pennsylvania, 382 West Street Road, Kennett Square, PA 19348, USA*

There are some instances in which infections of the heart are obvious. These infections may be bacterial, viral, fungal, or parasitic and can affect the endocardium (including valves), myocardium, pericardium, or vasculature. There are other instances in which the effect of an infection on the cardiovascular system is less obvious, especially if the primary site is distant from the heart itself. These cases could be more numerous and are likely underrecognized in equine practice. Although the effect of sepsis on the heart may be occult, it may not be insignificant. Better recognition and appropriate therapy, if required, might affect the outcome of critically ill patients.

Endocarditis

Endocarditis in horses is rare and is usually caused by a bacterial infection of the valves, although infections may also be caused by fungi, parasites, or viruses [1–3]. Infection of the mitral and aortic valves is more common than infection of the tricuspid and pulmonic valves [1–7]. Some bacteria are capable of colonizing the endocardium without predisposing factors, but other bacteria require certain predisposing conditions, such as a damaged endothelial surface, platelet aggregation, or high circulating agglutinins [7–10]. Microscopic tears or lesions are more prevalent on the valves of the left side of the heart because of the higher pressures, making these more likely sites for vegetative lesions [6,7]. Clinical signs are attributable to the infection (eg, fever, weight loss, anorexia, lethargy) and the valve dysfunction (eg, murmur, tachycardia, signs of heart failure) [5–7]. It is most

---

* Corresponding author. Cornell University Hospital for Animals, PO Box 34, Ithaca, NY 14853.
 E-mail address: saj2@cornell.edu (S.A. Jesty).

likely that the affected valve becomes regurgitant, although stenosis also occurs [2]. Occasionally, horses with endocarditis do not have a murmur. This could be because of a pulmonic valve lesion, a mural lesion, a lesion small enough not to allow for regurgitation or stenosis, or a lesion large enough to no longer allow for regurgitation [5,7]. Many animals affected by bacterial endocarditis are young, and most are male, as is the case in people and dogs [2,5].

A working diagnosis of endocarditis can be made in a horse with characteristic clinical signs and a new murmur, but definitive diagnosis is made using echocardiography and blood culture [2,5,7,11–13]. Vegetative lesions may appear hypoechoic and "shaggy" when immature and smoother and more echogenic when more mature (Fig. 1) [14]. Occasionally, endocarditis cannot be visualized on echocardiography, although this is unusual. Blood work may show leukocytosis, hyperfibrinogenemia, hyperproteinemia, and anemia [5–7]. Ideally, blood culture also yields positive results, but this should not be used as an absolute criterion for diagnosis if clinical signs and echocardiography are consistent with a vegetative lesion. If possible, blood culture should be performed two to three times before the initiation of antimicrobial therapy. The most common isolates include *Streptococcus* spp and *Actinobacillus* spp, but a large number of isolates have now been reported [2,4–7,15–22].

Ideally, treatment should include intravenous bactericidal antimicrobials at a dose rate to achieve serum concentrations of at least four times the minimum inhibitory concentration (MIC) for a specific organism [6]. While blood culture results are pending, empiric therapy should be initiated, including penicillin and an aminoglycoside. A constant rate infusion of penicillin may be more efficacious than bolus dosing. Intravenous antimicrobials should be

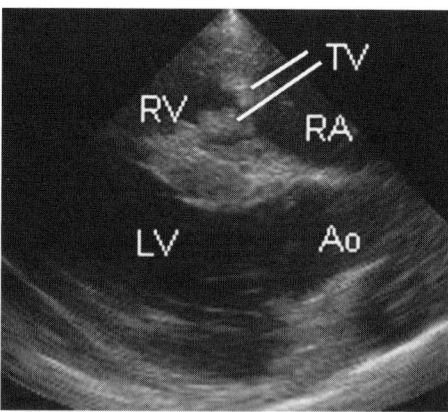

Fig. 1. Echocardiogram of a horse with bacterial endocarditis of the tricuspid valve. The lesions are large, smooth, and echoic. The horse had a significant amount of tricuspid regurgitation. Ao, aorta; LV, left ventricle; RA, right atrium; RV, right ventricle; TV, tricuspid valve.

used for a minimum of 10 to 14 days; at that time, oral antimicrobials can be substituted for at least an additional 4 to 6 weeks of therapy [5,7,8]. Often, a longer course of intravenous antimicrobials is needed (4–6 weeks) before switching to oral therapy. The switch to oral antimicrobials should be made when clinical signs have abated, clinicopathologic data have neared normal, blood culture is negative, and the echocardiogram is consistent with a healing lesion (smooth and more echogenic than younger lesions) [5]. During this period, the horse should be treated with an antithrombotic agent, such as aspirin (10 mg/kg administered orally once daily). The prognosis for left-sided bacterial endocarditis is grave [5–7]. These horses usually succumb to the infection itself (which is difficult to resolve) or to heart failure secondary to valve incompetence [5,7]. Sterilization of lesions on the mitral and aortic valves occurs only rarely [6,23,24]. Heart failure may occur months or years later depending on the severity of colonization of the valve and the subsequent valvular damage. Even when a bacteriologic cure is achieved, the damaged valve usually becomes more deformed as it heals, allowing for continued, or even exacerbated, regurgitation [5]. Right-sided bacterial endocarditis is rarer but carries a better prognosis, because right-sided regurgitation tends to be more forgiving than left-sided regurgitation [5]. Tricuspid valve endocarditis occurs most frequently secondary to septic jugular vein thrombophlebitis [3,5,14]. Additional sequelae of bacterial endocarditis include thromboembolic disease and immune-mediated synovitis [7].

In human medicine, transesophageal echocardiography (TEE) has become the diagnostic tool of choice for bacterial endocarditis [25,26]. Transthoracic echocardiography has high specificity (98%) but fairly low sensitivity (60%–70%), whereas TEE has similarly high specificity and significantly higher sensitivity (75%–95%) [26–28]. TEE requires a probe long enough to reach the base of the heart via the esophagus and would need to be custom made for equine practice. It requires considerable expertise, as is necessary for standard echocardiography. The image set obtained via TEE is quite distinct from that which can be obtained transthoracically.

Myocarditis

Myocarditis is often a diagnosis of exclusion in the horse. Myocardial injury subsequent to localized or systemic infections can result in nonspecific cardiac inflammation and fibrosis [14,29]. Infectious causes include viruses (equine influenza, equine infectious anemia, and equine viral arteritis), bacteria (*Staphylococcus aureus*, *Streptococcus equi*, and *Borrelia burgdorferi* or Lyme disease), and parasites (*Strongylus vulgaris* and *Onchocerca* spp) [1,29–31]. Clinical signs of myocarditis are quite variable, ranging from none with a subclinical infection to sudden death. Many horses show poor performance or have signs associated with infection (eg, fever, lethargy, tachycardia). Electrocardiography may reveal arrhythmias, and focal lesions in the myocardium, dilation of the ventricles, or poor systolic function may be imaged echocardiographically. Biochemical markers for cardiac injury have been used in equine medicine for a long time. The cardiac isozyme of creatinine kinase (CKMB) has been used to evaluate cardiomyocyte damage in the past, but it lacks specificity [30,32,33]. More recently, cardiac troponin I (cTnI) has mostly replaced CKMB as the cardiac biochemical marker of choice in equine medicine. cTnI is a component of the tropomyosin-troponin complex, and the cardiac and skeletal muscle forms can be differentiated [34]. A small proportion of cTnI is found in the cardiomyocyte cytosol, and cellular disruption leads to increased serum concentration of the protein compared with normal [34]. A reference range has been reported for normal Thoroughbreds [35], and increases of cTnI compared with normal have been documented in myocarditis and aortic root rupture cases [36,37]. cTnI should be measured in horses in which myocarditis is suspected; indeed, an increase in cTnI might be enough to support a diagnosis in the absence of other diagnostic clues. In human medicine, there have been recent studies showing that cTnI is an indicator of many types of myocardial insult, including myocardial infarction, heart failure, myocarditis, and myocardial trauma [38,39]. Additionally, increases have been seen with sepsis, hypertension, renal disease, liver disease, and pulmonary embolism [39]. These more recent reports have led to a decrease in the specificity of cTnI as a marker for cardiac disease in human beings. Perhaps the increase in cTnI in noncardiac cases reflects subtle cardiomyocyte strain that cannot be ascertained using other diagnostic approaches [39]. There are no reports to date in the veterinary literature of increased cTnI in noncardiac cases, but its use is relatively recent in equine medicine.

Pericarditis

Pericarditis is an inflammation of the pericardial sac, which is usually caused by bacterial or viral infections. Other causes include fungal, parasitic, immune-mediated, or neoplastic pericarditis; however, a cause is not identified in many cases, and it is termed *idiopathic* [40–43]. Horses that are presented with pericarditis often have a vague history of respiratory illness within the preceding few weeks. Pericarditis may be further defined as effusive (fluid accumulation with or without cardiac tamponade), fibrinous (fibrin is found with the pericardial sac, with or without fluid accumulation), or constrictive (fibrosis of the pericardium that reduces distensibility and affects diastolic filling) [40]. The effusive and fibrinous types of pericarditis are more common than the constrictive type, with the exception of the epidemic of pericarditis cases seen associated with mare reproductive loss syndrome in Kentucky in 2001 [44,45].

The most common clinical signs are not specific for pericarditis but are similar to the clinical signs associated with other infections, including fever, anorexia, and lethargy. Often, horses with pericarditis are presented with signs of colic. Signs specific for pericarditis include pericardial friction rubs, tachycardia, and muffled heart sounds. Pericardial friction rubs are heard when the inflamed epicardial and pericardial surfaces rub against one another (as occurs in cases of fibrinous pericarditis). Classically, pericardial friction rubs are triphasic, occurring during atrial systole, ventricular systole, and at the end of early ventricular filling. If cardiac tamponade is a component of the pathophysiology, clinical signs of right-sided heart failure (jugular and peripheral vein distention, jugular pulses, ventral edema, and ascites or hepatomegaly) and left-sided output failure (weakness, lethargy, collapse, oliguria, and cardiogenic shock) develop. The diagnosis is best made using echocardiography [40,42,43]. An echocardiogram can reveal the amount of pericardial fluid, the presence of cardiac tamponade (as evidenced by right atrial and right ventricular diastolic collapse), the character of the pericardial fluid, and the structure and function of the heart. Cardiac tamponade is a hemodynamically important condition in which high intrapericardial pressure decreases cardiac filling compared with normal [44,45]. Pleural effusion is also common in cases of pericarditis in horses [40].

Treatment, if at all possible, should include pericardial drainage and lavage and should be performed as soon as possible. There should be at least 5 cm of fluid surrounding the heart to use a large-bore argyle catheter (24 French). Pericardiocentesis should be performed with continual electrocardiographic monitoring. The fluid should be completely drained, with some of the fluid collected for cytologic evaluation, bacterial culture and sensitivity testing, and virus isolation. Viral titers can be performed as well, although despite efforts, a specific cause is not identified in many cases of presumed infectious pericarditis. Drainage of the fluid improves cardiac filling and cardiac output. The pericardial space should be lavaged with at least the same volume as that removed. This serves to remove debris (eg, fibrin, inflammatory cells, infectious organisms, immune complexes) [41]. Antimicrobials should then be instilled and left within the pericardial space, and an indwelling catheter should remain for repeat drainage and lavage until no longer necessary [40]. Sodium penicillin and gentamicin have been instilled in the pericardial space safely.

Other treatments given concurrently should include systemic antimicrobials (one should assume septic pericarditis until proven otherwise) and nonsteroidal anti-inflammatory drugs. *Streptococcus* spp have traditionally been considered the most likely bacteria to infect the pericardium because they are the most common bacterial isolates cultured from pericardial fluid; however, both gram-positive and gram-negative bacteria have been seen cytologically [41]. More recently, horses affected by the fibrinous pericarditis associated with the mare reproductive loss syndrome seen in Kentucky during 2001 had other species isolated, including *Actinobacillus* spp, *Escherichia coli*, and *Enterococcus faecalis* [46,47]. Antimicrobial selection should initially be broad spectrum until results of culture can guide further therapy. Intravenous fluids can also be given before pericardial drainage to increase preload and after pericardial drainage to replace losses from urination once cardiac output surges. Diuretics, such as furosemide, are contraindicated in cases of pericardial effusion and cardiac tamponade because they decrease preload further, exacerbating the situation.

In the event that constrictive pericarditis is causing diastolic dysfunction and signs of right-sided heart failure, surgical partial or total pericardectomy might be indicated. In these scenarios, medical management consists of broad-spectrum antimicrobials and nonsteroidal anti-inflammatory drugs, but this is unlikely to improve the clinical course.

Vasculitis

Infections can affect the vasculature in a number of ways. Thrombophlebitis refers to occlusion of the vein by a thrombus and is often associated with bacterial infection [48]. Arterial thrombosis often affects the cranial mesenteric artery or the aortoiliac quadrification in horses and is sometimes associated with parasitic migration [49–51]. Finally, activation of the clotting cascade by sepsis can predispose horses to developing thrombi, especially in the limbs, even in the absence of organisms at the site [52,53].

Jugular vein thrombosis is a risk for any animal with a jugular intravenous catheter [48,54,55]. Several studies have examined the factors associated with jugular vein thrombosis and have found catheter-related factors (eg, catheter material, size of the catheter, type of fluid being administered, duration of catheterization) and patient-related factors (eg, hypercoagulable state like anemia, hypotension, fever, diarrhea, colitis, protein-losing disease, sepsis, endotoxemia) [30,48,55]. Clinical signs of septic jugular thrombophlebitis include fever, lethargy, anorexia, swelling, heat, and pain over the site and possible congestion and swelling of the head. A diagnosis can be made on the basis of history and clinical signs and confirmed with ultrasonography, blood culture, and culture of the catheter tip [30,48,54–56]. Ultrasonography has become the diagnostic tool of choice to characterize thrombosis. The thrombus is more likely to have cavitary hypoechoic or anechoic regions if it is septic, as opposed to nonseptic jugular thrombophlebitis (Fig. 2). Ultrasonography should also be used to choose a site for fluid collection within the thrombus itself for culture and sensitivity testing [14,30,48,56]. Treatment includes removing the intravenous catheter, warm compresses or hydrotherapy, appropriate antimicrobials, nonsteroidal anti-inflammatory drugs, and antithrombotic agents. Pending culture and sensitivity results, broad-spectrum bactericidal antimicrobials should be used, such as penicillin and an aminoglycoside. If possible, it would be prudent in these cases to use a lateral thoracic vein catheter rather than risk damaging the remaining jugular vein. Once the infection has stabilized (based on clinical signs, hematology, and ultrasonography), the horse can be switched to treatment with appropriate oral antimicrobials for longer term therapy (6–8 weeks). Continued antimicrobial therapy is recommended until the

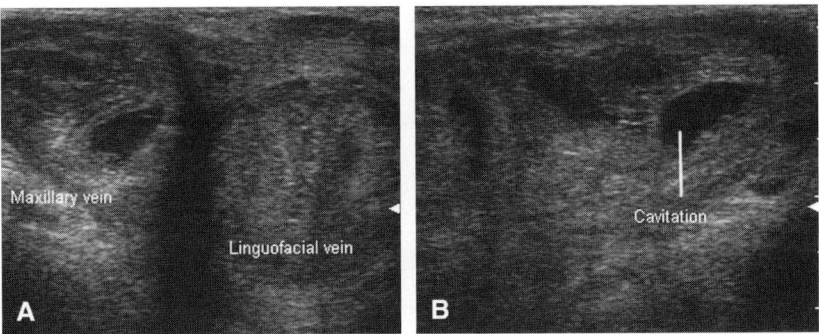

Fig. 2. Sonogram of septic thrombophlebitis. The left image is a short-axis view, and the right image is a long-axis view. Notice the layering of the thrombotic material (so-called "onion skin" appearance) and the cavitary lesions (fluid) that are associated with a septic process. The layered heterogeneous appearance is associated with chronicity. Fluid collection for cytology and bacterial culture and sensitivity testing should be guided by ultrasound.

cavitary lesion is no longer distinctly visible ultrasonographically. Despite lengthy treatment, severe septic thrombophlebitis may be difficult to resolve; in these cases, thrombectomy, resection of the jugular vein, or jugular reconstruction can be attempted [30,57,58]. Resection requires that the surgeon be able to ligate the vein proximal and distal to the thrombus. Reconstruction can be attempted using the horse's saphenous vein or synthetic materials but is contraindicated in the face of an active infection. The prognosis for complete resolution of septic thrombophlebitis is guarded. A major sequela of jugular thrombophlebitis is bacterial endocarditis, specifically of the tricuspid valve [14,30,48].

Aortoiliac (saddle) and cranial mesenteric thromboses have been closely associated with verminous arteritis, especially the migration of *Strongylus vulgaris* [30,49,50,59]. The damage caused by the migratory larvae produces endothelial disruption and allows for initiation of the clotting cascade. The resultant thrombi may be partially or completely occlusive. The most likely clinical sign associated with aortoiliac thrombosis is claudication or pain associated with exercise. This occurs as the oxygen demand of the hind limb musculature increases beyond the level to which the artery can supply oxygen. The pain and lameness resolve with rest but reappear with renewed exercise. The clinical signs associated with cranial mesenteric thrombosis are those associated with infarction of the large colon, including colic and severe sepsis. Unfortunately, the latter diagnosis is often made at surgery, when the damage is too great to be treated. At this time, euthanasia is often necessary. Diagnosis of aortoiliac thrombosis can be made on examination per rectum, ultrasonography per rectum, arteriography, and nuclear scintigraphy [49,51,60–63]. The first two diagnostic tests are the most likely to be used, and ultrasonography per rectum has high sensitivity and specificity for diagnosis of thrombosis (Fig. 3) [14,51,60–62]. Often, the thrombus is sterile, and

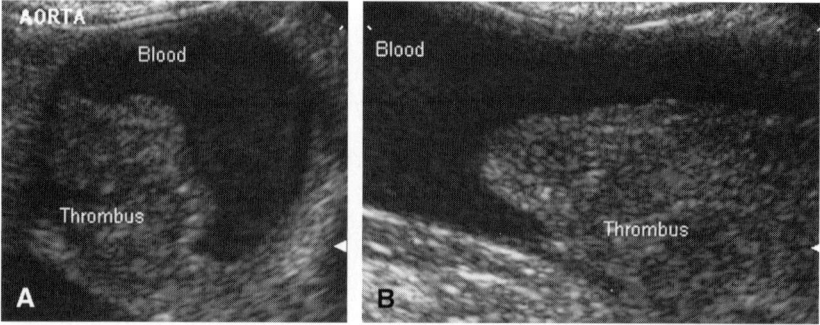

Fig. 3. Sonogram of aortoiliac thrombosis. The left image is a short-axis view, and the right image is a long-axis view. In this image, the thrombus is more homogeneous and hypoechoic, making it more likely to be acute or subacute.

treatment includes antithrombotics and a good deworming program [50]. The prognosis for a horse with aortoiliac thrombosis to recover enough to resume the previous level of exercise is poor. Recently, surgery has been investigated as a means to improve the prognosis of these horses. Partial or total removal of the thrombi has been performed using a Fogarty thrombectomy catheter, with varying results [64]. Although recurrence of thrombosis is likely, it might be less severe or collateral circulation might become adequate in the meantime. Since the advent of widespread anthelmintic use, the incidence of aortoiliac thrombosis has declined significantly; however, the disease persists, making it likely that parasitic migration is not the only predisposition [49,50].

Finally, more widespread thrombosis of smaller peripheral vessels can be encountered in cases of sepsis, even if the organism that has initiated the sepsis does not have direct effects on the vessel [30,48,49,54,55]. Hemostasis requires a delicate balance between procoagulant and anticoagulant factors. This balance is often upset by diseases that cause septicemia, endotoxemia, and sepsis. Sepsis has been associated with hypercoagulability and thrombosis in horses [52,53,65]. A coagulation profile should be performed in any horse with serious gastrointestinal disease, including enterocolitis, protein-losing enteropathy or nephropathy (because of the loss of antithrombin III [ATIII]), and hemoconcentration. The diagnosis of disseminated intravascular coagulopathy (DIC) is often concomitant with thrombosis [48,53,66–68]. Peripheral thrombosis is often suspected based on physical examination (eg, cold extremities, no limb pulse). Confirmation of the diagnosis can be provided using Doppler ultrasonography, scintigraphy, arteriography, and digital subtraction angiography (Fig. 4) [52,53]. CT and MRI of the extremities could also provide valuable information. Treatment should include broad-spectrum antimicrobial therapy if infection or bacteremia is suspected, intravenous fluids to ensure adequate perfusion to the extremities, and hyperimmune heparinized plasma to neutralize endotoxin and

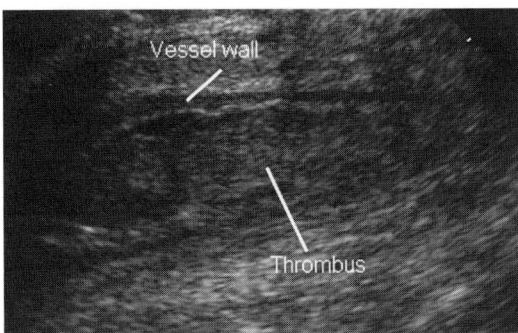

Fig. 4. Sonogram of a saphenous vein thrombus in a septic horse.

provide activated ATIII [52,53]. Thrombolytic therapy is used in the early stages of thrombosis in human beings and small animals (<6 hours after thrombosis has occurred). These "clot busters" include streptokinase, urokinase, and tissue plasminogen activator. Thrombolytic therapy has been tried without success in a foal [52]. It is uncommon to see the horse so quickly after thrombus formation, and delivering enough of the thrombolytic agent to the necessary site has proven difficult; however, this therapy might prove more useful in the future [53].

Septicemia

Whereas endocarditis, myocarditis, and pericarditis are examples of overt cardiac infections, there are likely more numerous instances in which other underlying disease processes (eg, infection, septicemia, endotoxemia) can have important covert effects on the heart. Sepsis is a major cause of mortality in critically ill patients, and cardiac disease is just one aspect of multiple organ dysfunction [69].

Horses experimentally given endotoxin develop a myriad of clinical signs, including pulmonary hypertension, lactic acidosis, hemoconcentration, neutropenia, initial vasoconstriction followed by vasodilation, increased cardiac output compared with normal (secondary to the decrease in systemic vascular resistance), and increased vascular permeability compared with normal [70]. These various clinical signs are closely associated with the complex cascade of proinflammatory and anti-inflammatory mediators triggered by infectious organisms or endotoxin. Myocardial dysfunction has been repeatedly documented in septic human patients. Despite a hyperdynamic overcirculatory state incurred by the low systemic vascular resistance, human patients have biventricular dilation, decreased systolic function, decreased diastolic function, and a blunted response to fluid resuscitation [69,71–73]. In the past, it was hypothesized that myocardial hypoxia could be the cause of the dysfunction; however, this theory has recently been proven false, because it has become clear that global myocardial perfusion is normal or increased compared with normal in septic patients [69,72,73]. Now, it is believed that cardiac dysfunction in these patients is attributable to the presence of myocardial depressant substances, including (among others) tumor necrosis factor-α (TNFα) and interleukin-1β [71–73]. Changes in multiple other cellular mechanisms are likely involved as well, including ATP preservation, myocardial nitric oxide interactions, intracellular calcium release from the sarcoplasmic reticulum, adhesion molecule expression, and apoptotic pathways [69].

Evaluating myocardial function remains a difficult task in human medicine, and it is even more elusive in equine practice. Biochemical markers can be used to infer the state of myocardial function by evaluating perfusion (eg, blood lactate, blood urea nitrogen [BUN], creatinine concentrations), but these indices are certainly not specific for cardiac function.

Measurements of cardiac output can provide information about cardiac function, but cardiac output is not routinely measured, even in critically ill horses. Also, cardiac output depends not only on contractility but on preload, afterload, and heart rate. Multiple methods of determining cardiac output have been used in horses, and they have recently been reviewed in an excellent article by Corley and colleagues [74]. Briefly, the "gold standard" for cardiac output determination is calculation using the Fick principle; however, this is not likely to be used in a clinical setting, because the data collection is obtrusive and tedious. Indicator dilution methods show promise for clinical use, especially those utilizing lithium chloride [74–76]. Doppler echocardiography can also be used. Cardiac output is the product of Πr^2 (or the cross-sectional area of the aorta) $\times$ TVI $\times$ HR, where r is the radius of the aorta, TVI is the area under the curve or time velocity integral for the aortic stroke volume, and HR is the heart rate. Unfortunately, accurate Doppler measurements require that the ultrasound beam be in parallel with the interrogated flow, and this is often difficult in horses, making this calculation less accurate. Although this method still has fair a correlation with dye dilution, TEE yields more accurate information compared with transthoracic echocardiography [74,75]. Finally, pulse contour analysis is used to calculate cardiac output directly from the arterial pressure wave forms using the area under the arterial pressure tracing during systole. Pulse contour analysis can provide continuous beat-to-beat assessment of cardiac output, which might provide valuable information about critically ill septicemic patients in the future. Pulse contour analysis was recently shown to have a good correlation with cardiac output as determined by lithium dilution in anesthetized horses [75].

There are a number of other diagnostics performed in human medicine to assess cardiac function. Tissue Doppler echocardiography is an important recent development in cardiology. The principles of tissue Doppler imaging (TDI) are similar to those of color Doppler imaging, which has been used in echocardiography for some time. Reflected sound waves shift to lower frequencies if the fluid or tissue is moving away from the ultrasound beam and to a higher frequency if the fluid or tissue is moving toward the ultrasound beam. Because tissue shifts of the myocardium are of a higher amplitude and slower velocity than blood flow, they can be evaluated separately from blood flow in the heart using threshold and filter algorithms [77,78]. In human patients, TDI is increasingly being used to assess ventricular systolic and diastolic function. During disease states, the myocardium moves differently than normal, and abnormal myocardial motion during contraction and relaxation can be characterized using TDI. This modality has strong predictive power in a variety of cardiac diseases in people [79,80]. TDI is available on many of the newer ultrasound machines that would be in use in referral hospitals for standard echocardiography in horses. Although the modality has been tested in small animals, we are not aware of any data available yet in horses at the time of this writing.

Heart rate variability (HRV) is another modality used in human medicine to assess the balance of autonomic tone affecting the heart. Normally, the sympathetic and parasympathetic systems are in constant balance and flux with one another. Continual changes in heart rate reflect this system and are indicators of cardiac physiology [81,82]. The ability of the heart to respond to minute-to-minute changes in demand is a vital aspect of normal function. Sepsis affects autonomic balance so that there is a continually high sympathetic tone at the expense of parasympathetic tone. Associated with this is a loss of HRV, which can be depicted on power spectral analysis of the heart rate over time [81]. Decreased HRV compared with normal precedes the development of septic shock and is a useful tool in the human intensive care unit to evaluate patient risk [81,82]. HRV software is available on most continual electrocardiography Holter analyzer programs; thus, all that would be necessary to gain information on HRV in horses is a Holter unit.

Treatment for sepsis has many aspects; it is almost as complex as the pathophysiology itself. We do not try to cover all aspects of treatment here but do touch on the aspects of treatment that pertain directly to the cardiovascular system. During sepsis, systemic vascular resistance decreases compared with normal, which actually promotes a hyperdynamic state in which cardiac output can increase, although perfusion of organs often decreases compared with normal [71]. The main objectives of treatment with regard to the cardiovascular system include fluid resuscitation, pressors, and inotropes. Combined, this support may improve hemodynamics and allow for more appropriate tissue perfusion. Dobutamine and dopamine are the infusions most commonly used to increase cardiac output via their positive inotropic effects [70,83]. Catecholamines are usually used to restore blood pressure, although septic human patients have a blunted response to norepinephrine and epinephrine [71,84]. The store of endogenous vasopressin becomes exhausted fairly quickly, and, recently, exogenous vasopressin has become more popular as a vasoconstrictor. Vasopressin is often used in combination with norepinephrine or epinephrine [85].

Summary

Continual progress is being made in equine medicine with regard to the understanding of infections of cardiac structures and the effect of sepsis on the heart. It is likely that myocardial depression is underrecognized in patients with serious infection, endotoxemia, or septicemia. Many of our advances take root in human medicine; thus, it is here that we can look for guidance with regard to new diagnostics and therapy. Included in this article are a number of modalities not yet in widespread use in equine practice. Some may never take hold, and others may prove unhelpful, but some might become more important, and perhaps even widespread, as we continue to improve clinical veterinary science.

References

[1] Brown CM. Acquired cardiovascular disease. Vet Clin North Am Equine Pract 1985;2: 371–82.
[2] Buergelt CD, Cooley AJ, Hines SA, et al. Endocarditis in six horses. Vet Pathol 1985;22: 333–7.
[3] Pipers FS, Hamlin RL, Reef V. Echocardiographic detection of cardiovascular lesions in a horse. J Equine Med Surg 1979;3:68–77.
[4] Wagenaar G, Kroneman J, Breukink H. Endocarditis in the horse. Blue Book for the Veterinary Professional 1967;12:38–45.
[5] Maxson AD, Reef VB. Bacterial endocarditis in horses: ten cases (1984–1995). Equine Vet J 1997;29:394–9.
[6] Dedrick P, Reef VB, Sweeney RW, et al. Treatment of bacterial endocarditis in a horse. J Am Vet Med Assoc 1988;193:339–42.
[7] Ball MA, Weldon AD. Vegetative endocarditis in an Appaloosa gelding. Cornell Vet 1992; 82:301–9.
[8] Physick-Sheard PW. Diseases of the endocardium and valves. In: Colahan PT, Mayhew IG, Merritt AM, et al, editors. Equine medicine and surgery. 4th edition. Goleta (CA): American Veterinary Publications; 1991. p. 295–314.
[9] Weinstein L, Schlesinger JJ. Pathoanatomic, pathophysiologic, and clinical correlations in endocarditis (first of two parts). N Engl J Med 1974;291:832–6.
[10] Kasari TR, Roussel AJ. Bacterial endocarditis. Part I. Pathophysiologic, diagnostic, and therapeutic considerations. Compend Contin Educ Pract Vet 1989;11:655–9.
[11] Dillon JC. Echocardiography in valvular vegetations. Am J Med 1977;62:856–62.
[12] Bonagura JD, Herring DS, Welker F. Echocardiography. Vet Clin North Am Equine Pract 1985;2:311–33.
[13] Rantanen NW. Diseases of the heart. Vet Clin North Am Equine Pract 1986;2:33–47.
[14] Reef VB. Cardiovascular ultrasonography. In: Equine diagnostic ultrasound. Philadelphia: WB Saunders; 1998. p. 215–73.
[15] Ewert S, Brown C, Derksen F, et al. *Serratia marcescens* endocarditis in a horse. J Am Vet Med Assoc 1992;200:961–3.
[16] Travers CW, Van den Berg JS. *Pseudomonas spp* associated vegetative endocarditis in two horses. S Afr Vet 1995;66:172–6.
[17] Church S, Harrigan KE, Irving AE, et al. Endocarditis caused by *Pasteurella caballi* in a horse. Vet J 1998;76:528–30.
[18] Peet RL, McDermott J, Williams JM, et al. Fungal myocarditis and nephritis in a horse. Aust Vet J 1981;57:439–40.

[19] Innes JR, Berger J, Francis J. Subacute bacterial endocarditis with pulmonary embolism in a horse associated with *Shigella equirulis*. Br Vet J 1950;106:245–50.
[20] McCormick BS, Peet RL, Downes K. *Erysipelothrix rhusiopathiae* vegetative endocarditis in a horse. Aust Vet J 1985;61:392.
[21] Nilsfors L, Lombard CW, Weckner D, et al. Diagnosis of pulmonary valve endocarditis in a horse. Equine Vet J 1991;23:479–82.
[22] Pace LW, Wirth NR, Foss RR, et al. Endocarditis and pulmonary aspergillosis in a horse. J Vet Diagn Invest 1994;6:504–6.
[23] Collatos C, Clark S, Reef VB, et al. Septicemia, atrial fibrillation, cardiomegaly, left atrial mass and *Rhodococcus equi* septic osteoarthritis in a foal. J Am Vet Med Assoc 1990;197: 1039–42.
[24] Hillyer MH, Mair TS, Holmes JR. Treatment of bacterial endocarditis in a Shire mare. Equine Vet Educ 1990;2:5–7.
[25] Horstkotte D. Endocarditis: epidemiology, diagnosis and treatment. Z Kardiol 2000;89: IV2–V11.
[26] Mylonakis E, Calderwood SB. Infective endocarditis in adults. N Engl J Med 2001;345: 1318–30.
[27] Shivley BK, Gurule FT, Roldan CA, et al. Diagnostic value of transesophageal compared with transthoracic echocardiography in infective endocarditis. J Am Coll Cardiol 1991;18: 391–7.
[28] Heidenreich PA, Masoudi FA, Maini B, et al. Echocardiography in patients with suspected endocarditis: a cost effective analysis. Am J Med 1999;107:198–208.
[29] Sleeper MM. Myocardial disease. In: Robinson NE, editor. Current therapy in equine medicine. 5th edition. Philadelphia: WB Saunders; 2003. p. 620–1.
[30] Fregin GF. The cardiovascular system. In: Mansmann RA, McAllister ES, editors. Equine medicine and surgery. 3rd edition. Santa Barbara (CA): America Veterinary Publications; 1982. p. 645–701.
[31] Reef VB, McGuirk SM. Diseases of the cardiovascular system. In: Smith BP, editor. Large animal internal medicine. 3rd edition. St. Louis (MO): Mosby; 2002. p. 443–78.
[32] Slack J, McGuirk SM, Erb HN, et al. Biochemical markers of cardiac injury in normal, surviving septic, or nonsurviving septic neonatal foals. J Vet Intern Med 2005;19: 577–80.
[33] Apple FS. Tissue specificity of cardiac troponin I, cardiac troponin T and creatinine kinase-MB. Clin Chem Acta 1999;284:151–9.
[34] Muir J. Progress in myocardial damage detection: new biochemical markers for clinicians. Crit Rev Clin Lab Sci 1997;34:1–66.
[35] Phillips W, Giguere S, Franklin RP, et al. Cardiac troponin I in pastured and race training Thoroughbred horses. J Vet Intern Med 2003;17:597–9.
[36] Schwarzwald CC, Hardy J, Bucellato M. High cardiac troponin I serum concentration in a horse with multiform ventricular tachycardia and myocardial necrosis. J Vet Intern Med 2003;17:364–8.
[37] Cornelisse CJ, Schott HC, Olivier NB, et al. Concentration of cardiac troponin I in a horse with a ruptured aortic regurgitation jet lesion and ventricular tachycardia. J Am Vet Med Assoc 2000;217:231–5.
[38] Jeremias A, Gibson CM. Narrative review: alternative causes for elevated cardiac troponin levels when acute coronary syndromes are excluded. Ann Intern Med 2005;142: 786–91.
[39] Nunes JP. Cardiac troponin I in systemic diseases. A possible role for myocardial strain. Rev Port Cardiol 2001;20:785–8.
[40] Worth CT, Reef VB. Pericarditis in horses: 18 cases (1986–1995). J Am Vet Med Assoc 1998; 212:248–53.
[41] Bernard W, Reef VB, Clark ES, et al. Pericarditis in horses: six cases (1982–1986). J Am Vet Med Assoc 1990;196:468–71.

[42] Robinson J, Marr CM, Reef VB, et al. Idiopathic, aseptic, effusive, fibrinous, nonconstrictive pericarditis with tamponade in a Standardbred filly. J Am Vet Med Assoc 1992;201: 1593–8.
[43] Freestone JF, Thomas WP, Carlson GP, et al. Idiopathic effusive pericarditis with tamponade in the horse. Equine Vet J 1987;19:38–42.
[44] Bolin DC, Donahue JM, Vickers ML, et al. Microbiologic and pathologic findings in an epidemic of equine pericarditis. J Vet Diagn Invest 2005;17:38–44.
[45] Seahorn JL, Slovis NM, Reimer JM, et al. Case-controlled study of factors associated with fibrinous pericarditis among horses in central Kentucky during spring 2001. J Am Vet Med Assoc 2003;223:832–8.
[46] Kittleson MD, Kienle RD. Pericardial disease and cardiac neoplasia. In: Kittleson MD, Kienle RD, editors. Small animal cardiovascular medicine. St. Louis (MO): Mosby; 1998. p. 413–31.
[47] Spodick DH. Pericardial diseases. In: Braunwald E, editor. Heart disease: a textbook of cardiovascular medicine. 5th edition. Philadelphia: WB Saunders; 1997. p. 1823–72.
[48] Dolente BA, Beech J, Lindborg S, et al. Evaluation of risk factors for development of catheter-associated jugular thrombophlebitis in horses: 50 cases (1993–1998). J Am Vet Med Assoc 2005;227:1134–41.
[49] Maxie MG, Physick-Sheard PW. Aortoiliac thrombosis in horses. Vet Pathol 1985;22: 238–49.
[50] DeLay J, Peregrine AS, Parsons DA. Verminous arteritis in a 3-month old Thoroughbred foal. Can Vet J 2001;42:289–91.
[51] Edwards GB, Allen WE. Aorto-iliac thrombosis in two horses: clinical course of the disease and use of real-time ultrasonography to confirm diagnosis. Equine Vet J 1988;20:384–7.
[52] Forrest LJ, Cooley AJ, Darien BJ. Digital arterial thrombosis in a septicemic foal. J Vet Intern Med 1999;13:382–5.
[53] Brianceau P, Divers TJ. Acute thrombosis of limb arteries in horses with sepsis: five cases (1988–1998). Equine Vet J 2001;33:105–9.
[54] Divers TJ. Prevention and treatment of thrombosis, phlebitis, and laminitis in horses with gastrointestinal disease. Vet Clin North Am Equine Pract 2003;19:779–90.
[55] Traub-Dargatz JL, Dargatz DA. A retrospective study of vein thrombosis in horses treated with intravenous fluids in a veterinary teaching hospital. J Vet Intern Med 1994;8:264–6.
[56] Gardner SY, Reef VB, Spencer PA. Ultrasonographic evaluation of horses with thrombophlebitis of the jugular vein: 46 cases (1985–1988). J Am Vet Med Assoc 1991; 199:370–3.
[57] Rijkenhuizen ABM, van Swieten HA. Reconstruction of the jugular vein in horses with post thrombophlebitis stenosis using saphenous vein graft. Equine Vet J 1998;30:236–9.
[58] Wiemer P, Gruys E, van Hoeck B. A study of seven different types of grafts for jugular vein transplantation in the horse. Res Vet Sci 2005;79:211–7.
[59] Cranley JJ, McCullagh KG. Ischemic myocardial fibrosis and aortic strongylosis in the horse. Equine Vet J 1981;13:35–42.
[60] Duggan VE, Holbrook TC, Dechant JE, et al. Diagnosis of aorto-iliac thrombosis in a quarter horse foal using Doppler ultrasound and nuclear scintigraphy. J Vet Intern Med 2004;18: 753–6.
[61] Tithof PK, Rebhun WC, Dietze AE. Ultrasonographic diagnosis of aorto-iliac thrombosis. Cornell Vet 1985;75:540–4.
[62] Reef VB, Roby KA, Richardson DW, et al. Use of ultrasonography for the detection of aorto-iliac thrombosis in horses. J Am Vet Med Assoc 1987;190:286–8.
[63] Boswell JC, Marr CM, Cauvin ER, et al. The use of scintigraphy in the diagnosis of aorto-iliac thrombosis in a horse. Equine Vet J 1999;31:537–41.
[64] Brama PA, Rijkenhuizen AB, van Swieten HA, et al. Thrombosis of the aorta and the caudal arteries in the horse; additional diagnostics and a new surgical treatment. Vet Q 1996;18: S85–9.

[65] Triplett EA, O'Brien RT, Wilson DG, et al. Thrombosis of the brachial artery in a foal. J Vet Intern Med 1996;10:330–2.
[66] Barton MH, Morris DD, Norton N, et al. Hemostatic and fibrinolytic indices in neonatal foals with presumed septicemia. J Vet Intern Med 1998;12:26–35.
[67] Weiss DJ, Rashid J. The sepsis-coagulant axis: a review. J Vet Intern Med 1998;12:317–24.
[68] Darien BJ, Williams AM. Possible hypercoagulation in 3 foals with septicemia. Equine Vet Educ 1993;5:19–22.
[69] Levy RJ, Deutschman CS. Evaluating myocardial depression in sepsis. Shock 2004;22:1–10.
[70] Trim CM, Moore JN, Hardee MM, et al. Effects of an infusion of dopamine on the cardiopulmonary effects of *Escherichia coli* endotoxin in anesthetized horses. Res Vet Sci 1991;50: 54–63.
[71] Young JD. The heart and circulation in severe sepsis. Br J Anaesth 2004;93:114–20.
[72] Krishnagopalan S, Kumar A, Parrillo JE, et al. Myocardial dysfunction in the patient with sepsis. Curr Opin Crit Care 2002;8:376–88.
[73] Kumar A, Haery C, Parrillo JE. Myocardial dysfunction in septic shock. Crit Care Clin 2000; 16:251–87.
[74] Corley KTT, Donaldson LL, Durando MM, et al. Cardiac output technologies with special reference to the horse. J Vet Intern Med 2003;17:262–72.
[75] Hallowell GD, Corley KTT. Use of lithium dilution and pulse contour analysis cardiac output determination in anesthetized horses: a clinical evaluation. Vet Anesth Analgesia 2005;32:201–11.
[76] Linton RA, Young LE, Marlin DJ, et al. Cardiac output measured by lithium dilution, thermodilution, and transesophageal Doppler echocardiography in anesthetized horses. Am J Vet Res 2000;61:731–7.
[77] Sengupta PP, Mohan JC, Pandian NG. Tissue Doppler echocardiography: principles and applications. Indian Heart J 2002;54:3–16.
[78] Brodin LA. Tissue Doppler, a fundamental tool for parametric imaging. Clin Physiol Funct Imaging 2004;24:147–55.
[79] Sanderson JE, Wang M, Yu CM. Tissue Doppler imaging for predicting outcome in patients with cardiovascular disease. Curr Opin Cardiol 2004;19:458–63.
[80] Nikitin NP, Witte KK. Application of tissue Doppler imaging in cardiology. Cardiology 2004;101:170–84.
[81] Moriguchi T, Hirasawa H, Oda S, et al. Analysis of heart rate variability is a useful tool to predict the occurrence of septic shock in patients with severe sepsis. Nippon Rinsho 2004;62: 2285–90.
[82] Schmidt HB, Werdan K, Muller-Werdan U. Autonomic dysfunction in the ICU patient. Curr Opin Crit Care 2001;7:314–22.
[83] Raisis AL, Young LE, Blissitt KJ. Effect of a 30-minute infusion of dobutamine hydrochloride on hind limb blood flow and hemodynamics in halothane-anesthetized horses. Am J Vet Res 2000;10:1282–8.
[84] Ruokonen E, Parviainen I, Uusaro A. Treatment of impaired perfusion in septic shock. Ann Med 2002;34:590–7.
[85] Wenzel V, Lindner KH. Employing vasopressin during cardiopulmonary resuscitation and vasodilatory shock as a lifesaving vasopressor. Cardiovasc Res 2001;51:529–41.

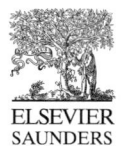

Pathophysiology, Diagnosis, and Management of Urinary Tract Infection in Horses

Melinda A. Frye, DVM, MS, PhD

Department of Clinical Sciences, Colorado State University Veterinary Medical Center, 300 West Drake, Fort Collins, CO 80526, USA

Clinical disease resulting from bacterial colonization of the equine urinary tract remains an uncommon occurrence [1,2]. Equine urinary tract infection (UTI) is rarely a primary event, most often occurring subsequent to mechanical obstructions or functional impairments that impede normal urine flow. In contrast to the less prominent role of UTIs in equine patients, bacterial infections of the urinary tract represent one of the most common reasons prompting human patients to seek medical attention [3]. Because of this, much investigative effort has been devoted to the pathophysiology, diagnosis, and treatment of human bacterial UTIs. Although etiology, causative organisms, and available antimicrobials are partly specific to human beings, much can be learned about bacterial virulence and the urinary tract immune defenses that is likely to be relevant, in some form, across species.

As with all infections, attributes of the environment, host, and infectious agent combine to increase or decrease the opportunity for development of clinical disease. A host with weakened resistance to bacterial colonization may be susceptible to infection by strains with low virulence, whereas colonization by highly pathogenic strains may be required to cause clinical disease in an immunocompetent host [4]. Studies in human beings have greatly expanded our knowledge of host-agent interactions at the level of the uroepithelium as well as local urinary tract defenses that prevent bacterial colonization. Resultant advances in the understanding of virulence factors and host responses are described. Although no remarkable previously unidentified uropathogens in Equidae have been identified and no novel antimicrobial classes for treatment of UTIs have evolved [5], investigations in human beings and equids have assisted in better defining and validating current

E-mail address: melinda.frye@colostate.edu

approaches. New information regarding normal urinary parameters in horses is reviewed. Bacterial resistance to commonly used antimicrobials is an emerging problem in veterinary medicine; thus, current guidelines for use of antimicrobial therapy are discussed. In light of antimicrobial resistance, alternative interventions aimed at long-term prevention of UTIs are also described.

Host-agent interactions in the urinary tract

In order for an ascending UTI to manifest in the horse, there is usually identifiable impairment of host factors designed to act as a deterrent to the initial entry and continued presence of potentially uropathogenic bacteria. Briefly, this may include obstruction of normal urine flow by masses or strictures; disruption of the uroepithelium by trauma or neoplasia; or diminished numbers of normal urethral, vulvar, or preputial flora [1,2]. In women, individual factors like epithelial cell adherence and perineal conformation are additional factors that influence susceptibility to UTIs [6,7].

Once the infectious agent enters the urinary tract, bacterial factors favoring attachment and colonization are engaged. Uropathogenic *Escherichia coli* exhibits such factors, making it particularly suited to colonize the uroepithelium successfully and to contribute to clinical disease (Fig. 1). Consistent with this, *E coli* is commonly isolated from urine in normal horses [8] and is one of the most common isolates obtained from human beings and horses with bacterial UTI [1,2,4,9]. Uropathogenic strains of *E coli* are phenotypically different from less virulent strains [9] and selectively emerge from the population of fecal flora to produce disease because of the presence of virulence factors [10]. Phenotypic variation may be attributed to mutations arising as a result of antimicrobial exposure or altered environmental conditions, such as infection [11,12].

A principal virulence factor that contributes to initial binding of the bacterium to the uroepithelium and adherence in the face of urine flow is the presence of fimbriae [2–4,9]. Uropathogenic bacteria have surface fimbriae that attach to uroepithelial glycolipid receptors [2]. Great variation is seen in fimbrial antigenicity, receptor specificity, and function [4]. Additionally, transcriptional control is exerted to alter the temporal expression of fimbrial protein so that *E coli* strains isolated from cases of cystitis display patterns of fimbrial expression that are distinct from those strains isolated in pyelonephritis [9]. Presumably, pyelonephritis isolates with low initial fimbrial expression progress more readily to the kidneys [9]. Thus, variations in fimbrial expression not only determine virulence but influence the localization of epithelial colonization. Fimbrial vaccines administered to mice and people have been effective in UTI prophylaxis, boosting innate resistance and offering an alternative to antimicrobial therapy when bacterial resistance, persistent outflow anomalies, or unexplained recurrence exists [13,14].

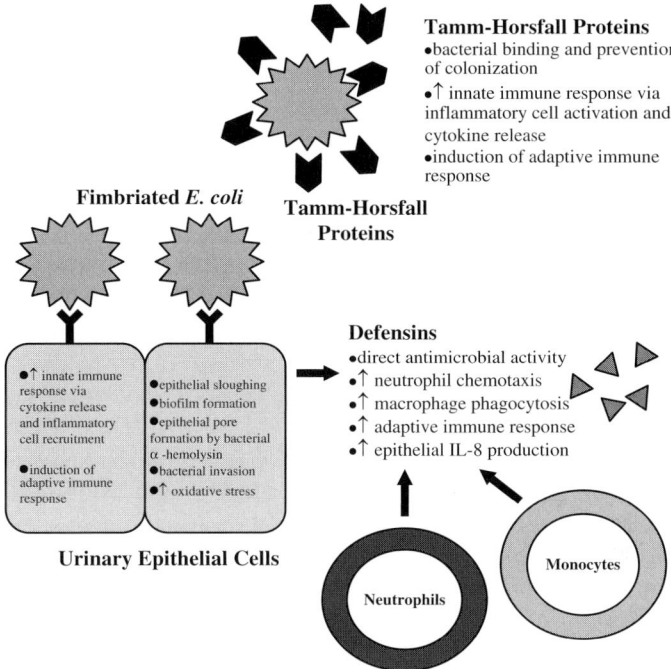

Fig. 1. Schematic representation of the proposed uroepithelial, inflammatory cell, and secreted protein response on exposure to uropathogenic *Escherichia coli*. IL, interleukin.

In addition to aiding in bacterial attachment, fimbriae activate host signaling that mediates the uroepithelial response to bacterial presence. A subset of uropathogenic *E coli* fimbriae, type 1 fimbria, facilitates bacterial invasion of the uroepithelium [15]. Yet another type, F1C fimbriae, modulates renal defenses by stimulating epithelial interleukin (IL)-8 production [16] and subsequent neutrophil chemotaxis. The lipopolysaccharide (LPS) portion of the outer membrane of gram-negative bacteria also influences the host inflammatory response. When LPS is released from the bacterial cell membrane, it binds to LPS binding protein (LBP). By binding to toll-like receptor (TLR)-4 on macrophages and activating nuclear factor-κB, LPS-LBP promotes transcription of a host of inflammatory response genes, with subsequent production of chemokines and cytokines [17]. Specifically, LPS exposure of murine urinary tract mucosal cells resulted in IL-6 activation [18]. The cytokine IL-6 activates macrophages and increases the generation of acute-phase proteins, thus contributing to the inflammatory response to bacteria [17]. Further evidence for the protective role of TLRs is the use of TLR ligands, such as the LPS constituent lipid A, as an adjuvant in amplifying the adaptive immune response [19]. Not surprisingly, dysfunction in TLR-4 signaling can cause increased susceptibility to UTI because of the lack of neutrophil chemotaxis [20].

Exposure to LPS exerts deleterious effects on the epithelium via oxidant-mediated cytotoxicity [54]. In a rodent model, antioxidants (butylated hydroxytoluene, N,N'-diphenyl-L-phenylenediamine, and superoxide dismutase) aimed at reducing nitric oxide and superoxide were shown to attenuate oxidant injury to renal tubular cells. The pro-oxidant nature of UTIs has been documented clinically in diabetic human beings [21]. Although administration of antioxidants has been shown to alleviate renal scarring attributable to experimental pyelonephritis [22], the beneficial effects of antioxidants in altering early cytotoxicity in vivo have yet to be demonstrated.

In addition to fimbriae and LPS, approximately 50% of uropathogenic E coli produce the pore-forming α-hemolysin [17]. α-Hemolysins exert cytopathic effects on the uroepithelium by generating pores in the cell membrane, thereby easing passage of bacteria into the cell and subsequent mucosal invasion [23,24].

After attachment to the uroepithelium, pathogenic bacteria may form a biofilm to protect against host defenses [25]. A biofilm is defined as a collection of cells that are permanently attached to a scaffold or to each other and are fixed in extracellular polymeric material [26]. The biofilm milieu is far from inert, and a collection of studies describes bacterial interactions with the biofilm matrix, phenotypic heterogeneity, and the presence of water channels [26,27]. Biofilm affords bacteria the opportunity for development of antimicrobial resistance, protection from antimicrobial activity, and defense against the host immune system [26].

On interaction of the uroepithelium with microbes, events aimed at prevention of further invasion and colonization commence. These include sloughing of the superficial epithelial layer as a strategy to reduce the microbial population [3]. Secretory IgA is the principal immunoglobulin type in the vagina, and it exists in small amounts in urine [28]. IgA has been shown to bind fimbriated E coli by interactions between specific receptors, and subsequent bacterial agglutination was postulated to be the mechanism of IgA-induced antibacterial activity at mucosal surfaces [29]. Further, urinary epithelial cells, lacking protective mucus or cilia, respond to the presence of bacteria by secreting soluble proteins that attract immunocompetent cells and enhance the expression of proinflammatory cytokines [3].

Tamm-Horsfall protein (THP) is one such soluble mediator that is only produced in the renal tubular cells of the distal loop of Henle, and it is the most plentiful protein in mammalian urine [3,30]. Recent investigations incorporating a THP-knockout murine model revealed the importance of THP in protecting against bacterial colonization of the uroepithelium [31]. Mice lacking the THP gene demonstrated increased susceptibility to cystitis attributed to type 1 fimbriated E coli. It has been proposed that a principal mechanism by which THP exerts this effect is through binding of type 1 fimbriae, thereby preventing attachment of E coli to uroepithelial receptors [31,32]. In addition to this antimicrobial action, THP enhances innate immunity by inducing monocyte proliferation and tumor necrosis factor

(TNF)-α secretion [33] as well as IL-8 expression by neutrophils [34] in human beings. Further, THP facilitates the maturation, and therefore the antigen-presenting capabilities, of myeloid dendritic cells [35].

Renal defensins are another class of molecules that contribute to the innate immune response of the uroepithelium [36,37]. Mammalian defensins are produced by neutrophils and monocytes or by mucosal epithelial cells of various body systems [38]. Like THP, defensins act on all levels of the protective response, exerting direct antimicrobial effects [38,39], enhancing innate immunity by promoting phagocytosis by macrophages and neutrophil chemotaxis [40,41], and contributing to the adaptive immune response by augmented T-cell chemotaxis [42]. In people, the group of defensins originating from urogenital, pulmonary, and gastrointestinal mucosal epithelial cells are called β-defensins [39]. Analysis of equine liver, heart, spleen, gastrointestinal, and renal tissue revealed diffuse β-defensin mRNA expression [37]. The presence of β-defensin in the equine kidney, along with peptide conservation and homology with other mammals, suggests that equine β-defensin is likely to contribute to the local urinary immune response in horses [37]. In multiple models of rodent diabetes, kidney β-defensin gene expression was reduced, and it was suggested that the paucity of defensins may partly contribute to the increased incidence of UTIs in diabetic individuals [43]. Interestingly, the rare phenomenon of clinical or occult UTI in the absence of structural or functional anomalies in equids has been observed in cases of hyperadrenocorticism [44–46], a condition accompanied by hyperglycemia and insulin resistance (ie, secondary diabetes mellitus). Because β-defensin has not been measured in horses with hyperadrenocorticism, it is currently unknown whether this condition is associated with reduced β-defensin expression.

Human uroepithelial cells secrete IL-8 constitutively in vivo, and it has been hypothesized that this enables a rapid host response to the introduction of microorganisms [47]. In addition to basal IL-8 secretion, urinary epithelial cells stimulated by *E coli* and other bacteria increase IL-8 production and IL-8 receptor expression [48,49]. Increased IL-8 activity contributes to the host immune defense by localizing extravasated neutrophils and facilitating migration across the uroepithelial barrier [50].

It is now evident that the uroepithelium generates a complex immune response on exposure to uropathogenic bacteria. Although activation of the innate and adaptive immune responses is clearly necessary for bacterial clearance and inhibition of colonization, the same cells and mediators that destroy microorganisms may also be cytotoxic to uroepithelial cells. One example of this phenomenon is that of IL-6, the aforementioned cytokine that activates macrophages and increases the generation of acute-phase proteins [17]. The urinary IL-6 response is correlated with the severity of infectious disease in human beings [51,52], reflecting an appropriate proinflammatory response to an increasingly larger pathogenic stimulus. Greater IL-6 production is not entirely without detriment, however, because cytokine concentration is correlated with renal scarring in children [52]. In contrast, IL-6–deficient mice displayed greater bacterial growth and increased mortality when compared with wild-type mice, suggesting impaired bacterial clearance [53]. As discussed previously, a similar balance must be achieved in LPS signaling. Although LPS exerts oxidant-meditated cytotoxicity [54] and deleterious systemic effects [4], a reduced response to LPS impairs neutrophil chemotaxis, thus increasing susceptibility to UTIs [20]. As a result, it is evident that tight regulation of the uroepithelial response to bacterial invasion is essential to optimize clearance of microbes while minimizing renal cell necrosis and fibrosis. Consistent with this, use of anti-inflammatory agents in the treatment of uncomplicated UTIs is generally not indicated but has been recommended for management of selective cases of chronic cystitis in women [55] and in noninfectious inflammatory conditions of the renal system (ie, bladder irrigation with dimethyl sulfoxide [DMSO]) [56].

Infectious agents

The organisms most commonly isolated from horses with ascending cystitis include *E coli, Proteus, Klebsiella, Enterobacter, Corynebacterium, Streptococcus, Staphylococcus,* and *Pseudomonas* [1,2]. Except for *Klebsiella* and *Corynebacterium*, all these organisms were identified in cultures of normal equine urine [8], lending validity to the notion that weakened host defenses allow virulent strains of normal flora to contribute opportunistically to ascending UTI in the equid. Although methicillin-resistant *Staphylococcus aureus* is being isolated from equids in the United States and abroad, sources of the isolate have thus far been limited to nasal secretions, wounds, and an abdominal granuloma [57–59]. This author is unaware of any emerging strains of uropathogenic bacteria in the equine population. In normal equids and those with cystitis, it is not uncommon to isolate multiple organisms from the urine [2,8]. In addition to the microorganisms commonly associated with ascending cystitis, growth of *Actinobacillus equuli, Streptococcus equi, Rhodococcus equi,* and *Salmonella* spp has been observed in septic foals and may presumably contribute to the incidence of septic nephritis of hematogenous origin [60].

Fluorescent antibody isolation of *Leptospira interrogans* in equine urine has been described, and associated with elevated *Leptospira* serum titers, pyuria, negative urine cultures, elevated serum creatinine, fever, and bilaterally enlarged kidneys on ultrasound examination [61]. Equine leptospirosis has been well described, with novel findings being limited to a recent report of nonulcerative keratouveitis in an affected horse in Japan [62].

Parasitic infections of the equine urinary tract have been well characterized [2]. Recently, the nematode *Halicephalobus deletrix* was identified as the causative organism in three horses with severe and progressive neurologic signs accompanied by granulomatous nephritis or overt renal granulomas

[63,64]. Diagnosis was confirmed by microscopic identification of adults, larvae, and eggs within the granulomas; larvae within the renal tubules; and adults and eggs in the urine sediment [63,64].

Diagnosis

The complete blood cell count (CBC) may be normal in equids with lower UTIs, and although an inflammatory leukogram may be present in horses with pyelonephritis [65], this finding alone is nonspecific. Thus, although the CBC may assist in detecting renal involvement and determining disease severity, urinalysis remains the least expensive and most definitive test for diagnosing bacterial UTIs. A high suspicion of UTI should be present with visualization of more than 20 microorganisms and more than 10 white blood cells (WBCs) per high-power field during examination of the urine sediment [2,65]. A definitive diagnosis and isolation of causative organisms can be obtained by urine culture. Bacterial growth of more than 10,000 colony-forming units (CFUs) per milliliter of urine, whether by urinary catheterization or voided midstream sample, has traditionally been diagnostic for UTI in equids [2,65,66]. This has been extrapolated from other species [66], however, and urinalysis reference ranges that are diagnostic for clinically relevant UTI in equids are just beginning to be defined.

Investigation of urinalysis parameters in 6 mares was conducted nearly 20 years ago [66]. Urine was obtained from 6 normal mares by bladder catheterization, and four of six samples exhibited no bacterial growth on culture. Minimal growth of *Streptococcus* spp was observed in one sample, and more than 30,000 CFUs/mL of *Streptococcus* spp grew in the other sample. The authors postulated that the latter mare had bacterial infection in the absence of pyuria or that the urine was contaminated during catheterization. More recently, analysis of voided midstream urine obtained from 22 normal horses revealed that 1 or fewer WBCs per high-power field was present in all samples, and bacteria were visualized in only 2 of 22 samples [8]. With regard to quantitative urinary culture in normal equids, this study revealed that collection method and gender should be considered when establishing reference ranges. Urine culture revealed a significant difference between catheterized and voided samples. Female equids had a mean growth of 6054 CFUs/mL in voided urine and 172 CFUs/mL in catheterized urine, whereas male equids had respective means of 490 and 82 CFUs/mL. It should be noted that the presence of large numbers of squamous epithelial cells in a voided sample suggests that perineal contamination may have occurred, and culture results should be interpreted accordingly [4]. It is also evident that a significant difference exists between genders when voided samples are compared, with female equids having greater bacterial growth. Based on the results of this study, the authors proposed revised values of CFU/mL for equine urine, based on collection method, that should be interpreted as contamination, suspicion of UTI, and clinically relevant UTI

(Table 1) [4]. The investigators proposed that 40,000 or more CFUs/mL should be observed in voided midstream samples and 1000 or more CFUs/mL should be observed in catheterized samples before a diagnosis of UTI is made in either gender [4]. The authors acknowledge that further evaluation of urine from clinically affected horses is warranted to confirm the recommended reference ranges; however, these initial data suggest that traditional values may promote false-positive results when voided urine is examined and false-negative results when catheterized samples are assessed [4].

In human patients with UTI and unknown renal involvement, serum markers of inflammation are used to assist in diagnosing pyelonephritis. Concentrations of IL-6 and IL-8 have been shown to be elevated in urine and serum of patients with acute pyelonephritis [67], and this profile was distinct from those individuals with asymptomatic bacteriuria only, who were less likely to have an elevated level of serum IL-6 [68]. Serum and urine proinflammatory cytokines are reduced in human beings after successful antimicrobial management of pyelonephritis, thereby providing a measure of treatment efficacy [69]. Procalcitonin, a product of the thyroid gland that is produced by the macrophage-monocyte system under conditions of sepsis, has recently been proposed as a specific serum marker to aid in the differentiation of acute pyelonephritis from lower UTI [70,71]. The usefulness of this marker in human beings is currently debated, with some investigators reporting low test sensitivity and specificity and others reporting significant accuracy in determining renal involvement [70,71]. Presently, it would seem prudent to use traditional measures of systemic inflammation and renal dysfunction in the diagnosis of pyelonephritis in the horse, including the CBC and chemistry profile, respectively [2].

Endoscopy of the urinary tract has emerged as one of the more useful tools in localizing inflammation and identifying conditions that contribute to the development of UTIs. A flexible endoscope with a minimum length of 100 cm and outside diameter of less than 12 mm is appropriate for visualization of the bladder in adult horses of either gender [72]. As the endoscope is advanced from the distal urethra proximally toward the bladder,

Table 1
Bacteriuria in male and female horses

	Clinically relevant (CFU/mL)	Suspicious (CFU/mL)	Contamination (CFU/mL)
Midstream voided urine	>40,000	20,000–40,000	<20,000
Catheterized urine	>1,000	500–1,000	<500

Abbreviation: CFU/mL, colony-forming units per milliliter of urine.
Data from MacLeay JM, Kohn CW. Results of quantitative cultures of urine by free catch and catheterization from healthy horses. J Vet Intern Med 1998;12:76–8.

the urethral mucosa can be observed for strictures, adhesions, uroliths, or mucosal defects [72]. Cystoscopy is beneficial for visualizing mucosal irritation (ie, cystitis) or masses [72,73], cystic calculi (Fig. 2) [73], sabulous urolithiasis attributable to bladder paralysis [74], and dilated ureteral openings associated with vesicoureteral reflux [2]. Incompetent ureteral apertures may be present in equids with ectopic ureter or bladder distention or paralysis and may increase the risk for ascending pyelonephritis, because the normally protective ureteral opening is dilated and loses the ability to serve as a barrier against urine reflux [2]. Cystoscopy may also aid in characterization of the urine leaving individual ureters by observation (ie, gross hematuria) as well as by microscopic examination of samples obtained by ureteral catheterization [72,73]. In addition to localizing the origin of abnormal urine, cystoscopy can establish ureteral patency by observing for regular discharge of urine into the bladder approximately once every minute [72].

Although application of ultrasonography to examination of the lower urinary tract is limited compared with endoscopy, it is a cost-effective, minimally invasive, and accessible modality for visualization of the equine kidneys. Ultrasonography can aid in localization of pathologic findings (ie, calculi, obstruction) as well as chronicity (ie, renal fibrosis) [75,76]. Additionally, this modality can often be used to distinguish renal abscesses from noninfectious masses [75]. Additional imaging techniques used in human patients, such as urograms, CT, MRI, and radionuclide studies [4], are not widely available to equine patients. At equipped referral institutions, CT and MRI can be performed in small foals and nuclear studies can be performed in adult horses and foals. Radiography without contrast rarely provides information that cannot be obtained by the more informative

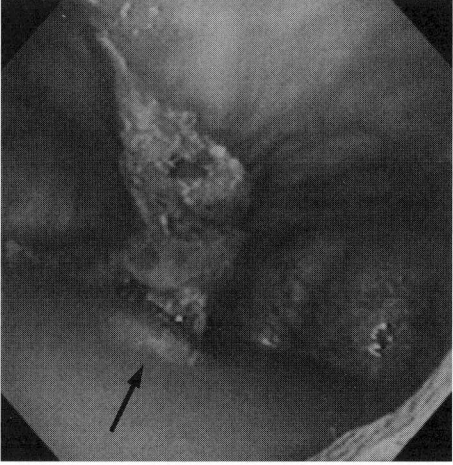

Fig. 2. Cystitis secondary to urolithiasis. The urolith is visible ventrally, protruding slightly from the urine (*arrow*).

modalities of endoscopy and ultrasound, although the diagnostic yield is greater in young horses and miniature breeds [77].

Management

Antimicrobials

Because the cause of UTIs in equids is most often a structural or functional resistance to urine flow, it is critical to resolve the primary problem before, or concomitant to, the initiation of antimicrobial treatment. This may include removal or dissolution of uroliths, surgical correction of congenital anomalies, traumatic sequelae (ie, fibrous adhesions after foaling) or masses, or treatment of neurologic disease underlying detrusor muscle atony.

Once the inciting pathologic condition is addressed, use of antimicrobials aimed at eradication of causative organisms remains the basis of treatment of UTI in equids. In addition to bacterial susceptibility and urine drug concentration, ease of administration must be a primary consideration so that owner compliance is maximized. For cases of uncomplicated cystitis (ie, no structural or functional anomalies), at least 1 week of antimicrobial treatment is recommended; length of treatment may increase to 6 weeks for recurrent UTI or 2 months for renal abscesses [1,2,78]. In addition to these general guidelines, it is prudent to assess for resolution of bacteriuria or clinical signs before cessation of treatment. In human patients, 10 to 14 days of antimicrobial therapy is recommended for treatment of persistent or repeated infections attributable to structural or functional anomalies or to infection with resistant bacterial strains [5,79].

Two unconventional populations of patients are worth noting. First, women may have symptoms of a UTI (ie, dysuria, frequency of urination) but fail to have positive dipstick results for nitrites and leukocytes, or bacterial growth on culture, on testing of voided midstream urine [80]. Treatment of these women with trimethoprim-sulfa for 3 days reduced the duration of symptoms when compared with women who received placebo treatment, suggesting that the decision to treat with antimicrobials should be based on patient signs and symptoms rather than strictly on laboratory analysis [80]. In contrast, it is not uncommon for individuals who are elderly or have spinal cord trauma to have asymptomatic bacteriuria [81,82], defined as more than 100,000 CFUs/mL of voided urine without accompanying signs or symptoms of UTI [5]. It is generally believed that this latter condition does not induce adverse sequelae in otherwise healthy people with controlled bladder pressures, and antibiotic treatment is not routinely indicated [81,82].

Penicillins, cephalosporins, and potentiated sulfonamides are excreted by glomerular filtration with active tubular secretion [83]. Because of this, these antimicrobials reach high concentrations in the urine and are excellent choices for treatment of UTIs [2]. Additional water-soluble agents include aminoglycosides and fluoroquinolones (amphipathic). Consistent with this, most UTIs in equids can be treated successfully with ampicillin, penicillin with an aminoglycoside, trimethoprim-sulfonamides, ceftiofur, or enrofloxacin [1,2,84]. In vitro bacterial resistance to the penicillins and trimethoprim-sulfonamides should be interpreted with the understanding that the same organisms may be sensitive to these agents in vivo, given the high urinary concentrations achieved [1,83].

Trimethoprim-sulfonamides are an excellent choice for treatment of UTIs in equids because of their broad antibacterial activity, low cost, and ease of administration [85]. Pyrimidines, such as trimethoprim, and the sulfonamides are bacteriostatic alone but act synergistically to have a bactericidal effect when combined [84]. Many uropathogenic bacteria, including *Streptococcus* spp, *Staphylococcus* spp, and *E coli*, are sensitive to trimethoprim-sulfonamides [85]. In people and horses, sulfonamides have been associated with crystalluria and hematuria [83,85,86]. This is rarely a complication with newer preparations, although horses with acidic urine, dehydration, or poor renal perfusion should be considered at risk for these sequelae [83,85,86]. Given the ease of long-term administration of trimethoprim-sulfonamides and high urinary concentrations achieved, one might use these agents for UTI prophylaxis in cases of bladder atony or outflow obstruction. Trimethoprim-sulfamethoxazole prophylaxis significantly reduced the incidence of bacteriuria and UTI in human patients with spinal cord injury, although emergence of drug-resistant bacterial strains was not an uncommon complication [87]. Whether for treatment or prophylaxis, use of trimethoprim-sulfonamides requires that care be taken so that the aforementioned complications as well as the occurrence of diarrhea or colitis [83,85,88–90] are minimized.

The penicillin and cephalosporin classes of drugs, collectively termed β-lactams, are frequently used to treat equine UTIs. Penicillins are often the initial drugs used (ie, before or without culture and sensitivity testing) because of high concentrations of these drugs in urine. Benzylpenicillins (ie, procaine penicillin G, potassium penicillin) may be combined with aminoglycosides [2] to enhance activity against gram-negative uropathogens. Alternatively, aminopenicillins (ie, ampicillin) may be used, because this group better penetrates the LPS layer of gram-negative bacteria [83]. These agents may only be administered parenterally, and this may prohibit the use of penicillins for prolonged treatment. A study examining the use of orally (ie, via nasogastric tube) administered penicillin G sodium in equids demonstrated poor systemic availability and high cecal concentrations, which may augment the risk for development of colitis [91]. Indeed, the more customary parenteral route of β-lactam administration has been associated with *Clostridium difficile* colitis [92].

Ceftiofur is an extended-spectrum cephalosporin that, unlike other third-generation cephalosporins, is effective against a wide range of gram-positive and gram-negative organisms [93]. Although it is generally considered to be safe in equids [93], ceftiofur has been associated with diarrhea [83]. Interstitial nephritis and tubular necrosis are associated with large doses or chronic use of cephalosporins; however, the risk for development of nephrotoxicity with approved doses in patients with normal renal function is low [94]. In equine patients, use of cephalosporins uncommonly affords additional treatment benefit over that achieved with use of penicillins or potentiated sulfonamides [95]. Ceftiofur, however, because of a wide spectrum of activity, may offer an advantage in treating UTIs attributable to bacteria that are resistant to more commonly used antimicrobials [95]. Some gram-negative bacteria may be resistant to ceftiofur at approved doses (reported as ranging from 2.2 mg/kg administered intramuscularly every 12 hours [93] to 4.4 mg/kg administered intramuscularly or intravenously every 24 hours [83]). In this case, two options exist. First, a higher dose of ceftiofur may be given (ie, 5.5 mg/kg administered intramuscularly every 8 to 12 hours in adults) for treatment of infections attributable to gram-negative enteric bacteria [93]. Injection site tenderness and reduced appetite are the primary adverse sequelae observed in horses administered high doses of ceftiofur intramuscularly [93]. An alternative to use of high doses of ceftiofur is use of the fourth-generation cephalosporin cefepime. This agent has a wider spectrum of activity than third-generation cephalosporins and is efficacious in treating infection attributable to many gram-negative bacteria that are resistant to third-generation drugs [96]. Cefepime has been used in human patients to treat UTI and is favored over other antimicrobials because of a low rate of emergence of antimicrobial resistance and efficacy against bacteria that are resistant to other antibacterial agents [97,98]. In adult horses, colic was observed with intramuscular (two of six cases) and oral (four of six cases) cefepime administration, but no serious or long-term sequelae resulted [99]. For treatment of adult horses, a dose of 2.2 mg/kg administered intravenously or intramuscularly every 8 hours has been recommended [99]; in foals, a dose of 11 mg/kg administered intravenously every 8 hours has been advised [96].

Use of cefepime should be reserved for treatment of bacteria that are proven sensitive and are resistant to more conventional antimicrobials. Although one attribute of cefepime is resistance to β-lactamases [96], extended-spectrum β-lactamase (ESBL)–producing *E coli, Klebsiella* spp, *Enterobacter* spp, and *Pseudomonas* spp have been identified in the urine of human patients [100]. Of the antimicrobials chosen to treat these infections, cefepime was the least efficacious [100]. Another drug developed for use with β-lactamase–associated antimicrobial resistance is imipenem [83]. This agent has extremely broad activity and is highly concentrated in urine when combined with cilastatin [83]. Imipenem is expensive, however, and pharmacokinetic data in horses are lacking; therefore, extrapolation from small animal doses is necessary [83]. These factors, combined with practices designed to reduce drug resistance, limit the practical use of this drug.

Although enrofloxacin has acceptable bioavailability (50%–60%) with oral administration in horses [83,101], its use should be restricted to the treatment of urinary pathogens with sole susceptibility to this drug [84] because of the significant correlation between the development of *E coli* resistance and frequency of use [102]. Additionally, in human patients, ESBL production was observed significantly more often in ciprofloxacin-resistant strains of *E coli* than in those strains susceptible to ciprofloxacin [103], suggesting a positive correlation between the emergence of ciprofloxacin resistance and subsequent ESBL formation. Advantages to the use of enrofloxacin include oral bioavailability, a broad spectrum of activity that includes many uropathogens, inactivity against anaerobes (thus, less perturbation of normal gastrointestinal flora), and few adverse sequelae in adult horses [93].

Lactobacillus

Equine patients with persistent structural impediments to normal urine flow or those with chronic functional impairments that prohibit bladder emptying may experience chronic intermittent ascending UTIs. In women with recurrent UTIs, vaginal suppositories containing *Lactobacillus* spp or *Lactobacillus* growth factor were shown to reduce the infection rate and increase the time to first infection [104]. The number of adherent lactobacilli per vaginal cell was highest after 6 months of weekly treatment, and higher lactobacilli counts correlated with the reduced rate of infection [104]. Most recurrent UTIs were attributable to typical uropathogens, primarily *E coli* [104]. More recently, a murine strain of *Lactobacillus* was shown to prevent and treat ascending bladder colonization with *Proteus mirabilis* in mice [105].

Application of probiotics for UTI prophylaxis has benefits over long-term antimicrobial use in that side effects (ie, colitis) and antimicrobial resistance are curtailed [106]. Additionally, probiotic treatment uses organisms that remain viable and exert beneficial effects for longer durations than those attributable to antimicrobials; thus, frequency of treatment is reduced [104]. Finally, the use of probiotics is aimed at restoration rather than disruption of host flora [106].

To be therapeutic, the selected *Lactobacillus* strain must adhere to the uroepithelium and colonize the host, interfere with pathogen binding to the uroepithelium (ie, by creating a biosurfactant), inhibit pathogen growth (ie, through hydrogen peroxide, acid, or bacteriocin production), and be free of adverse sequelae [106,107]. Further, the chosen strain must be permissive for the normal flora specific to the species to which it is administered [107]. In human beings, *Lactobacillus crispatus*, *Lactobacillus rhamnosus*, and *Lactobacillus fermentum* have demonstrated promise for use in UTI prophylaxis [106].

Cranberry

Cranberry products have long been used to prevent and treat UTIs in people. Traditionally believed to exert bacteriostatic effects through urine acidification, it is now known that cranberry, in quantities that could reasonably be consumed, does not lead to sufficient hippuric acid secretion to reduce urine pH remarkably and render the urine bacteriostatic [108]. Subsequently, a different mechanism of urinary tract protection was identified. Ingestion of cranberry juice inhibited adherence of *E coli* to the uroepithelium of mice and people [109]. More specifically, cranberry juice was shown to alter the conformation and adhesion of *E coli* p-fimbriae in vitro, and these changes occurred independently of pH [110]. Clinical studies have revealed mixed results. Although cranberry juice has shown potential in preventing UTIs in certain populations (ie, sexually active women with a history of UTI), no benefit has been observed in populations at high risk for UTIs (ie, individuals with neurogenic bladder) [108]. Dried cranberry is available as capsules or tablets and has been shown to reduce recurrent UTIs as well as antimicrobial use in women in a cost-effective manner [111]. The safety and efficacy of cranberry products in equids have not been explored; however, these findings highlight the potential efficacy of nonpharmacologic intervention in the long-term prevention of UTIs in susceptible populations, a trend that must continue in light of adverse sequelae and resistance associated with chronic antimicrobial use.

Vaccinations

Future treatments aimed at preventing UTIs in those with bacterial resistance, persistent outflow anomalies, or unexplained recurrence may include the use of vaccines directed against bacterial virulence factors. Fimbrial vaccines administered to mice, monkeys, and human beings have proven effective in UTI prophylaxis, boosting innate resistance and offering an alternative to chronic antimicrobial therapy [13,14,112].

Special considerations

Urinary catheterization

Long-term urinary catheterization is rarely used in equids. Chronic urinary catheterization contributes to UTIs in human patients, partly by development of a biofilm externally and intraluminally [113], which promotes bacterial adhesion with subsequent colonization [114]. Bacteria inhabiting the biofilm are resistant to mechanical removal by urine flow and are protected from host immune defenses and antimicrobials [114]. Additionally, urinary catheters, whether indwelling or intermittently placed, provide a means by which bacteria can travel from the perineum to the bladder [114]. In the intensive care setting, only 5.1% of dogs developed a UTI after

3 days of indwelling urinary catheterization; however, the probability of developing a UTI increased with the length of time the catheter was in place (ie, increased to 10.3% on day 4) [115]. Additionally, care was taken to insert and maintain catheters aseptically [115], and this may not be feasible to the same extent in equine patients. Because of the association of UTIs with indwelling urinary catheters, the use of intermittent catheterization in human patients is the subject of much study. Elderly individuals with incomplete bladder evacuation because of detrusor muscle weakness experienced a lower rate of UTIs and improved urinary continence when catheterized intermittently compared with those who were not catheterized [116]. This suggests that management of chronic bladder atony by intermittent catheterization may actually reduce the incidence of UTIs by improving bladder emptying and restoring detrusor muscle tone.

The practice of administering prophylactic antimicrobials concomitantly with intermittent catheterization was recently challenged when a study revealed a higher incidence of UTIs in people given antimicrobials when compared with those who were not [117]. It was suggested that the increased incidence of *E coli*–related UTI may have been attributable to antimicrobial-induced expansion of resistant strains [117]. Antimicrobial treatment of asymptomatic bacteriuria in catheterized patients is reserved for those at high risk (ie, immunosuppressed) or for those in whom development of a UTI could have serious adverse sequelae (ie, pregnant women) [118]. Intermittent bladder irrigation with antibacterial solutions has not been shown to reduce bacteriuria in catheterized people [118]. Recently, investigations into the use of hydrophilic- and silver alloy/hydrogel-coated urinary catheters have revealed fewer UTIs in human patients with neurogenic bladder dysfunction and in those in the acute care setting (ie, no primary bladder or urinary dysfunction) [119,120]. Moreover, use of these catheters was deemed cost-effective when measured against reduced UTI treatment costs [120].

Hematogenous bacterial nephritis

As noted previously, rare cases of equine infectious nephritis may occur as a sequela to primary sepsis [60]. Some clinicians hold the view that complete obstruction of urine flow or preexisting renal trauma must be present for pyelonephritis or renal abscesses of hematogenous origin to occur [4,121]. Regardless of the cause, prolonged antimicrobial treatment is indicated and has been described in equids [2]. In cases of refractory unilateral pyelonephritis or renal abscessation, when the alternative kidney is verified functional by analysis of ureteral urine, serum chemistry, and ultrasound examination, a unilateral nephrectomy may be indicated [2,122,123]. In people, there is evidence that small (<3 cm in diameter) renal abscesses may be managed with parenteral antimicrobials if diagnosed promptly and that medium (3 to 5 cm in diameter) and large (>5 cm in diameter) abscesses (Fig. 3) may be

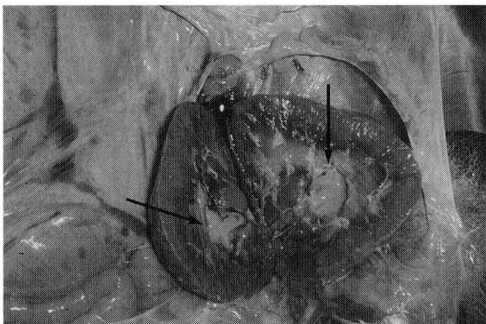

Fig. 3. Abscess in the renal pelvis (*arrows*).

successfully managed by open or percutaneous drainage [4,124]. Evacuation of renal abscesses has not been described in equids.

Summary

Interest in the pathophysiology, diagnosis, and management of UTIs in human patients is high because of the high disease prevalence in this population. Although not all information can be reliably extrapolated to equine patients, much can be learned about pathophysiologic mechanisms that are likely to be relevant to both species, as in the case of β-defensins. Investigation of bacterial isolates in urine of normal horses has improved the ability to interpret urine sediment and culture results reliably. Although causative bacteria and antimicrobial treatment options have not remarkably changed over recent years, emergence of antimicrobial resistance in human beings and equids demands that a prudent and informed approach be adopted. Further, care must be taken to avoid the adverse sequelae specific to equids. Future investigative efforts should be directed at innovative preventive efforts that are amenable to long-term use, reduce the emergence of resistant bacterial strains, and minimize adverse side effects.

References

[1] Schott H. Urinary tract infection and bladder displacement. In: Robinson N, editor. Current therapy in equine medicine. 5th edition. Philadelphia: WB Saunders; 2003. p. 837–9.
[2] Schott H. Urinary tract infections. In: Reed S, Bayly W, Sellon D, editors. Equine internal medicine. 2nd ed. Philadelphia: WB Saunders; 2004. p. 1253–8.
[3] Saemann MD, Weichhart T, Horl WH, et al. Tamm-Horsfall protein: a multilayered defence molecule against urinary tract infection. Eur J Clin Invest 2005;35:227–35.
[4] Schaeffer A. Infections of the urinary tract. In: Walsh P, Retik A, Vaughan E, et al, editors. Campbell's urology. 8th edition. Philadelphia: WB Saunders; 2002. p. 515–602.
[5] Williams DH, Schaeffer AJ. Current concepts in urinary tract infections. Minerva Urol Nefrol 2004;56:15–31.
[6] Schaeffer AJ, Jones JM, Dunn JK. Association of vitro Escherichia coli adherence to vaginal and buccal epithelial cells with susceptibility of women to recurrent urinary-tract infections. N Engl J Med 1981;304:1062–6.

[7] Hooton TM, Stapleton AE, Roberts PL, et al. Perineal anatomy and urine-voiding characteristics of young women with and without recurrent urinary tract infections. Clin Infect Dis 1999;29:1600–1.
[8] MacLeay JM, Kohn CW. Results of quantitative cultures of urine by free catch and catheterization from healthy adult horses. J Vet Intern Med 1998;12:76–8.
[9] Guyer DM, Gunther NW IV, Mobley HL. Secreted proteins and other features specific to uropathogenic Escherichia coli. J Infect Dis 2001;183(Suppl):S32–5.
[10] Yamamoto S, Tsukamoto T, Terai A, et al. Genetic evidence supporting the fecal-perineal-urethral hypothesis in cystitis caused by Escherichia coli. J Urol 1997;157:1127–9.
[11] Labat F, Pradillon O, Garry L, et al. Mutator phenotype confers advantage in *Escherichia coli* chronic urinary tract infection pathogenesis. FEMS Immunol Med Microbiol 2005;44:317–21.
[12] Taddei F, Matie I, Godelle B, et al. To be a mutator, or how pathogenic and commensal bacteria can evolve rapidly. Trends Microbiol 1997;5:427–8.
[13] Hopkins WJ, Uehling DT. Vaccine development for the prevention of urinary tract infections. Curr Infect Dis Rep 2002;4:509–13.
[14] Li X, Lockatell CV, Johnson DE, et al. Development of an intranasal vaccine to prevent urinary tract infection by Proteus mirabilis. Infect Immun 2004;72:66–75.
[15] Martinez JJ, Mulvey MA, Schilling JD, et al. Type 1 pilus-mediated bacterial invasion of bladder epithelial cells. EMBO J 2000;19:2803–12.
[16] Backhed F, Alsen B, Roche N, et al. Identification of target tissue glycosphingolipid receptors for uropathogenic, F1C-fimbriated Escherichia coli and its role in mucosal inflammation. J Biol Chem 2002;277:18198–205.
[17] Jahnukainen T, Chen M, Celsi G. Mechanisms of renal damage owing to infection. Pediatr Nephrol 2005;20:1043–53.
[18] de Man P, van Kooten C, Aarden L, et al. Interleukin-6 induced at mucosal surfaces by gram-negative bacterial infection. Infect Immun 1989;57:383–8.
[19] Hoebe K, Janssen E, Beutler B. The interface between innate and adaptive immunity. Nat Immunol 2004;5:971–4.
[20] Haraoka M, Hang L, Frendeus B, et al. Neutrophil recruitment and resistance to urinary tract infection. J Infect Dis 1999;180:1220–9.
[21] Gul M, Kurutas E, Ciragil P, et al. Urinary tract infection aggravates oxidative stress in diabetic patients. Tohoku J Exp Med 2005;206:1–6.
[22] Matsumoto T, Mitzunoe Y, Ogata N, et al. Antioxidant effect on renal scarring following infection of mannose-sensitive-piliated bacteria. Nephron 1992;60:210–5.
[23] Trifillis AL, Donnenberg MS, Cui X, et al. Binding to and killing of human renal epithelial cells by hemolytic P-fimbriated E. coli. Kidney Int 1994;46:1083–91.
[24] Warren JW, Mobley HL, Hebel JR, et al. Cytolethality of hemolytic Escherichia coli to primary human renal proximal tubular cell cultures obtained from different donors. Urology 1995;45:706–10.
[25] Seno Y, Kariyama R, Mitsuhata R, et al. Clinical implications of biofilm formation by Enterococcus faecalis in the urinary tract. Acta Med Okayama 2005;59:79–87.
[26] Donlan RM, Costerton JW. Biofilms: survival mechanisms of clinically relevant microorganisms. Clin Microbiol Rev 2002;15:167–93.
[27] Anderson GG, Palermo JJ, Schilling JD, et al. Intracellular bacterial biofilm-like pods in urinary tract infections. Science 2003;301:105–7.
[28] Tizard I. Veterinary immunology. 7th edition. Philadelphia: WB Saunders; 2004. p. 494.
[29] Wold AE, Mestecky J, Tomana M, et al. Secretory immunoglobulin A carries oligosaccharide receptors for Escherichia coli type 1 fimbrial lectin. Infect Immun 1990;58:3073–7.
[30] Weichhart T, Zlabinger GJ, Saemann MD. The multiple functions of Tamm-Horsfall protein in human health and disease: a mystery clears up. Wien Klin Wochenschr 2005;117:316–22.

[31] Mo L, Zhu XH, Huang HY, et al. Ablation of the Tamm-Horsfall protein gene increases susceptibility of mice to bladder colonization by type 1-fimbriated Escherichia coli. Am J Physiol Renal Physiol 2004;286:F795–802.
[32] Pak J, Pu Y, Zhang ZT, et al. Tamm-Horsfall protein binds to type 1 fimbriated Escherichia coli and prevents E. coli from binding to uroplakin Ia and Ib receptors. J Biol Chem 2001; 276:924–30.
[33] Su SJ, Chang KL, Lin TM, et al. Uromodulin and Tamm-Horsfall protein induce human monocytes to secrete TNF and express tissue factor. J Immunol 1997;158:3449–56.
[34] Kreft B, Jabs WJ, Laskay T, et al. Polarized expression of Tamm-Horsfall protein by renal tubular epithelial cells activates human granulocytes. Infect Immun 2002;70: 2650–6.
[35] Saemann MD, Weichhart T, Zeyda M, et al. Tamm-Horsfall glycoprotein links innate immune cell activation with adaptive immunity via a Toll-like receptor-4-dependent mechanism. J Clin Invest 2005;115:468–75.
[36] Donovan KL, Topley N. What are renal defensins defending? Nephron Exp Nephrol 2003; 93:125–8.
[37] Davis EG, Sang Y, Blecha F. Equine beta-defensin-1: full-length cDNA sequence and tissue expression. Vet Immunol Immunopathol 2004;99:127–32.
[38] Yang D, Chertov O, Oppenheim JJ. The role of mammalian antimicrobial peptides and proteins in awakening of innate host defenses and adaptive immunity. Cell Mol Life Sci 2001;58:978–89.
[39] Ganz T. Defensins in the urinary tract and other tissues. J Infect Dis 2001;183(Suppl 1): S41–2.
[40] Ichinose M, Asai M, Imai K, et al. Enhancement of phagocytosis by corticostatin I (CSI) in cultured mouse peritoneal macrophages. Immunopharmacology 1996;35:103–9.
[41] Van Wetering S, Mannesse-Lazeroms SP, Van Sterkenburg MA, et al. Effect of defensins on interleukin-8 synthesis in airway epithelial cells. Am J Physiol 1997;272:888–96.
[42] Chertov O, Michiel DF, Xu L, et al. Identification of defensin-1, defensin-2, and CAP37/azurocidin as T-cell chemoattractant proteins released from interleukin-8-stimulated neutrophils. J Biol Chem 1996;271:2935–40.
[43] Hiratsuka T, Nakazato M, Date Y, et al. Nucleotide sequence and expression of rat beta-defensin-1: its significance in diabetic rodent models. Nephron 2001;88:65–70.
[44] Schott II HC. Pituitary pars intermedia dysfunction: equine Cushing's disease. Vet Clin North Am Equine Pract 2002;18:237–70.
[45] Allen J, Barbee D, Crisman M. Diagnosis of equine pituitary tumors by computed tomography—part 1. Compend Contin Educ Pract Vet 1988;10:1103–6.
[46] Hillyer M, Taylor F, Mair T, et al. Diagnosis of hyperadrenocorticism in the horse. Equine Vet Educ 1992;4:131–4.
[47] Hang L, Wullt B, Shen Z, et al. Cytokine repertoire of epithelial cells lining the human urinary tract. J Urol 1998;159:2185–92.
[48] Otto G, Burdick M, Strieter R, et al. Chemokine response to febrile urinary tract infection. Kidney Int 2005;68:62–70.
[49] Agace W, Hedges S, Andersson U, et al. Selective cytokine production by epithelial cells following exposure to Escherichia coli. Infect Immun 1993;61:602–9.
[50] Godaly G, Proudfoot AE, Offord RE, et al. Role of epithelial interleukin-8 (IL-8) and neutrophil IL-8 receptor A in Escherichia coli-induced transuroepithelial neutrophil migration. Infect Immun 1997;65:3451–6.
[51] Otto G, Braconier J, Andreasson A, et al. Interleukin-6 and disease severity in patients with bacteremic and nonbacteremic febrile urinary tract infection. J Infect Dis 1999; 179:172–9.
[52] Benson M, Jodal U, Agace W, et al. Interleukin (IL)-6 and IL-8 in children with febrile urinary tract infection and asymptomatic bacteriuria. J Infect Dis 1996;174: 1080–4.

[53] Khalil A, Tullus K, Bartfai T, et al. Renal cytokine responses in acute Escherichia coli pyelonephritis in IL-6-deficient mice. Clin Exp Immunol 2000;122:200–6.
[54] Traylor LA, Mayeux PR. Nitric oxide generation mediates lipid A-induced oxidant injury in renal proximal tubules. Arch Biochem Biophys 1997;338:129–35.
[55] Loran OB, Zaitsev AV, Godunov BN, et al. Current aspects in the diagnosis and treatment of chronic cystitis in women. Urol Nefrol (Mosk) 1997:7–14.
[56] Hanno P. Interstitial cystitis and related disorders. In: Walsh P, editor. Campbell's urology. 8th edition. Philadelphia: WB Saunders; 2002. p. 631–70.
[57] O'Mahony R, Abbott Y, Leonard FC, et al. Methicillin-resistant Staphylococcus aureus (MRSA) isolated from animals and veterinary personnel in Ireland. Vet Microbiol 2005; 109:285–96.
[58] Weese JS, Archambault M, Willey BM, et al. Methicillin-resistant Staphylococcus aureus in horses and horse personnel, 2000–2002. Emerg Infect Dis 2005;11:430–5.
[59] Weese JS, Rousseau J, Traub-Dargatz JL, et al. Community-associated methicillin-resistant Staphylococcus aureus in horses and humans who work with horses. J Am Vet Med Assoc 2005;226:580–3.
[60] Robinson JA, Allen GK, Green EM, et al. A prospective study of septicaemia in colostrum-deprived foals. Equine Vet J 1993;25:214–9.
[61] Divers TJ, Byars TD, Shin SJ. Renal dysfunction associated with infection of Leptospira interrogans in a horse. J Am Vet Med Assoc 1992;201:1391–2.
[62] Wada S, Yoshinari M, Katayama Y, et al. Nonulcerative keratouveitis as a manifestation of Leptospiral infection in a horse. Vet Ophthalmol 2003;6:191–5.
[63] Kinde H, Mathews M, Ash L, et al. Halicephalobus gingivalis (H. deletrix) infection in two horses in southern California. J Vet Diagn Invest 2000;12:162–5.
[64] Shibahara T, Takai H, Shimizu C, et al. Equine renal granuloma caused by Halicephalobus species. Vet Rec 2002;151:672–4.
[65] Divers T. Urinary tract infections. In: Smith B, editor. Large animal internal medicine. 3rd edition. St. Louis (MO): Mosby; 2002. p. 834–6.
[66] Kohn CW, Strasser SL. 24-hour renal clearance and excretion of endogenous substances in the mare. Am J Vet Res 1986;47:1332–7.
[67] Jacobson SH, Hylander B, Wretlind B, et al. Interleukin-6 and interleukin-8 in serum and urine in patients with acute pyelonephritis in relation to bacterial-virulence-associated traits and renal function. Nephron 1994;67:172–9.
[68] Hedges S, Stenqvist K, Lidin-Janson G, et al. Comparison of urine and serum concentrations of interleukin-6 in women with acute pyelonephritis or asymptomatic bacteriuria. J Infect Dis 1992;166:653–6.
[69] Horcajada JP, Velasco M, Filella X, et al. Evaluation of inflammatory and renal-injury markers in women treated with antibiotics for acute pyelonephritis caused by Escherichia coli. Clin Diagn Lab Immunol 2004;11:142–6.
[70] Tuerlinckx D, Vander Borght T, Glupczynski Y, et al. Is procalcitonin a good marker of renal lesion in febrile urinary tract infection? Eur J Pediatr 2005;164:651–2.
[71] Gurgoze MK, Akarsu S, Yilmaz E, et al. Proinflammatory cytokines and procalcitonin in children with acute pyelonephritis. Pediatr Nephrol 2005;10:1445–8.
[72] Schott H, Varner D. Urinary tract. In: Traub-Dargatz JL, Brown C, editors. Equine endoscopy. 2nd edition. St. Louis (MO): Mosby; 1997. p. 187–203.
[73] Sprayberry K. Cystoscopy. In: Slovis N, editor. Atlas of equine endoscopy. St. Louis (MO): Mosby; 2004. p. 169–82.
[74] Holt PE, Mair TS. Ten cases of bladder paralysis associated with sabulous urolithiasis in horses. Vet Rec 1990;127:108–10.
[75] Reimer J. Atlas of equine ultrasonography. St. Louis (MO): Mosby; 1998. p. 308.
[76] Traub-Dargatz J, Wrigley R. Ultrasonographic evaluation of the urinary tract. In: Rantanen N, McKinnon A, editors. Equine diagnostic ultrasonography. Baltimore (MD): Williams & Wilkins; 1998. p. 613–8.

[77] Schott II HC. Examination of the urinary system. In: Reed S, Bayly W, Sellon D, editors. Equine internal medicine. 2nd edition. Philadelphia: WB Saunders; 2004. p. 1200–20.
[78] Meyrier A. Diagnosis and management of renal infections. Curr Opin Nephrol Hypertens 1996;5:151–7.
[79] MacMillan RD. Complicated urinary tract infections in patients with voiding dysfunction. Can J Urol 2001;8:13–7.
[80] Richards D, Toop L, Chambers S, et al. Response to antibiotics of women with symptoms of urinary tract infection but negative dipstick urine test results: double blind randomised controlled trial. BMJ 2005;331:143–7.
[81] Nicolle LE. Asymptomatic bacteriuria in the elderly. Infect Dis Clin North Am 1997;11: 647–62.
[82] Sotolongo JR Jr, Koleilat N. Significance of asymptomatic bacteriuria in spinal cord injury patients on condom catheter. J Urol 1990;143:979–80.
[83] Dowling P. Antimicrobial therapy. In: Bertone J, Horspool L, editors. Equine clinical pharmacology. Edinburgh: Saunders; 2004. p. 13–47, 369.
[84] McClure J, McClure J. Antimicrobial therapy. In: Savage C, editor. Equine medicine secrets. Philadelphia: Hanley and Belfus; 1999. p. 307–21.
[85] Van Duijkeren E, Vulto AG, Van Miert AS. Trimethoprim/sulfonamide combinations in the horse: a review. J Vet Pharmacol Ther 1994;17:64–73.
[86] Diaz F, Collazos J, Mayo J, et al. Sulfadiazine-induced multiple urolithiasis and acute renal failure in a patient with AIDS and Toxoplasma encephalitis. Ann Pharmacother 1996;30: 41–2.
[87] Gribble MJ, Puterman ML. Prophylaxis of urinary tract infection in persons with recent spinal cord injury: a prospective, randomized, double-blind, placebo-controlled study of trimethoprim-sulfamethoxazole. Am J Med 1993;95:141–52.
[88] Jones RL. Clostridial enterocolitis. Vet Clin North Am Equine Pract 2000;16:471–85.
[89] Ruff D, Jaffe J, London R, et al. Pseudomembranous colitis following low dose trimethoprim-sulfamethoxazole. J Urol 1985;134:1218–9.
[90] James AH, Katz VL, Dotters DJ, et al. Clostridium difficile infection in obstetric and gynecologic patients. South Med J 1997;90:889–92.
[91] Horspool LJ, McKellar QA. Disposition of penicillin G sodium following intravenous and oral administration to Equidae. Br Vet J 1995;151:401–12.
[92] Baverud V, Gustafsson A, Franklin A, et al. Clostridium difficile associated with acute colitis in mature horses treated with antibiotics. Equine Vet J 1997;29:279–84.
[93] Papich M. Antimicrobial therapy for horses. In: Robinson N, editor. Current therapy in equine medicine. 5th edition. Philadelphia: WB Saunders; 2003. p. 6–11.
[94] Plumb DC. Plumb's veterinary drug handbook. 5th edition. Ames (IA): Blackwell Publishing; 2005. p. 139–41.
[95] Schott HC. Drugs acting on the urinary system. In: Bertone J, Horspool L, editors. Equine clinical pharmacology. Edinburgh: Saunders; 2004. p. 155–75.
[96] Gardner SY, Papich MG. Comparison of cefepime pharmacokinetics in neonatal foals and adult dogs. J Vet Pharmacol Ther 2001;24:187–92.
[97] Sanders WE Jr, Tenney JH, Kessler RE. Efficacy of cefepime in the treatment of infections due to multiply resistant Enterobacter species. Clin Infect Dis 1996;23:454–61.
[98] Cunha BA, Gill MV. Cefepime. Med Clin North Am 1995;79:721–32.
[99] Guglick MA, MacAllister CG, Clarke CR, et al. Pharmacokinetics of cefepime and comparison with those of ceftiofur in horses. Am J Vet Res 1998;59:458–63.
[100] Kader AA, Angamuthu K. Extended-spectrum beta-lactamases in urinary isolates of Escherichia coli, Klebsiella pneumoniae and other gram-negative bacteria in a hospital in Eastern Province, Saudi Arabia. Saudi Med J 2005;26:956–9.
[101] Epstein K, Cohen N, Boothe D, et al. Pharmacokinetics, stability, and retrospective analysis of use of an oral gel formulation of the bovine injectable enrofloxacin in horses. Vet Ther 2004;5:155–67.

[102] Urbanek K, Kolar M, Strojil J, et al. Utilization of fluoroquinolones and Escherichia coli resistance in urinary tract infection: inpatients and outpatients. Pharmacoepidemiol Drug Saf 2005;14:741–5.
[103] Tolun V, Kucukbasmaci O, Torumkuney-Akbulut D, et al. Relationship between ciprofloxacin resistance and extended-spectrum beta-lactamase production in Escherichia coli and Klebsiella pneumoniae strains. Clin Microbiol Infect 2004;10:72–5.
[104] Reid G, Bruce A, Taylor M. Instillation of *lactobacillus* and stimulation of indigenous organisms to prevent recurrence of urinary tract infections. Microecology and Therapy 1995;23:32–45.
[105] Fraga M, Scavone P, Zunino P. Preventive and therapeutic administration of an indigenous Lactobacillus sp. strain against Proteus mirabilis ascending urinary tract infection in a mouse model. Antonie Van Leeuwenhoek 2005;88:25–34.
[106] Reid G, Bruce AW. Selection of lactobacillus strains for urogenital probiotic applications. J Infect Dis 2001;183(Suppl):S77–80.
[107] Reid G. The scientific basis for probiotic strains of Lactobacillus. Appl Environ Microbiol 1999;65:3763–6.
[108] Raz R, Chazan B, Dan M. Cranberry juice and urinary tract infection. Clin Infect Dis 2004; 38:1413–9.
[109] Sobota AE. Inhibition of bacterial adherence by cranberry juice: potential use for the treatment of urinary tract infections. J Urol 1984;131:1013–6.
[110] Liu Y, Black MA, Caron L, et al. Role of cranberry juice on molecular-scale surface characteristics and adhesion behavior of Escherichia coli. Biotechnol Bioeng 2005;93:297–305.
[111] Stothers L. A randomized trial to evaluate effectiveness and cost effectiveness of naturopathic cranberry products as prophylaxis against urinary tract infection in women. Can J Urol 2002;9:1558–62.
[112] Langermann S, Mollby R, Burlein JE, et al. Vaccination with FimH adhesin protects cynomolgus monkeys from colonization and infection by uropathogenic Escherichia coli. J Infect Dis 2000;181:774–8.
[113] Nicolle LE. Catheter-related urinary tract infection. Drugs Aging 2005;22:627–39.
[114] Trautner BW, Darouiche RO. Role of biofilm in catheter-associated urinary tract infection. Am J Infect Control 2004;32:177–83.
[115] Smarick SD, Haskins SC, Aldrich J, et al. Incidence of catheter-associated urinary tract infection among dogs in a small animal intensive care unit. J Am Vet Med Assoc 2004;224: 1936–40.
[116] Pilloni S, Krhut J, Mair D, et al. Intermittent catheterisation in older people: a valuable alternative to an indwelling catheter? Age Ageing 2005;34:57–60.
[117] Clarke SA, Samuel M, Boddy SA. Are prophylactic antibiotics necessary with clean intermittent catheterization? A randomized controlled trial. J Pediatr Surg 2005;40:568–71.
[118] Warren JW. Catheter-associated urinary tract infections. Int J Antimicrob Agents 2001;17: 299–303.
[119] De Ridder DJ, Everaert K, Fernandez LG, et al. Intermittent catheterisation with hydrophilic-coated catheters (SpeediCath) reduces the risk of clinical urinary tract infection in spinal cord injured patients: a prospective randomised parallel comparative trial. Eur Urol 2005;48:991–5.
[120] Rupp ME, Fitzgerald T, Marion N, et al. Effect of silver-coated urinary catheters: efficacy, cost-effectiveness, and antimicrobial resistance. Am J Infect Control 2004;32:445–50.
[121] Timmons JW, Perlmutter AD. Renal abscess: a changing concept. J Urol 1976;115:299–301.
[122] Trotter GW, Brown CM, Ainsworth DM. Unilateral nephrectomy for treatment of a renal abscess in a foal. J Am Vet Med Assoc 1984;184:1392–4.
[123] Irwin DH, Howell DW. Equine pyelonephritis and unilateral nephrectomy. J S Afr Vet Assoc 1980;51:235–6.
[124] Siegel JF, Smith A, Moldwin R. Minimally invasive treatment of renal abscess. J Urol 1996; 155:52–5.

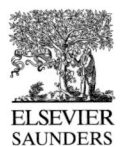

Reproductive Tract Infections in Horses

Kristina G. Lu, VMD[a],*, Peter R. Morresey, BVSc[b]

[a]Hagyard Equine Medical Institute, 4250 Iron Works Pike, Lexington, KY 40511, USA
[b]Rood and Riddle Equine Hospital, PO Box 12070, Lexington, KY 40580, USA

Female reproductive tract

Defense mechanisms

Anatomic barriers and physical uterine clearance

There are three anatomic barriers to infection of the female reproductive tract: (1) the labia, (2) the vestibulovaginal ring, and (3) the cervix. The normal cervix changes shape and consistency under the influence of reproductive hormones. This is particularly evident during diestrus and pregnancy. Cervical competence and physical uterine clearance of contaminants and bacteria have been considered the most important determinants of resistance to endometritis [1].

In addition to physical anatomic barriers, the reproductive tract has remarkable mechanisms for resisting infection and clearing microorganisms. Uterine contractility is important in the clearance of uterine fluid. Impaired uterine contractility contributes to the pathogenesis of persistent intromission-induced endometritis [2]. Mares susceptible to endometritis typically have delayed uterine clearance, which is manifested as reduced frequency, intensity, and duration of uterine myoelectrical activity [3–6]. Older mares susceptible to endometritis were found to have less active muscle tension compared with normal mares in response to muscle tension agonists, which is suggestive of an intrinsic uterine myometrial defect. This weaker response did not seem to be oxytocin or prostaglandin (PG) $F_{2\alpha}$–receptor mediated. Furthermore, less active tension was demonstrated with stimulation that was not receptor mediated. A similar calcium ion distribution occurred in both groups of mares, suggesting that alterations occur in muscle cell mechanics beyond receptor and calcium regulation [7]. Other explanations for poor mechanical clearance include decreased production or secretion

---

* Corresponding author.
E-mail address: luk@alumni.upenn.edu (K.G. Lu).

of $PGF_{2\alpha}$ in response to oxytocin stimulation, neurologic sequelae from repeated mechanical stretch of the multiparous uterus, and structural damage of collagen and elastin secondary to mechanical stretch of the multiparous uterus [7–9].

The endometrium of the mare is a ciliated mucosal surface. In this respect, it is similar in anatomy to the respiratory tract and, likewise, faces exogenous infectious and inflammatory challenges [10]. Pathologic changes of the endometrium lead to structural changes of the epithelial surface, including loss of the ciliated cells and the integrity of the mucosal barrier [11,12].

Mucus is an important part of infection defense of the reproductive tract. This is similar to the respiratory tract, where mucus aids in maintaining a sterile environment and defends against microbial invasion. Cervical mucus acts as a mechanical barrier and microfilter. In addition, it contains immunoglobulins, particularly secretory IgA, and proteins with antimicrobial activity. Lysozyme acts synergistically with IgA to induce bacteriolysis. In rabbits, the lysozyme concentration in secretory granules of cervical cells increases under estrogenic influence [13]. Similarly, in humans, the antibacterial activity of cervical mucus increases with estrogen administration [14]. In a study of human cervical mucus, the antibacterial effect of the mucus increased significantly secondary to sexual stimulation. Although the exact mechanism of this effect is unknown, the increased antibacterial effect may be attributable to the direct stimulation of mucosal cells, interaction with seminal proteins, or antibacterial proteins present in seminal plasma [15].

The human cervical mucus plug, which is present during gestation, also possesses broad-spectrum antibacterial activity. Examples of proteins found in the cervical mucus plug are lysozyme, secretory leukocyte protease inhibitor (SLPI), defensins, and lactoferrin [16].

Immunologic mechanisms

A critical component of the inflammatory response is an influx of polymorphonuclear cells (PMNs) in response to cytokines and chemoattractants. Comparing mares susceptible and resistant to chronic uterine infections, PMNs seemed to be fully functional in standardized environments in both groups of mares. Uterine secretions of susceptible mares seem to be a poorer source of opsonin, however. Thus, impaired PMN phagocytosis observed in susceptible mares may be attributable to dysfunctional opsonization. Furthermore, the chemotactic response of PMNs from susceptible mares seemed to be superior to that in normal mares, which may be reflective of enhanced chemoattraction provided by high concentrations of arachidonic acid metabolites [17].

Endogenous genetically encoded antimicrobial peptides have been shown to be key elements in the response to epithelial compromise and microbial invasion [18]. A major source of these host defense molecules is circulating phagocytic leukocytes. More recently, it has been shown that resident epithelial cells of the skin, respiratory, alimentary, and genitourinary tracts all synthesize and release antimicrobial peptides. The female reproductive tract is immunologically unique in its requirement for tolerance to allogenic sperm and to the conceptus. Additionally, it must be appropriately protected from and respond to a diverse array of sexually transmitted pathogens [19].

SLPI, a neutrophil elastase inhibitor, is produced by neutrophils, macrophages, and epithelial cells and has been found in the lung, cervix, seminal plasma, and endometrium. This protein has demonstrated antimicrobial functions, including bactericidal activity against gram-negative and gram-positive organisms as well as antiviral and antifungal properties. Evidence also suggests that SLPI inhibits proinflammatory systems, such as the cyclooxygenase (COX)-2 inflammatory cascade as well as the effects of lipopolysaccharide and the nuclear factor-κB (NF-κB) signal transduction pathway [20,21]. Interestingly, the production of SLPI may be associated with menstrual status. In a study investigating the antibacterial properties of human endometrial cells, endometrial cells from premenopausal women inhibited bacterial growth, whereas cells from postmenopausal women were unable to inhibit bacterial growth [22]. This result is potentially attributed to the association of SLPI with the endometrial glandular epithelial cells that are no longer present in postmenopausal women [20,22].

Lactoferrin is a broad-spectrum antimicrobial protein found in the endometrial epithelium and cervical mucus [23,24]. Lactoferrin is an iron-binding protein, and it is surmised that the protein's bacteriostatic properties are secondary to the sequestration of iron that is necessary for bacterial growth. Lactoferrin is produced and stored by neutrophils, along with a wide range of tissues, including reproductive tissue under estrogen control [25]. Lactoferrin may be produced by the amnionic epithelium, because the protein is present in amnionic fluid with concentrations increasing with advancing gestational age. Furthermore, lactoferrin was found to be significantly increased in amnionic fluid associated with intra-amnionic infection compared with normal amnionic fluid [26].

Another group of antimicrobial molecules are defensins. α-Defensins are found in neutrophils and epithelial cells, whereas β-defensins are primarily present at epithelial surfaces, including the uterus. In humans, the β-defensins are expressed at different stages of the menstrual cycle, providing protection throughout the entire cycle [27,28]. Human β-defensin-2 expression is induced by inflammatory mediators, such as interleukin (IL)-1β, tumor necrosis factor-α (TNFα), and interferon-γ (IFNγ) [29]. Investigations into the regulation of these natural antimicrobial proteins suggest that some are constitutively expressed, whereas others are inducible [29]. In addition to their antimicrobial properties, β-defensins function as chemoattractants for inflammatory cells [28].

Uterine epithelial cells play an active role in immune protection. They express polymeric immunoglobulin receptors that transport IgA into the uterine lumen, release antimicrobial proteins (eg, SLPI, defensins), act as antigen-presenting cells as part of the adaptive immune response, and perform an important role in the innate immune response. The innate immune system uses receptors that recognize conserved pathogen-associated molecular patterns (PAMPs) associated with groups of organisms. Toll-like receptors that recognize PAMPs are expressed on many cell types, including epithelial cells, macrophages, and dendritic cells. In response to receptor binding to PAMPs, the cells of the innate immune system recruit an immune response via the production and release of chemokines and cytokines. Cytokines recently studied include CCL20 (in rats), transforming growth factor-β (TGFβ), and TNFα. Studies of rat endometrial cells using *Escherichia coli* along with isolated PAMPs demonstrated that PAMPs directly affect production of the chemokine CCL20 and TNFα. CCL20 has antimicrobial properties and is chemotactic for bone marrow–derived dendritic cell precursors, B cells, and memory T cells [30]. Estrogen plays a role in the regulation of chemokine and cytokine release by rat uterine endometrial cells. Estrogen was found to regulate the production of CCL20 and TNFα by uterine endometrial cells in the presence and absence of PAMPs [31].

The cytokines TNFα, IL-1β, and IL-6 are intercellular signaling proteins that modulate the acute-phase immune response and are also involved in other reproductive functions, such as inducing phospholipid metabolizing enzymes, stimulating further release of prostaglandins, and activating extracellular matrix remodeling enzymes [32]. In the uterus, leukocytes and endometrial cells produce these proinflammatory cytokines. In a comparison of mares susceptible and resistant to persistent postbreeding endometritis under basal conditions, susceptible mares were found to have significantly higher mRNA expression of all three cytokines during estrus and of IL-1β and TNFα during diestrus. After artificial insemination, mRNA expression of all three cytokines was high; however, this did not significantly differ between susceptible and resistant mares. During diestrus, resistant mares showed significantly lower IL-1β and TNFα mRNA expression than susceptible mares [33].

The NF-κB transcription signaling pathway seems to be involved in promoting the formation of inflammatory cytokines in human nongestational and gestational tissue (placenta, amnion, and choriodecidua) [34,35]. Microbial products activate NF-κB, enhancing proinflammatory cytokine production and release, which, in turn, activates NF-κB [36].

Nitric oxide (NO) is another inflammatory mediator produced and released in response to inflammation. A larger amount of NO was found in uterine secretions from mares susceptible to breeding-induced endometritis. Additionally, higher expression of NO synthase was found in susceptible mares. Although its exact role in endometritis has yet to be determined, NO's involvement in smooth muscle relaxation suggests a potential role in delayed uterine clearance [37].

Diagnosis of infection

Culture

Endometrial swabs for microbial culture and sensitivity testing are commonly used to diagnose uterine infections and to deem a mare uninfected before breeding. Traditional endometrial swab culture, when compared with culture from endometrial biopsy samples, is less diagnostic. When culture from a biopsy sample was used as the definitive method for diagnosing infection, the sensitivity of swab culture was reported to be 44%, the specificity was 98%, the positive predictive value was 95%, and the negative predictive value was 74% [38]. With endometrial histology used as the "gold standard" for diagnosing endometritis, culture from a biopsy sample, culture from an endometrial swab, and cytologic evaluation for diagnosis of endometritis (endometritis was defined histologically as >1 PMN per five 400× fields) were compared [38]. Culture from a biopsy sample yielded 82% sensitivity, 92% specificity, 97% positive predictive value, and 67% negative predictive value [38]. Culture from an endometrial swab yielded 34% sensitivity, 100% specificity, 100% positive predictive value, and 44% negative predictive value [38]. Growth likely attributable to contamination was classified as a negative culture [38].

Cytology

The literature contains guidelines for using endometrial cytology to diagnose endometritis [39]. There are several methods for obtaining the cytologic sample, including the use of a double-guarded swab or low-volume uterine lavage followed by centrifugation. The cytologic sample is typically assessed for eukaryotic cells, prokaryotic cells, and quantity of debris (Fig. 1). Inflammatory cell types are quantified by counting a minimum of 100 cells with 100× magnification using oil immersion (Fig. 2). Guidelines have been suggested for associating the percentage of neutrophils in a cytologic sample with the degree of endometrial inflammation: less than 5% neutrophils is considered noninflammatory, 5% to 15% neutrophils is considered mild inflammation, 15% to 30% neutrophils is considered moderate inflammation, and more than 30% neutrophils is considered severe inflammation [39,40].

Counting the number of intra- and extracellular microorganisms (bacterial and fungal) is also recommended. Additional evaluation for further organism identification may include Gram staining for bacterial organisms and Wright-Giemsa staining for fungal or yeast organisms (Fig. 3). Cytologic evaluation also includes assessment of debris that covers the 1000× (1000-power magnification) microscopic field [39].

Cytologic findings have been compared with the mare's reproductive stage and history. For an unbred mare 24 to 96 hours after ovulation, the cytologic sample may contain less than 5% neutrophils, 1 bacterium per 30 fields, and less than 25% debris per 1000× field using low-volume lavage

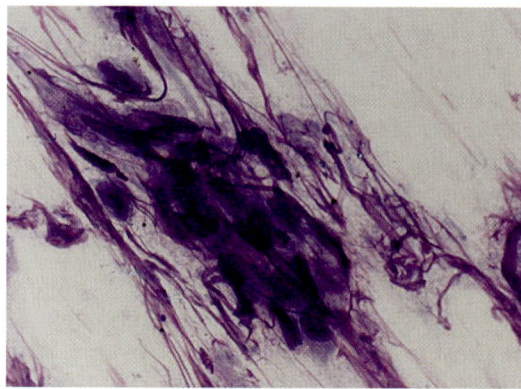

Fig. 1. Uterine cytology with epithelial cells and mucus from a normal mare. (*Courtesy of* Hagyard Equine Institute Laboratory, Lexington, KY).

and centrifugation to obtain the sample. Endometria 24 to 96 hours after breeding with frozen semen was found to have 5% or less neutrophils, less than 1 bacterium per 10 1000× fields, and 25% to 50% debris using low-volume lavage and centrifugation [41] to obtain the sample. Cytologic findings from mares susceptible to postbreeding endometritis but with no growth from culture of an endometrial swab revealed less than 5% neutrophils 96 hours after ovulation. Parameters for persistent inflammation after experimental infusion of *Streptococcus zooepidemicus* (subsp *equi*) were greater than 10% neutrophils, more than 1 bacterium per 30 fields at 1000×, and greater than 50% debris [42].

In the diagnostic study performed by Nielsen [38], cytologic evaluation was compared with histologic evidence of inflammation from an

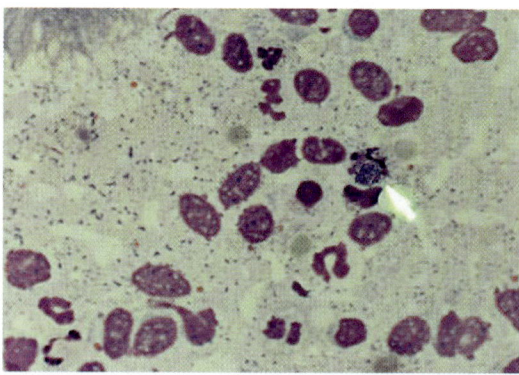

Fig. 2. Uterine cytology from a mare with bacterial endometritis. The arrow indicates a neutrophil with intracellular bacteria. (*Courtesy of* Hagyard Equine Institute Laboratory, Lexington, KY).

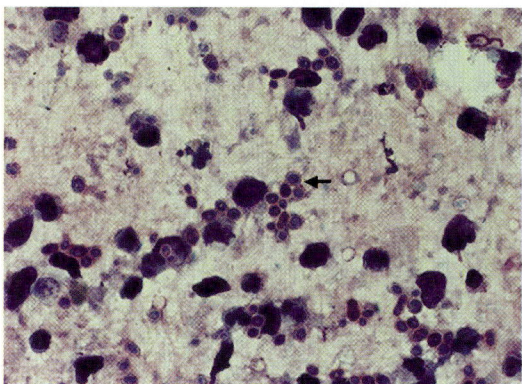

Fig. 3. Uterine cytology from a mare with fungal (yeast) endometritis. The arrow indicates organisms. (*Courtesy of* Hagyard Equine Institute Laboratory, Lexington, KY).

endometrial biopsy sample. Cytologic evaluation was 77% sensitive and 100% specific, with 100% positive predictive value and 62% negative predictive value [38].

Use of a cytobrush was compared with the traditional endometrial swab for obtaining samples [43]. Significantly more cells were obtained with less distortion of cells using the brush technique compared with the swab technique [43]. The cytobrush technique was deemed a more satisfactory method for cytologic evaluation [43]. The cytobrush technique was compared with uterine lavage for obtaining samples in postpartum cows [44]. The cytobrush was faster and more successful in obtaining a sufficiently large number of cells, particularly from an enlarged uterus, and resulted in less cellular distortion [44].

Biopsy

An endometrial biopsy histologic classification system has been described [45]. The histologic details of the endometrium reflect its functionality and ability to clear infection. A histologically normal endometrium (grade I) was associated with resistance to chronic uterine infection when challenged with intrauterine inoculation of *S equi* subsp *zooepidemicus* [46]. Mild to moderate histologic changes (grades IIa and IIb) were not consistently correlated with susceptibility to chronic infection [46]. Severe histopathologic changes (grade III) were associated with susceptibility to chronic uterine infection [46]. Endometrial biopsy may also aid in reaching a diagnosis of fungal infection by staining the sample with Gomori's methenamine silver stain [47].

In addition to the standard classification, it has been proposed to describe irregularities of endometrial differentiation more completely in an effort to elucidate causes of infertility. Histologic endometrial disturbances are found when some areas of the endometrium are differentiated appropriately for the estrus cycle in the presence of multifocal nonfibrotic glands that deviate from physiologic expectations. Endometrial differentiation disturbances were categorized into unequal endometrial differentiation affecting occasional glands, irregular endometrial differentiation that affected all or most glands, irregular proliferative differentiation involving distinct polymorphism of the glandular epithelia, irregular secretory differentiation, and completely irregular differentiation. It has been proposed that these histologically observed alterations may provide insight into the causes of infertility, such as hormonal imbalance or alterations involving hormonal receptors within the endometrium [48].

As mentioned previously, there is evidence that microbial culture directly from an endometrial biopsy specimen may be more revealing than culture from an endometrial swab for identifying a causative organism in cases of uterine infections [38].

Ultrasonography

Ultrasonography has been well established as an important diagnostic tool in equine medicine and reproduction. Highly fertile mares seldom have free intrauterine fluid after breeding [49]. In contrast, fluid present in the uterus after ovulation is often associated with susceptibility to endometritis [42,50]. Normal measurements of the uteroplacental thickness of pregnant mares have been established. The combined thickness of the uterus and placenta should not exceed 12 mm at any site. Cranial and ventral to the cervix, the combined thickness of the uterus and placenta should be less than 8 mm between 271 and 300 days of gestation, less than 10 mm between 301 and 330 days of gestation, and less than 12 mm after 330 days of gestation [51].

Doppler ultrasonography has been used for investigating uterine blood flow in mares [52]. The velocity of blood flow was evaluated after intrauterine infusion of skim milk extender, seminal plasma, and raw semen. Blood flow velocity increased compared with normal after infusion of seminal plasma and raw semen, potentially associated with an inflammatory reaction [52].

Endoscopy

Hysteroscopy has long been recognized as a diagnostic modality in mares with reproductive disease. The procedure allows direct observation of the reproductive tract as well as cytologic, microbial, and histologic sampling of specific sites under visual control. Endometrial abnormalities observed with hysteroscopy include endometrial degeneration, endometrial cysts, intraluminal fluid accumulation, transluminal adhesions, and masses [53,54]. Additionally, a correlation has been observed between the appearance of small arteries under the endometrium with age and the degree of endometrosis [55].

Various surgical procedures may also be performed hysteroscopically, including endometrial cyst removal via electrocautery, laser ablation, and synechiolysis [56–58].

In one study, the intrauterine inflammatory reaction and contamination induced by hysteroscopy in eight diestrus mares was investigated. Microbial growth of pathogenic organisms was obtained from endometrial swabs from 50% of the mares 5 days after hysteroscopy. No growth was obtained from endometrial swabs before hysteroscopy. In most cases, endometrial histopathologic examination revealed an acute inflammatory response with marked eosinophilia. During the estrous phase after hysteroscopy, 25% of the mares had persistent inflammation on histopathologic examination [59]. These findings provide guidance for intrauterine intervention after hysteroscopy.

Hormonal and peptide markers

A field that is developing in human and equine reproduction is the identification of protein markers indicative of gestational disease. Indicators of gestational disease include alterations of expected hormone levels and placental peptides.

In a study evaluating progestogens in the final trimester of normal and compromised equine pregnancies, 7 of 10 progestogens increased significantly in normal pregnancies as gestation progressed. Mares with placentitis had more marked increases in serum concentrations of progesterone or pregnenolone as well as in several metabolites compared with mares without placentitis. This was interpreted as a possible increase in fetal production of progestogens and increased metabolism in uteroplacental tissues in response to chronic stress. Placental pathologic findings other than placentitis were also associated with an increase compared with normal levels of progesterone and progesterone metabolites slightly different from that seen in mares with placentitis [60]. In severely compromised pregnancies with impending abortion, progesterone levels may decrease significantly, particularly during the first trimester [61].

Estrone sulfate is produced by the gonads of a viable fetus. Measurement of total estrogens has been described as useful for discerning between a normal and compromised fetus and may aid in developing diagnostic and treatment plans [62].

In human beings, various markers of intrauterine growth retardation (IUGR) have been investigated. These include growth factors, leptin, and vasoactive peptides. Insulin-like growth factor-1 (IGF-1) is important for fetal and placental development and late-gestation fetal growth [63]. A correlation has been observed between infants with IUGR and a low IGF-1 concentration; however, this is not seen in all cases of IUGR, and thus limits the use of IGF-1 as an indicator for IUGR in people. Epidermal growth factor (EGF) is necessary for implantation as well as for growth and differentiation of the placenta. Although a low EGF concentration is associated with IUGR, assaying for EGF may not be sufficiently accurate to be diagnostically valuable [64,65]. Leptin has also been investigated for its involvement in reproduction. Leptin is secreted from adipose and placental tissue and has been identified at other sites in various mammalian species [66]. Fetal leptin concentration is positively correlated with fetal growth [67]. Compared with normal pregnancies, maternal serum leptin concentrations tend to be increased with IUGR [68]. Thus, leptin may have the potential to be used as a marker of gestational abnormalities depending on the sample origin. Vasoactive peptides, such as endothelin, angiotensin II, and TNFα, may also be useful for early recognition of uteroplacental circulatory disturbances that can be associated with IUGR [64].

Intrauterine infection is associated with an increase in proinflammatory cytokine concentrations in uterine and cervical secretions compared with normal. In pregnant women, high IL-8 concentrations in cervical mucus as well as ultrasonographic evidence of a short cervix were associated with a high likelihood of microbial invasion of the amnionic cavity and chorioamnionitis [69]. Thus, a cervical mucus IL-8 assay has the potential to be used as an aid for selecting patients requiring antimicrobial therapy [69].

Disease syndromes

Endometritis

Endometritis has been labeled the third most common medical condition of horses [39,70]. Uterine infections are not limited to the horse. Estimates of the annual incidences of uterine infections in other species are 10% to 50% of dairy cattle, 20% to 75% of dairy buffaloes, and 5% to 10% of dairy sheep [71].

Persistent endometritis has been further categorized into sexually transmitted diseases, chronic infectious endometritis, persistent breeding-induced endometritis, and chronic degenerative endometritis, otherwise known as endometrosis [1].

Sexually transmitted diseases

Contagious equine metritis (CEM) is an equine sexually transmitted disease associated with infection by *Taylorella equigenitalis*. Thirty percent to 40% of mares bred by infected stallions develop the acute form of the disease, which is manifested as purulent metritis and cervicitis for 2 to 10 days, leading to at least temporary infertility. The organism is typically harbored in the clitoral sinus [72]. In 1997 and 1998, an organism similar to *T equigenitalis* was isolated from donkeys in California and Kentucky, respectively. The proposed name for this organism was *Taylorella asinigenitalis*. In a small study to characterize mares' response to infection with *T asinigenitalis*, an inability to infect mares with the California isolate was found. The Kentucky isolate did produce transient metritis and cervicitis and induced anti-*T equigenitalis* antibodies [73]. A real-time polymerase chain reaction

(PCR) assay has been developed for detection of *T equigenitalis* that distinguishes this organism from *T asinigenitalis* [74].

Other organisms associated with endometritis and thought to originate from the stallion's penis include *Pseudomonas aeruginosa* and *Klebsiella pneumoniae* capsule types 1, 2, and 5 [75]. These organisms are of particular concern because they can be refractory to traditional therapies.

Persistent breeding-induced endometritis

Breeding and breach of the normal anatomic barriers to infection may lead to uterine contamination. Semen induces an inflammatory response, and spermatozoa are chemotactic for neutrophils [76]. In most mares, the uterus is able to recover from the inflammatory event without intervention. Some mares, 15% of a Thoroughbred population in one study, develop persistent endometritis secondary to breeding. This is manifested as intrauterine fluid present beyond 12 hours after breeding [77]. Mares that typically fall into this category include aged multiparous mares as well as mature primiparous mares whose cervices have not yet been dilated from delivery of a foal. Mares with postbreeding endometritis have higher numbers of immunoglobulin-containing cells than normal mares in the face of potentially defective opsonization and generally poor uterine clearance as discussed previously. Other factors associated with persistent breeding-induced endometritis may include vascular degenerative changes as seen in older mares, a dependent uterus as seen in older and multiparous mares, and an inability to achieve sufficient cervical dilation in estrus as seen in mature primiparous mares [1].

Chronic infectious endometritis

Organisms typically associated with chronic infectious endometritis include *S equi* subsp *zooepidemicus*, *E coli*, *K pneumoniae*, *P aeruginosa*, and yeasts. *S equi* subsp *zooepidemicus* reportedly represents 66% of infections. This bacterium adheres to epithelial cells, and inflammatory and fibrotic changes associated with grade III endometrial changes were associated with bacterial adherence [12,78]. *E coli* is typically associated with fecal contamination; thus, the perineal conformation requires careful evaluation. *P aeruginosa* and *K pneumoniae* have been associated with previous intrauterine antimicrobial therapy [79].

Chronic degenerative endometritis

Chronic inflammation may predispose to the development of endometrial fibrosis. Degenerative endometrial changes (endometrosis) are considered irreversible and did not seem to alter the functional capacity of PMNs as compared with normal endometria when human recombinant IL-8 was used as an intrauterine chemoattractant [45,80]. Endometrosis must be differentiated from endometriosis, the human condition characterized by endometrial cellular explants.

Metritis

Methicillin-resistant *Staphylococcus aureus* (MRSA) is resistant to most β-lactam antimicrobials and, frequently, to other classes of antimicrobials. There is one report of a stud farm where multiple mares developed metritis secondary to MRSA [81]. The organism was thought to originate from a wound [81].

Placentitis and abortion

Infections are established in the fetal unit typically by ascending from the caudal reproductive tract or by a hematogenous route. Ascending placentitis is usually associated with compromise of at least one of the three physical barriers to infection: the labia, the vestibulovaginal sphincter, and the cervix.

In a review of causes of abortion, stillbirth, and perinatal death in horses, the most common cause was fetoplacental infection. Bacterial infection was diagnosed most frequently, with the three most frequent isolates being *S equi* subsp *zooepidemicus*, *E coli*, and *Leptospira* spp. The leptospiral serovar most associated with placentitis, abortion, stillbirth, and premature live birth in horses is Pomona type *kennewicki* [82]. Other organisms isolated include nocardioform actinomycetes, subsequently more specifically identified as several organisms, including *Crossiella equi* and *Amycolatopsis* spp [83,84]. *Pseudomonas* spp, *Streptococcus equisimilis*, *Enterobacter* spp, *Klebsiella* spp, α-hemolytic streptococci, *Staphylococcus* spp, and *Actinobacillus* spp were also isolated in cases of fetoplacental infection [85].

Rhodococcus equi is ubiquitous in some equine environments and is most frequently encountered in foal pneumonias. There are occasional reports of abortion associated with *R equi* isolated from the fetus and one report of placentitis associated with this gram-positive organism [86].

Four percent of all abortions or deaths and 17% of abortions or deaths in which a causative agent was discovered were attributed to equine herpesvirus (EHV). EHV was the only viral agent found to cause abortion, stillbirth, or perinatal death in this study. Abortion is primarily caused by EHV-1; however, there are occasional abortions associated with EHV-4 [87].

Herpesviruses are intracellular and disseminate to sites of secondary replication, which may include the uterus. Because of the intracellular nature of the virus, cytotoxic T lymphocytes are important for controlling infection and for devising immunization strategies. Naive mares, vaccinated mares, and mares exposed to EHV multiple times were compared for complement-fixing antibody titers, abortion after experimental infection, and cytotoxic T-lymphocyte frequency in blood samples. Antibody titers were low in naive mares, high in mares after vaccination, and low in previously infected mares. After experimental infection, all nine naive control mares aborted, one of the five vaccinated mares aborted, and none of the three previously infected mares aborted. Assessment of cytotoxic T-lymphocyte frequencies revealed that the cell frequencies were lower in mares that aborted compared with mares that did not abort, prompting the investigators to suggest that vaccine development be aimed toward inducing cytotoxic T lymphocytes, such as via mucosal immunization [88].

Seven percent of abortion cases with a definitive diagnosis were attributed to mycotic placentitis [85]. *Aspergillus* spp and mucoraceous fungi were most common [85].

Protozoal abortion is uncommon in horses, particularly in comparison to other domestic large animal species. There are sparse reports of isolation of *Neospora* spp from aborted fetuses. Serologic surveys show a higher prevalence of the disease in horses than those suggested by abortion results from investigations, with the serologic prevalence ranging from 2% to 23% in the United States and France. In an attempt to learn more about the prevalence of *Neospora* spp in association with abortion, investigators compared serology from mares that aborted, from mares routinely screened before breeding, and from randomly chosen horses. The prevalence of serum antibodies against *Neospora* spp was significantly higher in the group of mares that had recently aborted [89].

Treatment of the nonpregnant uterus

Resolution of female genital tract infections is predicated on the following: correction of anatomic defects, enhancement of uterine clearance, and treatment of specific infections.

Antibacterials

In a human proof-of-concept study, antimicrobial therapy was associated with improvement of histologic evidence of endometritis as well as with symptoms of endometritis regardless of whether organisms were grown from endometrial swabs [90]. The conclusion was that the focal presence of a small number of bacteria was sufficient to cause histologic evidence of endometritis yet elude discovery and that elimination of the bacteria led to clinical and histologic improvement [90].

Numerous reports exist of veterinary intrauterine antimicrobial use in domestic animals. Safety and efficacy may vary depending on the antimicrobial, patient species, pathogen species, and minimum inhibitory concentration (MIC) determined for the isolate. Intrauterine antimicrobial selection is directed by the safety of the drug in the uterus, sensitivity of the organism, and the MIC of the drug for the pathogenic organism. Although more information is available regarding the pharmacokinetics and safety of intrauterine therapies, drug choice is frequently empiric.

β-Lactam antimicrobials are time-dependent antimicrobials that interfere with cell wall formation by inhibiting the penicillin-binding proteins that catalyze polymer cross-linking necessary for cell wall formation. β-Lactams are bactericidal for growing cells. Differences in organism susceptibility are attributable to differences in penicillin-binding protein receptor sites, the amount of peptidoglycan present in the cell wall, drug penetration of the outer cell membrane of gram-negative bacteria, and β-lactamase–induced resistance [91]. Penicillins have long been used as intrauterine therapy. Evaluation of endometrial ampicillin concentration 24 hours after a 3-g intrauterine infusion of ampicillin revealed adequate drug concentrations to achieve the MIC for investigated isolates 24 hours after infusion [92]. One report described deposition of a white precipitate on the endometrium that persisted for 10 days after infusion of ampicillin [93]. Infusion of ticarcillin within 1 hour of breeding did not interfere with pregnancy rates [94]. The phagocytic ability of neutrophils was not affected by potassium benzylpenicillin or ticarcillin [95]. Investigations of intrauterine administration of ticarcillin revealed that a 6-g intrauterine infusion resulted in an endometrial concentration of 150 to 424 μg/g 60 minutes after infusion [96,97]. Ticarcillin clearance from plasma and the endometrium is rapid, thus potentially necessitating more frequent administration of ticarcillin to maintain concentrations greater than the MIC for this time-dependent antimicrobial [97] of tissue.

Cephalosporins are also β-lactam antimicrobials, but they have greater inherent resistance to β-lactamases because of molecular differences [98]. Pharmacokinetics and endometrial concentrations achieved from systemic therapy have been investigated. An endometrial tissue drug concentration of 2.2 μg/g (microgram of drug per gram of endometrial tissue) was achieved after four intramuscular doses of sodium cephapirin, a first-generation cephalosporin, at a dose of 20 mg/kg [99]. Simultaneous oral treatment with probenecid led to a significant increase in endometrial sodium cephapirin concentration [100]. After intramuscular administration of cefoxitin, a second-generation cephalosporin, endometrial concentrations of drug were 4.5 mg/g (milligrams of drug per gram of endometrial tissue) 4 hours after the fourth treatment at a dose of 20 mg/kg [101].

Intrauterine ceftiofur sodium, a third-generation cephalosporin, was found to be safe and equally as effective as penicillin mixed with another antimicrobial [102]. The endometrial ceftiofur sodium concentration was evaluated after intramuscular administration (2 mg/kg twice daily). Ceftiofur was not detected in endometrial tissue [103].

Aminoglycosides have also been used for intrauterine treatment for infection with gram-negative organisms and staphylococci. Amikacin, in particular, can be effective against *P aeruginosa*. These molecules are highly polar and are inhibited by divalent cations as well as by purulent and necrotic tissue. Aminoglycosides are rapidly bactericidal in a dose-related fashion by binding to the prokaryotic 30s ribosome and inhibiting protein synthesis [104].

Successful conception has been demonstrated after intrauterine infusion of gentamicin and amikacin in a buffered solution [105,106]. Various studies have been performed investigating the inflammatory response to intrauterine infusion of aminoglycosides. The phagocytic activity of neutrophils was found to be markedly decreased compared with normal after incubation with unbuffered gentamicin and amikacin solutions. This effect was less pronounced with buffered solutions [95]. Histologic evidence of inflammation was compared between mares receiving intrauterine gentamicin (2 g in 80 mL of saline) and intrauterine saline [107]. Gentamicin-treated mares had a less severe inflammatory response of shorter duration than saline-treated mares [107]. More recently, scanning electron microscopy was performed on the uterine epithelium of mares that received intrauterine gentamicin (2 g in 80 mL of saline) and mares that received intrauterine saline [108]. Endometrial epithelial cells had more cellular perforations and fewer and shorter microvilli, there were fewer ciliated cells, and more of the cilia were disrupted or drooping in the uterine epithelium treated with antimicrobials compared with the saline-treated uterine epithelium, suggesting that the effects of antimicrobial infusion on the endometrium require further study [108]. In an in vitro study using bovine endometrium, gentamicin sulfate inhibited spontaneous, oxytocin-induced, and $PGF_{2\alpha}$-induced myometrial contractions in a dose-dependent manner. Myometrial contractility was improved with the addition of calcium [109]. Previously, aminoglycoside antimicrobials had been shown to inhibit spontaneous myometrial activity of rat endometria [110].

Investigations of the tissue penetration of amikacin revealed that intrauterine infusion of amikacin was a more successful method of drug delivery than intramuscular administration to treat endometritis. The recommended dose for treatment of gram-negative endometritis was 4.4 mg/kg once daily [111]. A comparison of 2-g and 3-g infusions of amikacin revealed that the highest endometrial concentration occurred 1 hour after infusion, with minimal endometrial concentrations at 24 hours after infusion [112]. The 3-g infusion dose did not have a therapeutic advantage [112].

Enrofloxacin may be valuable for systemic treatment of reproductive tract infections caused by organisms, such as *K pneumoniae*, *E coli*, and *P aeruginosa*. Fluoroquinolones, such as enrofloxacin, inhibit DNA gyrase and are generally bactericidal to aerobic gram-negative bacteria. The safety of intrauterine infusion is not well documented, but efficacy studies have shown promising results. Intrauterine infusion of enrofloxacin at a dose of 2.5 mg/kg was studied for the histologic endometrial response and to measure the endometrial enrofloxacin concentration [113]. A statistically insignificant inflammatory response was observed with the infusion [113]. Enrofloxacin concentrations remained greater than the MIC for a sensitive *E coli* strain for 24 hours [113]. Investigation of intravenous administration of enrofloxacin at a dose of 5 mg/kg revealed adequate endometrial concentrations of enrofloxacin and its metabolite ciprofloxacin to treat infection with susceptible bacteria [114]. The systemic distribution of another fluoroquinolone, orbifloxacin, was also investigated [115]. Administration of a single oral dose of orbifloxacin at a rate of 7.5 mg/kg resulted in good distribution to body tissues, including endometrial tissue [115].

Tetracyclines are bacteriostatic antimicrobials that interfere with protein synthesis at the level of the prokaryotic 30s ribosome. There are anecdotal reports of intrauterine infusion of some tetracycline preparations causing severe inflammatory responses [116]. After intragastric administration of doxycycline (five doses of 10 mg/kg twice daily), the endometrial concentration was approximately 1.3 µg/mL. The MIC for the *S equi* subsp *zooepidemicus* strains that were evaluated was 1.0 µg/mL or less and less than 0.25 µg/mL for *S aureus* strains [117].

Sulfonamides interfere with the biosynthesis of folic acid by competing with para-aminobenzoic acid for the enzyme dihydropteroate synthetase [118]. Mares administered five doses of trimethoprim-sulfamethoxazole (trimethoprim, 2.5 mg/kg, and sulfamethoxazole, 12.5 mg/kg, given orally twice daily) had endometrial concentrations of both drugs that were equal to or exceeded the MIC of various bacteria, including strains of *S equi* subsp *zooepidemicus*, *Staphylococcus* spp, and *Corynebacterium pseudotuberculosis* as well as several obligate anaerobes [119].

In an evaluation of aerobic and anaerobic commensal bacteria and organisms associated with active endometritis, *Bacteroides fragilis* was found to be the predominant anaerobic bacterium in mixed intrauterine infections in the mare [120]. *B fragilis* commonly produces β-lactamases but is typically susceptible to metronidazole. In a study of metronidazole pharmacokinetics, intragastric administration of four maintenance doses of metronidazole (15-mg/kg loading dose, followed by 7.5 mg/kg every 6 hours) led to a mean endometrial metronidazole concentration of 0.9 µg/g of tissue [121]. Intravaginal metronidazole was demonstrated to reduce the incidence of postcesarean endometritis in women [122].

Tris-ethylenediaminetetraacetic acid (EDTA) has been shown to potentiate the effects of some antimicrobials. In vitro, Tris-EDTA acted synergistically with tetracycline, fluoroquinolone, aminoglycoside, macrolide, and β-lactam antimicrobials against resistant gram-positive and gram-negative bacteria. The combination of Tris-EDTA and antimicrobials has been successfully used to treat resistant pathogens in the soft tissues of small animals as well as for treatment of resistant bovine endometritis. EDTA acts by increasing the membrane permeability of gram-negative organisms, and Tris potentiates EDTA. Although gram-positive organisms are generally more resistant to the effects of Tris-EDTA, the combination of Tris-EDTA and antimicrobials has a synergistic deleterious effect on some gram-positive organisms [123].

Antifungals

The incidence of fungal endometritis is relatively low, with estimates ranging from 1% to 9% of mares diagnosed with endometritis. Fungal organisms may reside in the caudal reproductive tract or gain access to the reproductive tract secondary to poor conformation or iatrogenic means.

Intrauterine antimicrobial treatment, especially for an extended period, may be associated with fungal endometritis [124].

Treatment initially involves careful scrutiny of the caudal reproductive tract and perineal conformation. Large-volume uterine lavage may be beneficial for reducing organism numbers as well as for its counterirritant properties. Lavage additives proposed for fungal endometritis treatment include dimethyl sulfoxide (DMSO), dilute povidone-iodine, and acetic acid. In vitro, 10% to 20% DMSO reduced *Candida albicans* growth, whereas greater than 30% DMSO inhibited growth; however, 25% DMSO intrauterine infusion may cause reproductive epithelial cell ulceration [125]. Dilute acetic acid (20–30 mL of white vinegar in 1 L of normal saline) lowers the intrauterine pH, thus inducing prostaglandin release [126]. Some antifungal compounds may also be better absorbed with a lower environmental pH [124].

Intrauterine antifungal treatments include clotrimazole, nystatin, amphotericin B, and fluconazole [127,128]. Clotrimazole is a fungistatic azole drug that inhibits ergosterol synthesis, leading to fungal membrane and enzyme disruption. Nystatin and amphotericin B are polyene antifungal drugs that interfere with ergosterol binding and alter membrane permeability. Nystatin is fungicidal at four times the MIC. Amphotericin B is fungicidal; however, it also binds cholesterol in mammalian cells, and thus can be toxic to mammals. Fluconazole specifically inhibits fungal enzymatic synthesis of ergosterol, a component of fungal cell walls [129]. More recently, lufenuron has been used to treat fungal endometritis in mares. Lufenuron is a benzophenyl urea that disrupts chitin formation, a structural component of the fungal cell wall [130].

Uterotonics

Oxytocin has been used to induce uterine contractility to aid in fluid clearance. Administration of oxytocin in combination with intrauterine antimicrobials led to a significantly higher conception rate among treated mares than treatment with antimicrobials alone [131].

$PGF_{2\alpha}$ is commonly used for its luteolytic properties, leading to a decrease in progesterone and prompt return to estrus. Progesterone has been documented to be immunosuppressive; thus, decreasing the progesterone concentration acts as an indirect treatment for uterine infections.

$PGF_{2\alpha}$ also induces myometrial contractions. In cows administered the $PGF_{2\alpha}$ analogue cloprostenol, uterine contractility was enhanced for approximately 45 minutes; however, intrauterine pressure was only increased for 15 minutes [132]. In mares, uterine contractility may be beneficial in reducing fluid volume but not for reducing bacteria numbers [2]. Intrauterine bacterial challenges of sows in diestrus before prostaglandin susceptibility, progesterone-treated ewes, and control ewes suggested that administration of $PGF_{2\alpha}$ may be directly beneficial for the treatment of uterine infection by enhancing immune defenses and stimulating lymphocyte proliferation [71]. Results from in vitro studies indicate that $PGF_{2\alpha}$ enhances neutrophil chemotaxis and phagocytosis. Furthermore, $PGF_{2\alpha}$ is a proinflammatory molecule that may induce proinflammatory cytokines to enhance an immune response further [133,134].

Acupuncture may also be beneficial for re-establishing appropriate uterine contractility. Acupuncture has been recommended for use in the treatment of a retained placenta to improve uterine contractility and for dystocias to induce pelvic ligament relaxation, cervical softening, and coordinated strengthened uterine contractions [135]. The level of expression of COX-2 in the endometrium and myometrium was reduced with acupuncture in studies performed in pregnant rats. Measurement with pressure transducers revealed a significant decrease in uterine contractions with acupuncture when compared with controls [136].

Immunomodulation

Mycobacterium cell wall extract is typically used for immunomodulation in diseases involving chronic inflammation. Commercially available forms include an emulsion of a cell wall skeleton preparation purified from *Mycobacterium phlei*. Intravenous administration of mycobacterial cell wall extract to mares susceptible to persistent postbreeding endometritis led to downregulation of IL-1β mRNA expression compared with that in untreated susceptible mares [33]. It is postulated that mycobacterial cell wall extract aids in restoring homeostatic local inflammatory mechanisms.

Dexamethasone and IL-10 have been used to reduce amniotic prostaglandin synthesis in nonhuman primates with experimentally induced preterm labor [137]. Although the use of dexamethasone in pregnant mares may be controversial because of its potential to induce parturition in high doses, the use of immunomodulation as a treatment for placentitis or infection of the fetal unit has not been well documented in the horse.

In a study evaluating uterine PMNs, blood plasma was found to enhance phagocytic and chemotactic capabilities of uterine PMNs [17]. The efficacy of blood plasma as an intrauterine therapy has been debated [138,139].

Counterirritant therapy

Resolution of persistent inflammation and improvement of endometrial architecture have been shown to improve the reproductive prognosis [140]. Counterirritant therapy is aimed at stimulating endogenous acute inflammatory mechanisms so as to resolve chronic inflammatory and degenerative processes.

Intrauterine infusion of normal saline is a widely practiced technique for the physical removal of intrauterine detritus after foaling, removal of deleterious seminal fragments after breeding, and as a vehicle for other intrauterine therapeutic agents. Normal saline has been shown to initiate a mild endometritis [141,142]. Resultant prostaglandin production stimulates uterine myometrial activity and evacuation of endometrial glands. This effect is enhanced with warmed saline (40°C) [143].

Intrauterine use of DMSO has been investigated [125]. The hygroscopic action of DMSO results in dehydration and desquamation of superficial epithelial cells, leading to improvement in endometrial architecture. Endometrial fibrosis resulting from contact with DMSO is minimal because of the inhibitory effects of DMSO on collagen deposition. Overall improvements in reproductive performance as measured by foaling rates have been difficult to achieve, because improved conception rates are not matched by fetal survival [144].

Infusion of iodine preparations resulted in an acute inflammatory reaction in the superficial epithelial layer of the endometrium characterized by neutrophilia that lasted for up to 10 days and continuing as a chronic predominantly mononuclear cell reaction for up to 30 days [141]. Fibrosis may actually be increased after treatment [145]. Coadministered intrauterine drug absorption may be increased by iodine lavage; however, the potential for increased fibrosis should be considered [146].

Little information is available regarding the use of disinfectants on the equine endometrium. As assessed by histologic evaluation of endometrial biopsy samples, repeated uterine lavage using a 0.25% chlorhexidine solution did not injure the uterus [147]. By way of comparison, lavage of a synovial joint with 0.05% chlorhexidine, the lowest bactericidal concentration, was shown to be injurious [148].

Anecdotal reports of the intrauterine use of kerosene are common. The beneficial effects of kerosene are transient, and overall reproductive performance is unaffected. Aromatic components of kerosene are theorized to act as local irritants, causing local recruitment of leukocytes and expulsion of retained glandular secretions [80].

Infusion of autogenous plasma with the aim of resolving persistent endometrial inflammation has been widely practiced. Plasma has been shown to have a local inflammatory effect similar to that of normal saline, with PMN infiltration into the stratum compactum [142]. Improvement in posttreatment biopsy scores for mares infused with plasma has been shown, suggesting a counterinflammatory effect, although reproductive performance was not necessarily improved in all mares [138].

Mechanical curettage

There have been limited reports of mechanical endometrial curettage in the mare [149]. In a recent retrospective study, it was reported that in excess of 75% of mares improved one histopathologic grade in response to this technique [150]. Age was not considered to be a factor in the ability to favorably respond. Adverse effects, including the formation of transluminal adhesions, have been reported in human beings [151].

Treatment of the pregnant uterus

The treatments most commonly used for conditions like placentitis include antimicrobials, nonsteroidal anti-inflammatory drugs (NSAIDs), and progesterone supplementation. Strategies for treating mares with placentitis have been reviewed recently [152]. Treatment of the pregnant uterus necessitates considering the epitheliochorial placentation and transport of the antimicrobial into the fetal membranes. Several studies have evaluated the ability of some of the more commonly used antimicrobial drugs to cross equine fetal membranes. In a comparison of potassium penicillin G alone, gentamicin sulfate alone, penicillin and gentamicin in combination, and trimethoprim-sulfadiazine, only trimethoprim-sulfadiazine was present in sufficient concentrations in amnionic and allantoic fluid to treat a susceptible infection [153]. In another study performed with different drug assaying methods using in vivo microdialysis, the MICs of potassium penicillin G and gentamicin were reached for *S zooepidemicus* in allantoic fluid after intravenous administration [154]. In an additional study, the efficacy of trimethoprim-sulfamethoxazole with pentoxifylline for the treatment of induced placentitis was evaluated, and the results indicated that this drug combination may delay premature delivery of foals in mares with placentitis compared with uninfected and untreated pregnant mares. Four of five treated mares with induced placentitis aborted, but abortion occurred toward the end of a 2-week treatment period (n = 1) or after experimental treatment ceased (n = 3). Untreated mares with induced placentitis were not described [152].

Cytokines and prostaglandins produced in an inflammatory response also participate in the induction of parturition. Thus, anti-inflammatory therapy is an important component of placentitis treatment. NSAIDs used in cases of equine placentitis include flunixin meglumine and phenylbutazone. Pentoxifylline is a pharmacologic agent used as an adjunctive treatment for placentitis. Pentoxifylline is a xanthine derivative that increases red blood cell deformability, thus potentially improving perfusion. Pentoxifylline has also been shown to reduce TNFα concentrations in some cases of infection [155,156]. In nonhuman primates, indomethacin, a COX inhibitor, has been used to decrease prostaglandin secretion and uterine contraction in cases of induced preterm labor [157].

Progesterone supplementation is commonly recommended in cases of placentitis because of concerns that the placental function is compromised. Progesterone and altrenogest were shown to maintain pregnancy in ovariectomized mares [158]. Five progestogenic compounds were compared for efficacy in maintaining pregnancy in the face of $PGF_{2\alpha}$ administration between days 18 and 30 after ovulation. Four of the five compounds, medroxyprogesterone acetate, hydroxyprogesterone hexanoate, norgestomet, and megestrol acetate, were not able to maintain pregnancy when administered according to manufacturers' instructions. The fifth progestogen, altrenogest (0.044 mg/kg administered orally once a day) maintained pregnancy until day 30, which was the end of the experimental period [159]. There are anecdotal accounts of long-acting progesterone compounds being used successfully to maintain pregnancy.

Tocolytics have been used to inhibit uterine contractions in cases of premature labor in human beings. Mares with experimentally induced placentitis experienced altered myometrial contractility, including increased intensity and duration of large-spike myoelectrical bursts similar to contractures [160]. Clenbuterol, a β-sympathomimetic agent, has been used in mares in an attempt to induce uterine relaxation. A significant decrease in uterine tone was observed early in gestation [161]. The effects were less pronounced during late gestation [161]. Side effects included transient tachycardia in the mare and fetus [161].

Male reproductive tract

Infection of the male genital tract may have important consequences for male and female infertility. Direct effects on male fertility include impaired spermatogenesis, decreased sperm viability, and the potential for ductal obstruction. Accessory gland function may be impaired, altering seminal plasma composition and, potentially, sperm function [162]. Female fertility may be impaired by transference of the infection via semen or direct genital contact.

Infection of the accessory sex glands and internal tubular genitalia of the stallion is rarely reported [163]; however, reports of seminal vesiculitis [164,165] and ampullitis [166] do exist. Medical management and surgical vesiculectomy have been reported with varying success [164,166,167].

Defense mechanisms

Cellular and secretory defense mechanisms of the male genital tract share many common features with those detailed previously for the female genital tract. Anatomically, the male tubular tract is more resistant to ascending infection because of the greater distance between the constituent tissues and the external environment. Once established, however, infection of the male accessory sex glands can prove challenging to treat. This is because of the physiologically remote nature of the tissues, the tortuous glandular and ductal anatomy, the blood-testis barrier, and the pharmacokinetically unfavorable nature of the epithelial barriers and secretions of the tract.

Diagnosis of infection

Culture and cytology

A wide variety of microorganisms have been detected in the semen of breeding stallions [168]. Detection of bacteria in semen does not necessarily indicate infection, because sample contamination and transference of surface genital colonization can readily occur [169]. In cases in which bacteria have been detected, sperm morphology was deemed acceptable and few ejaculates contained inflammatory cells. Furthermore, in one study, there was no correlation between the occurrence of *P aeruginosa* in raw semen and pregnancy rates [168].

A heavy pure growth of pathogenic bacteria recovered after ejaculation is highly suggestive of infection of the internal genitalia [170]. In such cases, care should be taken to assess and remove the resident external flora of the genitalia before obtaining samples. Vesicular fluid can be collected by a cuffed tube passed to the colliculus seminalis concurrent with manual gland expression per rectum [170].

Cytologic evaluation of semen can be rewarding in cases of glandular infection. This is aided by fractionation of the ejaculate during collection. The presence of neutrophils, red blood cells, and bacteria is highly suggestive of seminal vesiculitis or ampullitis; however, this is not specific for the location of infection.

Ultrasonography

Ultrasonographic measurements of normal stallion accessory sex glands have been established [171]. The echogenic character of the ampullae and vesicular glands has been demonstrated to vary widely, even within the same animal. Recent sexual activity also has a marked influence on echodensity and homogeneity. Changes in the size of the gland, consistency of glandular fluids, and thickness of the muscular glandular wall are useful diagnostic aids [172].

Endoscopy

Fiberoptic endoscopy has been used diagnostically and therapeutically (Fig. 4). The capability to image the urethra and accessory sex gland openings [172] and the ability to instill medication intraluminally in the affected gland are valuable case management tools. Direct application of medication to the affected area bypasses unfavorable pharmacokinetic profiles of most

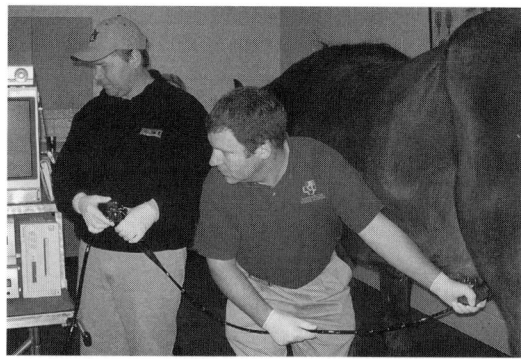

Fig. 4. Endoscopy of stallion reproductive tract. Diagnosis and treatment of accessory gland infections and pathologic findings are facilitated by this imaging modality.

drugs and ensures high local concentrations, allows assessment of the integrity of infected tissue, and facilitates the evacuation of cellular debris from the site of infection.

Biopsy

Excisional biopsy of the male reproductive tract is a useful tool to assess external and mucosal lesions, such as neoplasia (eg, squamous cell carcinoma, melanoma, fibrosarcoma), sarcoids, viral lesions (eg, papilloma, equine coital exanthema), and parasite-induced inflammatory reactions (eg, habronemiasis). Disruption of the blood-testis barrier and the potential for the introduction of infection should be considered when biopsies of the gonads and accessory sex glands, respectively, are contemplated.

Assessment of inflammatory mediators

Depending on their activation status, leukocytes in semen produce large quantities of cytokines, soluble cytokine receptors, and reactive oxygen metabolites [173–175]. Leukocyte population increases may also be associated with the formation of antisperm antibodies, which are detectable locally and systemically [176]. The magnitude of sperm damage depends on the location of the inflammatory response, duration of exposure, and ability of sperm to enable antilipoperoxidative mechanisms [177]. In one human study, the most specific marker for accessory gland infection was IL-6, meaning that this may be a useful tool to discriminate between physiologic and infectious leukocytospermia [175]. IL-6 was shown to correlate positively with the leukocyte count and negatively with the sperm motility count and morphology [178]. Reports on the efficacy of antimicrobial treatment are conflicting, with current investigation centering on neutralization of detrimental white blood cell secretory products.

Selected transmissible diseases

A limited number of infectious agents have been proven to be transmitted venereally from stallion to mare. Most are bacterial; however, viral and protozoal diseases also occur.

Contagious equine metritis

CEM was first identified in 1977 in Newmarket, England, with subsequent outbreaks in other countries, including the United States (Kentucky in 1978 and Missouri in 1979) [179]. The causative agent, *T equigenitalis*, is transmitted by carrier stallions or mares during intromission. Inapparent carrier mares or stallions are responsible for the spread of the disease.

With respect to the stallion, the bacteria may be isolated from the urethral fossa, urethral sinus, distal urethra, and preputial and penile surfaces [180]. In addition, *T equigenitalis* has been recovered at necropsy from the testis, epididymis, and seminal vesicles of an infected stallion [181].

Current measures to prevent reintroduction of CEM rely on the quarantine, culture, and treatment of imported horses [182]. This is complicated by the occurrence of false-negative bacterial culture results [182]. A further layer of protection consists of the test mating of candidate stallions to known CEM-negative mares. This does not consistently result in the colonization and seroconversion of test mares, however. A recent report highlights the potential for a breakdown in this control scheme [183]. It was suggested that bacterial cultures should be repeated over a 1- to 3-week time frame before stallions suspected of having CEM are mated to test mares and that additional cultures obtained more than 21 days after stallion treatment may aid in the detection of infection. Experimentally, PCR assay has proven to be a more sensitive method of *T equigenitalis* detection than culture [182]. This is further improved by a combined culture-PCR technique.

Equine viral arteritis

Equine viral arteritis can be diagnosed by virus isolation or serology. Equine arteritis virus (EAV) may be found in nasal secretions, blood, semen, placenta, and a number of tissues and fluids after death.

Paired serum samples can be collected for serology. Nasopharyngeal and conjunctival swabs and nonheparinized blood can be collected for virus isolation or PCR assay. Virus isolation samples should be taken early in the acute phase of illness. Carrier stallions can often be identified by virus isolation from semen; however, it must be noted that shedding is intermittent. Semen samples should be collected from suspect carrier stallions; these samples should contain the sperm-rich fraction of the ejaculate.

It is imperative that the negative status of a breeding stallion be established and documented before vaccination, because antibodies from field infection and vaccination are indistinguishable. Likewise, it is important to isolate vaccinated animals per the instructions of the vaccine manufacturer and federal regulations to ensure that shedding of vaccinal virus does not infect naive in-contact animals.

Pseudomonas aeruginosa *and* Klebsiella pneumoniae

It is commonly assumed that the stallion can be a lesionless penile carrier of pathogenic organisms that are readily transferable to the mare. It is prudent to serotype the organism involved, however, because there is likely no association between the colonizing organism of the stallion and the uterine invader of the mare [184]. *P aeruginosa* and *K pneumoniae* have been recognized to have an association with endometritis in the mare, particularly in those mares that have a defect in uterine clearance. Factors that predispose the penis and sheath to colonization are not known; however, it is surmised that washing and disinfection may be associated with the removal of commensal flora [169,184]. There also seems to be strain variation within the organisms involved, accounting for the variation in virulence.

All forms of cleansing have been shown to alter the bacterial flora of the stallion's penis. Soaps have been shown to favor the growth of coliforms, whereas iodine encouraged the growth of *P aeruginosa* and *K pneumoniae* [169]. A less disruptive approach may be the use of a dilute solution of hydrochloric acid (0.1%) [184]. The use of a 0.5% sodium hypochlorite solution, which is conveniently made with household bleach, has also been reported (R.M. Kenney, DVM, personal communication, 2006).

Treatment

Systemic antimicrobial administration may not achieve a bacteriologic cure, because the drug may fail to penetrate into infected tissues at a sufficient concentration for a sufficient time throughout the dosage interval. Few antimicrobial drugs pass readily across noninflamed epithelial cell borders present in the normal genital tract [185]. Those that do enter the genitourinary tract by an ion-trapping process. Lipid solubility and degree of ionization, which depend on the pH of plasma and seminal fluid, determine the extent of this process [186].

Seminal vesicle pH has been reported in the range of 7.5 to 7.8 [187]. Requirements for systemically administered drug penetration into the genital tract include bases with high lipid solubility and high pKa. Although not licensed for use in the horse, fluoroquinolones seem to have these favorable characteristics [114]. They have been shown to penetrate endometrial tissue and achieve concentrations sufficient to treat susceptible organisms.

Many antimicrobials have been demonstrated to have effects on spermatozoal motility in vitro [188], some at therapeutically achieved concentrations [189]. In addition, testicular spermatogenic function has been affected with antimicrobial use [190]. As such, antimicrobial treatment of asymptomatic leukocytospermia should be initiated with caution because of the doubtful clinical benefit and possible detrimental results on sperm function.

References

[1] Troedsson MH. Uterine clearance and resistance to persistent endometritis in the mare. Theriogenology 1999;52:461–71.
[2] Nikolakopoulos E, Watson ED. Uterine contractility is necessary for the clearance of intrauterine fluid but not bacteria after bacterial infusion in the mare. Theriogenology 1999;52: 413–23.
[3] Evans MJ, Hamer JM, Gason LM, et al. Factors affecting uterine clearance of inoculated materials in mares. J Reprod Fertil Suppl 1987;35:327–34.
[4] Troedsson MH, Liu IK. Uterine clearance of non-antigenic markers (51Cr) in response to a bacterial challenge in mares potentially susceptible and resistant to chronic uterine infections. J Reprod Fertil Suppl 1991;44:283–8.
[5] Neuwirth L, LeBlanc M, Maurgis D, et al. Scintigraphic measurement of uterine clearance in mares. Vet Radiol Ultrasound 1995;36:64–8.

[6] Troedsson MH, Liu IK, Ing M, et al. Multiple site electromyography recordings of uterine activity following an intrauterine bacterial challenge in mares susceptible and resistant to chronic uterine infection. J Reprod Fertil 1993;99:307–13.

[7] Rigby SL, Barhoumi R, Burghardt RC, et al. Mares with delayed uterine clearance have an intrinsic defect in myometrial function. Biol Reprod 2001;65:740–7.

[8] Nikolakopoulos E, Kindahl H, Watson ED. Oxytocin and PGF2α release in mares resistant and susceptible to persistent mating-induced endometritis. In: Proceedings of the Seventh International Symposium of Equine Reproduction, Pretoria, South Africa. 1998: 363–72.

[9] DeLille A, Silvers M, Cadario M, et al. Interaction of xylazine, acepromazine and oxytocin on intrauterine pressure in normal mares and those exhibiting a delay in uterine clearance. In: Proceedings of the Seventh International Symposium on Equine Reproduction, Pretoria, South Africa. 1998:373–9.

[10] Laurenzi GA, Guarneri JJ. Effects of bacteria and viruses on ciliated epithelium. A study of the mechanisms of pulmonary resistance to infection: the relationship of bacterial clearance to ciliary and alveolar macrophage function. Am Rev Respir Dis 1966;93:134–41.

[11] Ferreira-Dias GM, Nequin LG, King SS. Morphologic comparisons among equine endometrium categories I, II, and III, using light and transmission electron microscopy. Am J Vet Res 1999;60:49–55.

[12] Ferreira-Dias G, Nequin LG, King SS. Influence of estrous cycle stage on adhesion of Streptococcus zooepidemicus to equine endometrium. Am J Vet Res 1994;55:1028–31.

[13] Nicosia SV, Sowinski JM, Chilton BS, et al. Ultrastructural immunocytochemical localization of lysozyme in the mucociliary epithelium of the rabbit endocervix in different hormonal states. Anat Rec 1984;209:469–80.

[14] Schumacher GF, Kim MH, Hosseinian AH, et al. Immunoglobulins, proteinase inhibitors, albumin, and lysozyme in human cervical mucus. I. Communication: hormonal profiles and cervical mucus changes—methods and results. Am J Obstet Gynecol 1977;129:629–36.

[15] Eggert-Kruse W, Botz I, Pohl S, et al. Antimicrobial activity of human cervical mucus. Hum Reprod 2000;15:778–84.

[16] Hein M, Valore EV, Helmig RB, et al. Antimicrobial factors in the cervical mucus plug. Am J Obstet Gynecol 2002;187:137–44.

[17] Troedsson MH, Liu IK, Thurmond M. Function of uterine and blood-derived polymorphonuclear neutrophils in mares susceptible and resistant to chronic uterine infection: phagocytosis and chemotaxis. Biol Reprod 1993;49:507–14.

[18] Huttner KM, Bevins CL. Antimicrobial peptides as mediators of epithelial host defense. Pediatr Res 1999;45:785–94.

[19] Quayle AJ. The innate and early immune response to pathogen challenge in the female genital tract and the pivotal role of epithelial cells. J Reprod Immunol 2002;57:61–79.

[20] King AE, Critchley HO, Kelly RW. Presence of secretory leukocyte protease inhibitor in human endometrium and first trimester decidua suggests an antibacterial protective role. Mol Hum Reprod 2000;6:191–6.

[21] Jin FY, Nathan C, Radzioch D, et al. Secretory leukocyte protease inhibitor: a macrophage product induced by and antagonistic to bacterial lipopolysaccharide. Cell 1997;88:417–26.

[22] Fahey JV, Wira CR. Effect of menstrual status on antibacterial activity and secretory leukocyte protease inhibitor production by human uterine epithelial cells in culture. J Infect Dis 2002;185:1606–13.

[23] Masson P, Heremans J, Ferin J. Presence of an iron-binding protein (lactoferrin) in the genital tract of the human female. I. Its immunohistochemical localization in the endometrium. Fertil Steril 1968;19:679–89.

[24] Hiemstra PS, Maassen RJ, Stolk J, et al. Antibacterial activity of antileukoprotease. Infect Immun 1996;64:4520–4.

[25] Teng CT, Gladwell W, Beard C, et al. Lactoferrin gene expression is estrogen responsive in human and rhesus monkey endometrium. Mol Hum Reprod 2002;8:58–67.

[26] Pacora P, Maymon E, Gervasi MT, et al. Lactoferrin in intrauterine infection, human parturition, and rupture of fetal membranes. Am J Obstet Gynecol 2000;183:904–10.
[27] Fleming DC, King AE, Williams AR, et al. Hormonal contraception can suppress natural antimicrobial gene transcription in human endometrium. Fertil Steril 2003;79:856–63.
[28] King AE, Fleming DC, Critchley HO, et al. Differential expression of the natural antimicrobials, beta-defensins 3 and 4, in human endometrium. J Reprod Immunol 2003;59:1–16.
[29] King AE, Fleming DC, Critchley HO, et al. Regulation of natural antibiotic expression by inflammatory mediators and mimics of infection in human endometrial epithelial cells. Mol Hum Reprod 2002;8:341–9.
[30] Crane-Godreau MA, Wira CR. CCL20/macrophage inflammatory protein 3alpha and tumor necrosis factor alpha production by primary uterine epithelial cells in response to treatment with lipopolysaccharide or Pam3Cys. Infect Immun 2005;73:476–84.
[31] Crane-Godreau MA, Wira CR. Effects of estradiol on lipopolysaccharide and Pam3Cys stimulation of CCL20/macrophage inflammatory protein 3 alpha and tumor necrosis factor alpha production by uterine epithelial cells in culture. Infect Immun 2005;73:4231–7.
[32] Lappas M, Permezel M, Georgiou HM, et al. Nuclear factor kappa B regulation of proinflammatory cytokines in human gestational tissues in vitro. Biol Reprod 2002;67:668–73.
[33] Fumuso E, Giguere S, Wade J, et al. Endometrial IL-1beta, IL-6 and TNF-alpha, mRNA expression in mares resistant or susceptible to post-breeding endometritis. Effects of estrous cycle, artificial insemination and immunomodulation. Vet Immunol Immunopathol 2003; 96:31–41.
[34] Blackwell TS, Christman JW. The role of nuclear factor-kappa B in cytokine gene regulation. Am J Respir Cell Mol Biol 1997;17:3–9.
[35] Blackwell SC, Hassan SS, Wolfe HM, et al. Vaginal birth after cesarean in the diabetic gravida. J Reprod Med 2000;45:987–90.
[36] Barnes PJ, Karin M. Nuclear factor-kappaB: a pivotal transcription factor in chronic inflammatory diseases. N Engl J Med 1997;336:1066–71.
[37] Alghamdi AS, Foster DN, Carlson CS, et al. Nitric oxide levels and nitric oxide synthase expression in uterine samples from mares susceptible and resistant to persistent breeding-induced endometritis. Am J Reprod Immunol 2005;53:230–7.
[38] Nielsen JM. Endometritis in the mare: a diagnostic study comparing cultures from swab and biopsy. Theriogenology 2005;64:510–8.
[39] Card C. Post-breeding inflammation and endometrial cytology in mares. Theriogenology 2005;64:580–8.
[40] Brook D. Uterine cytology. In: McKinnon AO, Voss JL, editors. Equine reproduction. Baltimore (MD): Williams & Wilkins; 1993. p. 246–54.
[41] Card C, Carley S, Green J, et al. Endometrial cytology in mares bred with frozen semen. In: Proceedings of the 50th Conference of the American Association of Equine Practitioners, Denver, CO. 2004:505–9.
[42] Maloufi F, Pierson R, Otto S, et al. Mares susceptible or resistant to endometritis have similar endometrial echographic and inflammatory cell reactions at 96 hours after infusion with frozen semen and extender. In: Proceedings of the 48th Conference of the American Association of Equine Practitioners, Orlando, FL. 2002:51–7.
[43] Bourke M, Mills JN, Barnes AL. Collection of endometrial cells in the mare. Aust Vet J 1997;75:755–8.
[44] Kasimanickam R, Duffield TF, Foster RA, et al. The effect of a single administration of cephapirin or cloprostenol on the reproductive performance of dairy cows with subclinical endometritis. Theriogenology 2005;63:818–30.
[45] Kenney RM, Doig PA. Equine endometrial biopsy. In: Morrow DA, editor. Current therapy in theriogenology. Philadelphia: WB Saunders; 1986. p. 723–9.
[46] Troedsson MH, deMoraes MJ, Liu IK. Correlations between histologic endometrial lesions in mares and clinical response to intrauterine exposure with Streptococcus zooepidemicus. Am J Vet Res 1993;54:570–2.

[47] Freeman K, Rozel J, Slusher S, et al. Mycotic infections of the equine uterus. Equine Pract 1986;8:34–42.
[48] Schoon H, Wiegandt I, Schoon D, et al. Functional disturbances in the endometrium of barren mares: a histological and immunohistochemical study. J Reprod Fertil Suppl 2000;56:381–91.
[49] Burns T, Pierson R, Card C. Subjective and quantitative assessments of endometrial changes in mares inseminated with cryopreserved semen. In: Proceedings of the Society for Theriogenology, San Antonio, TX. 2000:47.
[50] Brinsko SP, Rigby SL, Varner DD, et al. A practical method for recognizing mares susceptible to post-breeding endometritis. In: Proceedings of the 49th Conference of the American Association of Equine Practitioners, New Orleans, LA. 2003:363–5.
[51] Troedsson MHT. Ultrasonographic evaluation of the equine placenta. Pferdeheilkunde 2001;17:583–8.
[52] Bollwein H, Mayer R, Stolla R. Transrectal Doppler sonography of uterine blood flow during early pregnancy in mares. Theriogenology 2003;60:597–605.
[53] Bracher V, Mathias S, Allen WR. Videoendoscopic evaluation of the mare's uterus: II. Findings in subfertile mares. Equine Vet J 1992;24:279–84.
[54] Santschi EM. Case presentation: uterine mass in a mare. Compend Contin Educ Pract Vet 2005;27:229–35.
[55] Inoue K, Ito K, Terada T, et al. Degenerative changes in the endometrial vasculature of the mare detected by videoendoscopic examination. In: Proceedings of the 46th Conference of the American Association of Equine Practitioners, Orlando, FL. 2002:325–9.
[56] Merkt H, Moura J, Klug E, et al. Treatment of endometrial cysts in mares. Arquivos da escola de medicina veterinaria da universidade federal da bahia 1996;18:197–203.
[57] Griffin J, Bennett S. Nd:YAG laser photoablation of endometrial cysts: a review of 55 cases (2000–2001). In: Proceedings of the 48th Conference of the American Association of Equine Practitioners, Orlando, FL. 2002:58–60.
[58] Schiemann V, Bartmann C. Transendoscopic synechiolysis of extensive intrauterine adhesions by repeated operative hysteroscopy in a mare—a case report. Pferdeheilkunde 2003;19:661–5.
[59] Schiemann V, Bartmann C, Kirpal G, et al. Diagnostic hysteroscopy in the mare—uterine contamination and endometrial reaction. Pferdeheilkunde 2001;17:557–64.
[60] Ousey JC, Houghton E, Grainger L, et al. Progestogen profiles during the last trimester of gestation in Thoroughbred mares with normal or compromised pregnancies. Theriogenology 2005;63:1844–56.
[61] Daels PF, Besognet B, Hansen B, et al. Effect of progesterone on prostaglandin F2 alpha secretion and outcome of pregnancy during cloprostenol-induced abortion in mares. Am J Vet Res 1996;57:1331–7.
[62] Riddle W. Preparation of the mare for normal parturition. In: Proceedings of the 49th Conference of the American Association of Equine Practitioners, New Orleans, LA. 2003:1–5.
[63] Hill DJ, Petrik J, Arany E. Growth factors and the regulation of fetal growth. Diabetes Care 1998;21(Suppl 2):B60–9.
[64] Page NM, Kemp CF, Butlin DJ, et al. Placental peptides as markers of gestational disease. Reproduction 2002;123:487–95.
[65] Lindqvist P, Grennert L, Marsal K. Epidermal growth factor in maternal urine—a predictor of intrauterine growth restriction? Early Hum Dev 1999;56:143–50.
[66] Henson MC, Castracane VD. Leptin in pregnancy. Biol Reprod 2000;63:1219–28.
[67] Varvarigou A, Mantzoros CS, Beratis NG. Cord blood leptin concentrations in relation to intrauterine growth. Clin Endocrinol (Oxf) 1999;50:177–83.
[68] Lepercq J, Challier JC, Guerre-Millo M, et al. Prenatal leptin production: evidence that fetal adipose tissue produces leptin. J Clin Endocrinol Metab 2001;86:2409–13.

[69] Rizzo G, Capponi A, Vlachopoulou A, et al. Ultrasonographic assessment of the uterine cervix and interleukin-8 concentrations in cervical secretions predict intrauterine infection in patients with preterm labor and intact membranes. Ultrasound Obstet Gynecol 1998;12: 86–92.
[70] Traub-Dargatz JL, Salman MD, Voss JL. Medical problems of adult horses, as ranked by equine practitioners. J Am Vet Med Assoc 1991;198:1745–7.
[71] Lewis GS. Steroidal regulation of uterine immune defenses. Anim Reprod Sci 2004;82–83:281–94.
[72] Simpson DJ, Eaton-Evans WE. Sites of CEM infection [letter]. Vet Rec 1978;102:488.
[73] Katz JB, Evans LE, Hutto DL, et al. Clinical, bacteriologic, serologic, and pathologic features of infections with atypical Taylorella equigenitalis in mares. J Am Vet Med Assoc 2000;216:1945–8.
[74] Premanandh J, George LV, Wernery U, et al. Evaluation of a newly developed real-time PCR for the detection of Taylorella equigenitalis and discrimination from T. asinigenitalis. Vet Microbiol 2003;95:229–37.
[75] Platt H, Atherton JG, Orskov I. Klebsiella and Enterobacter organisms isolated from horses. J Hyg (Lond) 1976;77:401–8.
[76] Troedsson MH, Scott MA, Liu IK. Comparative treatment of mares susceptible to chronic uterine infection. Am J Vet Res 1995;56:468–72.
[77] Rozeboom KJ, Troedsson MH, Shurson GC, et al. Late estrus or metestrus insemination after estrual inseminations decreases farrowing rate and litter size in swine. J Anim Sci 1997; 75:2323–7.
[78] Fowler JE Jr, Stamey TA. Studies of introital colonization in women with recurrent urinary infections. VII. The role of bacterial adherence. J Urol 1977;117:472–6.
[79] LeBlanc M. The equine endometrium and the pathophysiology of endometritis. In: Proceedings of the Reproductive Pathology Symposium, Montreal, Quebec, Canada. 1997:78–84.
[80] Allen WR. Proceedings of the John P. Hughes International Workshop on Equine Endometritis. Equine Vet J 1993;25:184–93.
[81] Anzai T, Kamada M, Kanemaru T, et al. Isolation of methicillin-resistant Staphylococcus aureus (MRSA) from mares with metritis and its zooepidemiology. J Equine Sci 1996;7: 7–11.
[82] Sheoran AS, Nally JE, Donahue JM, et al. Antibody isotypes in sera of equine fetuses aborted due to Leptospira interrogans serovar pomona-type kennewicki infection. Vet Immunol Immunopathol 2000;77:301–9.
[83] Donahue JM, Williams NM, Sells SF, et al. Crossiella equi sp. nov., isolated from equine placentas. Int J Syst Evol Microbiol 2002;52:2169–73.
[84] Labeda DP, Donahue JM, Williams NM, et al. Amycolatopsis kentuckyensis sp. nov., Amycolatopsis lexingtonensis sp. nov. and Amycolatopsis pretoriensis sp. nov., isolated from equine placentas. Int J Syst Evol Microbiol 2003;53:1601–5.
[85] Giles RC, Donahue JM, Hong CB, et al. Causes of abortion, stillbirth, and perinatal death in horses: 3,527 cases (1986–1991). J Am Vet Med Assoc 1993;203:1170–5.
[86] Patterson-Kane JC, Donahue JM, Harrison LR. Placentitis, fetal pneumonia, and abortion due to Rhodococcus equi infection in a Thoroughbred. J Vet Diagn Invest 2002;14:157–9.
[87] Smith KC, Blunden AS, Whitwell KE, et al. A survey of equine abortion, stillbirth and neonatal death in the UK from 1988 to 1997. Equine Vet J 2003;35:496–501.
[88] Kydd JH, Wattrang E, Hannant D. Pre-infection frequencies of equine herpesvirus-1 specific, cytotoxic T lymphocytes correlate with protection against abortion following experimental infection of pregnant mares. Vet Immunol Immunopathol 2003;96:207–17.
[89] Pitel PH, Romand S, Pronost S, et al. Investigation of Neospora sp. antibodies in aborted mares from Normandy, France. Vet Parasitol 2003;118:1–6.
[90] Eckert LO, Thwin SS, Hillier SL, et al. The antimicrobial treatment of subacute endometritis: a proof of concept study. Am J Obstet Gynecol 2004;190:305–13.

[91] Prescott JF. Beta-lactam antibiotics: penam penicillins. In: Prescott JF, Baggot JD, Walker R, editors. Antimicrobial therapy in veterinary medicine. Ames (IA): Iowa State University Press; 2000. p. 105–33.
[92] Love CC, Strzemienski PJ, Kenney RM. Endometrial concentrations of ampicillin in mares after intrauterine infusion of the drug. Am J Vet Res 1990;51:197–9.
[93] Mather EC, Refsal KR, Gustafsson BK, et al. The use of fiber-optic techniques in clinical diagnosis and visual assessment of experimental intrauterine therapy in mares. J Reprod Fertil Suppl 1979;2:293–7.
[94] LeBlanc M, Asbury AC, Rathwell A, et al. The effect of intrauterine infusion of ticarcillin disodium one hour post-coitus in reproductively normal mares. Equine Pract 1989;11:33–8.
[95] Fuller P, Asbury AC. In vitro effects of various antibiotics on phagocytosis by equine neutrophils: applications to intrauterine therapy in mares. In: Proceedings of the 32nd Conference of the American Association of Equine Practitioners, Nashville, TN. 2003:257–67.
[96] Spensley MS, Baggot JD, Wilson WD, et al. Pharmacokinetics and endometrial tissue concentrations of ticarcillin given to the horse by intravenous and intrauterine routes. Am J Vet Res 1986;47:2587–90.
[97] Van Camp SD, Papich MG, Whitacre MD. Administration of ticarcillin in combination with clavulanic acid intravenously and intrauterinely to clinically normal oestrous mares. J Vet Pharmacol Ther 2000;23:373–8.
[98] Prescott JF. Beta-lactam antibiotics: cephalosporins and cephamycins. In: Prescott JF, Baggot JD, Walker R, editors. Antimicrobial therapy in veterinary medicine. Ames (IA): Iowa State University Press; 2000. p. 134–59.
[99] Brown MP, Gronwall RR, Houston AE. Pharmacokinetics and body fluid and endometrial concentrations of cephapirin in mares. Am J Vet Res 1986;47:784–8.
[100] Juzwiak JS, Brown MP, Gronwall R, et al. Effect of probenecid administration on cephapirin pharmacokinetics and concentrations in mares. Am J Vet Res 1989;50:1742–7.
[101] Brown MP, Gronwall RR, Houston AE. Pharmacokinetics and body fluid and endometrial concentrations of cefoxitin in mares. Am J Vet Res 1986;47:1734–8.
[102] Ricketts SW. Treatment of equine endometritis with intrauterine irrigations of ceftiofur sodium: a comparison with mares treated in a similar manner with a mixture of sodium benzylpenicillin, neomycin sulphate, polymyxin B sulphate and furaltadone hydrochloride. Pferdeheilkunde 1997;13:486–9.
[103] Cervantes CC, Brown MP, Gronwall R, et al. Pharmacokinetics and concentrations of ceftiofur sodium in body fluids and endometrium after repeated intramuscular injections in mares. Am J Vet Res 1993;54:573–5.
[104] Prescott JF. Aminoglycosides and aminocyclitols. In: Prescott JF, Baggot JD, Walker R, editors. Antimicrobial therapy in veterinary medicine. Ames (IA): Iowa State University Press; 2000. p. 191–228.
[105] Houdeshell JW, Hennessey PW. Gentamicin in the treatment of equine metritis. Vet Med Small Anim Clin 1972;67:1348–52.
[106] Blue M, Oriol J. Conception in mares following intrauterine therapy with amikacin. J Equine Vet Sci 1982;2:200–2.
[107] Eilts BE, McCoy DJ, Taylor H, et al. Effect of repeated intrauterine infusions of gentamicin on the equine endometrium. Theriogenology 1988;29:1253–9.
[108] Al Bagdadi FK, Eilts BE, Richardson GF. Scanning electron microscopy of the endometrium of mares infused with gentamicin. Microsc Microanal 2004;10:280–5.
[109] Ocal H, Yuksel M, Ayar A. Effects of gentamicin sulfate on the contractility of myometrium isolated from non-pregnant cows. Anim Reprod Sci 2004;84:269–77.
[110] Paradelis AG. Aminoglycoside antibiotics and inhibition of uterine contractility. J Antimicrob Chemother 1982;9:328–9.
[111] Orsini JA, Park MI, Spencer PA. Tissue and serum concentrations of amikacin after intramuscular and intrauterine administration to mares in estrus. Can Vet J 1996;37:157–60.

[112] Caudle A, Purswell BJ, Williams D, et al. Endometrial levels of amikacin in the mare after intrauterine infusion of amikacin sulfate. Theriogenology 1983;19:433–9.
[113] Fumuso E, Checura C, Losinno L, et al. Endometrial tissue concentrations of enrofloxacin after intrauterine administration to mares. Vet Res Commun 2002;26:371–80.
[114] Papich MG, Van Camp SD, Cole JA, et al. Pharmacokinetics and endometrial tissue concentrations of enrofloxacin and the metabolite ciprofloxacin after i.v. administration of enrofloxacin to mares. J Vet Pharmacol Ther 2002;25:343–50.
[115] Haines GR, Brown MP, Gronwall RR, et al. Pharmacokinetics of orbifloxacin and its concentration in body fluids and in endometrial tissues of mares. Can J Vet Res 2001;65:181–7.
[116] Asbury AC, Lyle SK. Infectious causes of infertility. In: McKinnon AO, Voss JL, editors. Equine reproduction. Baltimore (MD): Williams & Wilkins; 1993. p. 381–91.
[117] Bryant JE, Brown MP, Gronwall RR, et al. Study of intragastric administration of doxycycline: pharmacokinetics including body fluid, endometrial and minimum inhibitory concentrations. Equine Vet J 2000;32:233–8.
[118] Prescott JF. Sulfonamides, diaminopyrimidines, and their combinations. In: Prescott JF, Baggot JD, Walker R, editors. Antimicrobial therapy in veterinary medicine. Ames (IA): Iowa State University Press; 2000. p. 290–314.
[119] Brown MP, Gronwall R, Castro L. Pharmacokinetics and body fluid and endometrial concentrations of trimethoprim-sulfamethoxazole in mares. Am J Vet Res 1988;49:918–22.
[120] Ricketts SW, Mackintosh ME. Role of anaerobic bacteria in equine endometritis. J Reprod Fertil Suppl 1987;35:343–51.
[121] Specht TE, Brown MP, Gronwall RR, et al. Pharmacokinetics of metronidazole and its concentration in body fluids and endometrial tissues of mares. Am J Vet Res 1992;53:1807–12.
[122] Pitt C, Sanchez-Ramos L, Kaunitz AM. Adjunctive intravaginal metronidazole for the prevention of postcesarean endometritis: a randomized controlled trial. Obstet Gynecol 2001;98:745–50.
[123] Farca AM, Nebbia P, Robino P, et al. Effects of the combination antibiotic-EDTA-Tris in the treatment of chronic bovine endometritis caused by antimicrobial-resistant bacteria. Pharmacol Res 1997;36:35–9.
[124] Dascanio J, Schweizer C, Ley WB. Equine fungal endometritis. Equine Vet Educ 2001;13:324–9.
[125] Frazer GS, Rossol TJ, Threlfall WR, et al. Histopathologic effects of dimethyl sulfoxide on equine endometrium. Am J Vet Res 1988;49:1774–81.
[126] Pascoe DR, Stabenfeldt GH, Hughes JP, et al. Endogenous prostaglandin F2 alpha release induced by physiologic saline solution infusion in utero in the mare: effect of temperature, osmolarity, and pH. Am J Vet Res 1989;50:1080–3.
[127] Ley WB. Current thoughts on the diagnosis and treatment of acute endometritis in mares. Veterinary Medicine 1989;89:648–60.
[128] Troedsson M. Diseases of the uterus. In: Robinson N, editor. Current therapy in equine medicine 4. Philadelphia: WB Saunders; 1997. p. 517–24.
[129] Prescott JF. Antifungal chemotherapy. In: Prescott JF, Baggot JD, Walker R, editors. Antimicrobial therapy in veterinary medicine. Ames (IA): Iowa State University Press; 2000. p. 367–95.
[130] Hess MB, Parker NA, Purswell BJ, et al. Use of lufenuron as a treatment for fungal endometritis in four mares. J Am Vet Med Assoc 2002;221:266–7.
[131] Ahmad M, Ahmad N, Mansoor M, et al. Synergistic effect of antibiotics and oxytocin in the treatment of endometritis in mares. Pakistan Veterinary Journal 2001;21:202–5.
[132] Hirsbrunner G, Knutti B, Kupfer U, et al. Effect of prostaglandin E2, DL-cloprostenol, and prostaglandin E2 in combination with D-cloprostenol on uterine motility during diestrus in experimental cows. Anim Reprod Sci 2003;79:17–32.
[133] Kelly RW, King AE, Critchley HO. Cytokine control in human endometrium. Reproduction 2001;121:3–19.

[134] Seals RC, Wulster-Radcliffe MC, Lewis GS. Uterine response to infectious bacteria in estrous cyclic ewes. Am J Reprod Immunol 2003;49:269–78.
[135] Chan WW, Chen KY, Liu H, et al. Acupuncture for general veterinary practice. J Vet Med Sci 2001;63:1057–62.
[136] Kim J, Shin KH, Na CS. Effect of acupuncture treatment on uterine motility and cyclooxygenase-2 expression in pregnant rats. Gynecol Obstet Invest 2000;50:225–30.
[137] Sadowsky DW, Novy MJ, Witkin SS, et al. Dexamethasone or interleukin-10 blocks interleukin-1beta-induced uterine contractions in pregnant rhesus monkeys. Am J Obstet Gynecol 2003;188:252–63.
[138] Adams GP, Ginther OJ. Efficacy of intrauterine infusion of plasma for treatment of infertility and endometritis in mares. J Am Vet Med Assoc 1989;194:372–8.
[139] Colbern G, Voss JL, Squires EL, et al. Intrauterine equine plasma as an endometritis therapy: use of an endometritis model to evaluate efficacy. J Equine Vet Sci 1987;7:66–8.
[140] Ricketts SW, Alonso S. Assessment of the breeding prognosis of mares using paired endometrial biopsy techniques. Equine Vet J 1991;23:185–8.
[141] Olsen LM, Al Bagdadi FK, Richardson GF, et al. A histological study of the effect of saline and povidone-iodine infusions on the equine endometrium. Theriogenology 1992;37:1311–25.
[142] Waelchli RO, Corboz L, Winder NC. Effect of intrauterine plasma infusion in the mare: histological, bacteriological and cytological findings. Theriogenology 1987;28:861–9.
[143] Threlfall W. Accurate diagnosis and appropriate therapy of uterine disease. In: Proceedings of the Mare Reproduction Symposium, Kansas City, MO. 1996:51–69.
[144] Ley WB, Bowen JM, Sponenberg DP, et al. Dimethyl sulfoxide intrauterine therapy in the mare: effects upon endometrial histological features and biopsy classification. Theriogenology 1989;32:263–76.
[145] Bennett DG, Poland HJ, Kaneps AJ, et al. Histologic effect of infusion solutions on the equine endometrium. Equine Pract 1981;3:37–42.
[146] Allen WE, Clarke AR. Absorption of sodium benzylpenicillin from the equine uterus after local Lugol's iodine treatment, compared with absorption after intramuscular injection. Equine Vet J 1978;10:174–5.
[147] Jackson PS, Allen WR, Ricketts SW, et al. The irritancy of chlorhexidine gluconate in the genital tract of the mare. Vet Rec 1979;105:122–4.
[148] Wilson DG, Cooley AJ, MacWilliams PS, et al. Effects of 0.05% chlorhexidine lavage on the tarsocrural joints of horses. Vet Surg 1994;23:442–7.
[149] Ricketts SW. Endometrial curettage in the mare. Equine Vet J 1985;17:324–8.
[150] Ricketts SW, Barrelet A. The ability of mares to respond to treatment for uterine abnormalities diagnosed by endometrial biopsy and some causes for failure to respond—a review of 1099 cases. Pferdeheilkunde 2001;17:644–9.
[151] March CM. Intrauterine adhesions. Obstet Gynecol Clin North Am 1995;22:491–505.
[152] Macpherson ML. Treatment strategies for mares with placentitis. Theriogenology 2005;64:528–34.
[153] Sertich PL, Vaala WE. Concentrations of antibiotics in mares, foals and fetal fluids after antibiotic administration in late pregnancy. In: Proceedings of the 38th Conference of the American Association of Equine Practitioners, Orlando, FL. 1992:727–36.
[154] Murchie T, Macpherson ML, LeBlanc M, et al. A microdialysis model to detect drugs in the allantoic fluid of pregnant pony mares. In: Proceedings of the 49th Conference of the American Association of Equine Practitioners, New Orleans, LA. 2003:118–21.
[155] Lauterbach R, Zembala M. Pentoxifylline reduces plasma tumour necrosis factor-alpha concentration in premature infants with sepsis. Eur J Pediatr 1996;155:404–9.
[156] Lauterbach R, Pawlik D, Zembala M, et al. Pentoxifylline in and prevention and treatment of chronic lung disease. Acta Paediatr Suppl 2004;93:20–2.

[157] Sadowsky DW, Haluska GJ, Gravett MG, et al. Indomethacin blocks interleukin 1beta-induced myometrial contractions in pregnant rhesus monkeys. Am J Obstet Gynecol 2000;183:173–80.
[158] Shideler RK, Squires EL, Voss JL, et al. Progestogen therapy of ovariectomized pregnant mares. J Reprod Fertil Suppl 1982;32:459–64.
[159] McKinnon AO, Lescun TB, Walker JH, et al. The inability of some synthetic progestogens to maintain pregnancy in the mare. Equine Vet J 2000;32:83–5.
[160] McGlothlin JA, Lester GD, Hansen PJ, et al. Alteration in uterine contractility in mares with experimentally induced placentitis. Reproduction 2004;127:57–66.
[161] Card C, Wood M. Effects of acute administration of clenbuterol on uterine tone and equine fetal and maternal heart rates. In: Biology of reproduction monograph 1. Caxambu, Brazil; 1995. p. 7–11.
[162] Purvis K, Christiansen E. The impact of infection on sperm quality. Hum Reprod 1996;11: 31–41.
[163] Cooper W. Methods of determining the site of bacterial infections in the stallion reproduction tract. In: Proceedings of the Annual Meeting of the Society for Theriogenology, Mobile, AL. 1979:1–4.
[164] Klug E, Deegen E, Liesk R, et al. The effect of vesiculectomy on seminal characteristics in the stallion. J Reprod Fertil Suppl 1979;27:61–6.
[165] Sojka JE, Carter G. Hemospermia and seminal vesicle enlargement in a stallion. Compend Contin Educ Pract Vet 1985;7(Suppl):S587–8.
[166] Blanchard TL, Varner DD, Hurtgen JP, et al. Bilateral seminal vesiculitis and ampullitis in a stallion. J Am Vet Med Assoc 1988;192:525–6.
[167] Blanchard TL, Woods JA, Brinsko SP, et al. Theriogenology question of the month. Treatment options for erosive seminal vesiculitis caused by Acinetobacter calcoaceticus. J Am Vet Med Assoc 2002;221:793–5.
[168] Malmgren L, Olsson EE, Engvall A, et al. Aerobic bacterial flora of semen and stallion reproductive tract and its relation to fertility under field conditions. Acta Vet Scand 1998;39: 173–82.
[169] Bowen JM, Tobin N, Simpson RB, et al. Effects of washing on the bacterial flora of the stallion's penis. J Reprod Fertil Suppl 1982;32:41–5.
[170] Varner DD, Blanchard TL, Brinsko SP, et al. Techniques for evaluating selected reproductive disorders of stallions. Anim Reprod Sci 2000;60–61:493–509.
[171] Pozor MA, McDonnell SM. Ultrasonographic measurements of accessory sex glands, ampullae, and urethra of normal stallions of various size types. Theriogenology 2002;58: 1425–33.
[172] Freestone JF, Paccamonti DL, Eilts BE, et al. Seminal vesiculitis as a cause of signs of colic in a stallion. J Am Vet Med Assoc 1993;203:556–7.
[173] Anderson DJ, Hill JA. Cell-mediated immunity in infertility. Am J Reprod Immunol Microbiol 1988;17:22–30.
[174] Huleihel M, Lunenfeld E, Levy A, et al. Distinct expression levels of cytokines and soluble cytokine receptors in seminal plasma of fertile and infertile men. Fertil Steril 1996;66:135–9.
[175] Huleihel M, Levy A, Lunenfeld E, et al. Distinct expression of cytokines and mitogenic inhibitory factors in semen of fertile and infertile men. Am J Reprod Immunol 1997;37:304–9.
[176] Witkin SS, Toth A. Relationship between genital tract infections, sperm antibodies in seminal fluid, and infertility. Fertil Steril 1983;40:805–8.
[177] Storey BT. Biochemistry of the induction and prevention of lipoperoxidative damage in human spermatozoa. Mol Hum Reprod 1997;3:203–13.
[178] Paradisi R, Mancini R, Bellavia E, et al. T-helper 2 type cytokine and soluble interleukin-2 receptor levels in seminal plasma of infertile men. Am J Reprod Immunol 1997;38: 94–9.
[179] Swerczek TW. Contagious equine metritis—outbreak of the disease in Kentucky and laboratory methods for diagnosing the disease. J Reprod Fertil Suppl 1979;27:361–5.

[180] Powell D. Contagious equine metritis. In: Morrow DA, editor. Current therapy in theriogenology. Philadelphia: WB Saunders; 1986. p. 786–92.
[181] Schluter H, Kuller H, Friedrich U, et al. Epizootiology and treatment of contagious equine metritis (CEM) with particular reference to treatment of infected stallions. Prakt Tierarzt 1991;72:503–11.
[182] Bleumink-Pluym NM, Werdler ME, Houwers DJ, et al. Development and evaluation of PCR test for detection of Taylorella equigenitalis. J Clin Microbiol 1994;32:893–6.
[183] Kristula MA, Smith BI. Diagnosis and treatment of four stallions, carriers of the contagious metritis organism—case report. Theriogenology 2004;61:595–601.
[184] Kenney R, Cummings M, Zierdt C, et al. Pseudomonas aeruginosa—somatic typing of genital tract isolates and colonization of the stallion penis: significance, diagnosis and treatment. In: Proceedings of the 38th Conference of the American Association of Equine Practitioners, Orlando, FL. 1992:601–8.
[185] Stamey TA, Bushby SR, Bragonje J. The concentration of trimethoprim in prostatic fluid: nonionic diffusion or active transport? J Infect Dis 1973;128:686–92.
[186] Pichini S, Zuccaro P, Pacifici R. Drugs in semen. Clin Pharmacokinet 1994;26:356–73.
[187] Pickett BW, Amann R, McKinnon AO. Management of the stallion for maximum reproductive efficiency: II. Animal reproduction laboratory general series bulletin [1005], 1. Fort Collins (CO): Colorado State University; 1989.
[188] Varner DD, Scanlan CM, Thompson JA, et al. Bacteriology of preserved stallion semen and antibiotics in semen extenders. Theriogenology 1998;50:559–73.
[189] Hargreaves CA, Rogers S, Hills F, et al. Effects of co-trimoxazole, erythromycin, amoxicillin, tetracycline and chloroquine on sperm function in vitro. Hum Reprod 1998;13:1878–86.
[190] Crotty KL, May R, Kulvicki A, et al. The effect of antimicrobial therapy on testicular aspirate flow cytometry. J Urol 1995;153:835–8.

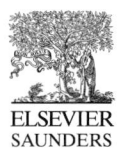

Meningitis and Encephalomyelitis in Horses

Alessandra Pellegrini-Masini, DMV, PhD[a],*, Leanda C. Livesey, BVM&S, MRCVS[b]

[a]*Equine Section, Department of Clinical Sciences, College of Veterinary Medicine, Auburn University, Auburn, AL 36849, USA*
[b]*J.T. Vaughan Teaching Hospital, College of Veterinary Medicine, 1500 Wire Road, Auburn University, Auburn, AL 36849, USA*

Neurologic diseases represent an important cost for the equine industry; even mild deficits may result in loss of use of athletic horses, whereas severe clinical signs may not only be critical for the horse but may expose owners and care providers to significant risks. Early diagnosis may increase the likelihood of a positive outcome (eg, bacterial meningitis) and be the key to prevention of large-scale outbreaks (eg, equine herpesvirus myeloencephalitis [EHM]). Some diseases are difficult to diagnose or to rule out (eg, equine protozoal myeloencephalitis [EPM]), with the consequence of time and cost wasted in unnecessary treatments. This article does not purport to be a review of meningitis and encephalomyelitis in horses; rather, it provides an overview of diagnostic tests, treatment developments, and preventative measures reported in the equine and human medical literature of the past few years.

Meningitis

Meningitis may arise from a disseminated bacterial infection of the meninges and subarachnoid space (SAS; bacterial meningitis), or it may reflect inflammation secondary to a primary infection localized within the nervous tissue (eg, brain abscess). Because of the closed-space localization of the infection and the proximity to the control centers of the central nervous system (CNS), bacterial meningitis carries a high risk of fatality [1,2]. The condition has been reported as a complication of septicemia in as many as 8% to 10% of septic foals [2–6]. Predisposing factors in foals

---

* Corresponding author.
E-mail address: pelleal@auburn.edu (A. Pellegrini-Masini).

include failure of adequate passive transfer of humoral immunity [2,4] and increased permeability of the blood-brain barrier in the neonate [2]. The pathogens most frequently isolated from septic foals with bacterial meningitis were gram-negative enteric bacteria [6–8], *Streptococcus* spp, and *Staphylococcus aureus* [8].

Infectious meningitis is considered to be a rare occurrence in adult horses. A retrospective study of horses with neurologic diseases presented over a period of 12 years to a referral hospital identified fungal and bacterial meningitis in 2 and 3 of 450 horses, respectively [7]. The pathogens isolated from adult horses with meningitis include *Cryptococcus neoformans* [9–11], *Streptococcus equi* subsp *equi* [7,12–15], *Streptococcus equi* subsp *zooepidemicus* [12,16,17], *Streptococcus suis* [18], *Actinomyces* spp [19], *Klebsiella pneumoniae* [12,20], *Escherichia coli* [7,15], *Actinobacillus equuli* [12], and *Pasteurella caballi* [12]. Reported routes of CNS infection of adult horses include hematogenous dissemination [7,19,20], direct contamination secondary to skull fractures [7,15], or extension from an adjacent site of infection (eg, paranasal sinuses, periorbital tissues, retropharyngeal lymph nodes, guttural pouch) [12,21]. Meningitis secondary to brain abscess has been reported in horses [14,15,19,21]. Pituitary abscesses are highly represented [19,21,22], possibly because the pituitary gland (as well as the median eminence, preoptic recess, pineal gland, and endothelium of the choroid plexus) lacks a complete blood-brain barrier and the capillaries have discontinuous tight junctions, plasmalemmal vesicles, and fenestrations resembling the characteristics of the systemic vasculature [23]. In some cases, the cause of meningitis remains unknown [24,25].

Diagnosis

Historical and physical examination findings, in association with laboratory and diagnostic test results, contribute to reaching a diagnosis of meningitis.

History and physical examination

The history of horses affected by meningitis may include a previous diagnosis of an infectious disease involving the head (particularly strangles) [12,14,15], nasal discharge [19,21,24], lameness [9,25], fever of unknown origin [21], or trauma [15].

Systemic clinical signs are common and consist of lethargy, fever, anorexia, and generalized weakness. Other abnormalities on physical examination include weight loss [10,25], cervical pain or stiffness and reluctance to flex the neck [10,21,25], an erratic breathing pattern [21], epistaxis [15,19,21], exophthalmus [19,21], enophthalmos and third eyelid protrusion [16], nasal discharge [12,19,21], and muscle fasciculations [10,21,25]. A wide range of neurologic signs have been described. Most commonly, affected horses display ataxia that ranges in severity [9–12,14–17,19,21,24,25]. The mental status of the horse may be altered, and excitement [11,14,24], disorientation [21], and aggressive behavior [21] have been reported. Unwillingness to walk forward [21] or backward [10], leaning toward one side [15], compulsive circling [15,21,24], and a head tilt [10,15,16,24] may indicate the presence of a localized lesion. Head pressing was reported in one horse [21]. Some horses have hyperesthesia [9,24,25], and others may be hypoesthetic [24]. During examination of the cranial nerves, blindness [10,14,15,17,19,21,24], strabismus [3,16], anisocoria [3], facial nerve paralysis [15–17,21,24], dysphagia [12], and nystagmus [3,21] were observed. Opisthotonus and seizures can be observed in adult horses [15,20,21,25] and even more commonly in neonatal foals [3,6,16]. Gluteal muscle atrophy [9,10] and signs consistent with cauda equina syndrome [9–11] were reported in horses affected by cryptococcal meningitis.

Hematology and blood culture

Early diagnosis and avoidance of delays in initiating antimicrobial treatment are of primary importance in the management of meningitis, and some authors advocate the use of an algorithmic approach [1,26]. In the presence of clinical signs suggesting meningitis, a blood sample should be collected immediately after stabilization of the patient for hematology and chemistry as well as for bacterial blood culture [1,27]. Mature neutrophilia (with or without a left shift) and hyperfibrinogenemia are the most common clinicopathologic abnormalities in horses with infectious meningitis [12,19,21,24]. Some horses only have neutrophilia [10,14,18] or hyperfibrinogenemia [21,24,25], or only hyperglobulinemia [15,24]. The results of the hemogram may also be normal [24,25]. Hypoglobulinemia and lymphopenia were observed in three horses with bacterial meningitis and immunodeficiency [25]; in the presence of these findings, further workup to evaluate immune function (including lymphocyte flow cytometry and immunoglobulin levels) may be warranted.

Forty percent to 60% of human patients with bacterial meningitis have a positive blood culture [23,28]; blood cultures may be positive even though cerebrospinal fluid (CSF) cultures are negative [23,26,28]. Because of the low number of blood cultures submitted for horses with bacterial meningitis (only 4 of 24 reviewed cases), it is difficult to comment on the utility of this test for the diagnosis of meningitis in the horse. Three of the four cultures were negative, and the only positive one [16] yielded an isolate different from the one recovered from the brain during postmortem examination. Blood culture may be particularly useful in foals, where bacterial meningitis is typically a complication of bacteremia.

Cerebrospinal fluid analysis

CSF cytology and culture should subsequently be performed for all horses suspected of having meningitis. Cytology and evaluation of total protein and glucose concentrations are routinely performed for human patients suspected of having meningitis, even though these values are poorly correlated with prognosis [1]. Most human patients exhibit a neutrophilic pleocytosis; in the presence of a normal nucleated cell count, the differential examination may show a high percentage of neutrophils [1,26,29]. Human patients with bacterial meninigitis may have a lymphocytic predominance in 10% of the early cases [29], however, and there are reports of normal CSF values in human patients with bacterial meningitis [30,31]. Neutrophilic pleocytosis and an increased protein concentration compared with normal are the most common findings in horses with infectious meningitis. Among the reviewed cases, two horses had a normal cell count but increased neutrophils compared with normal on the differential examination [12,15]. One horse had an initial lymphocytic pleocytosis that became neutrophilic on a subsequent CSF sample [25]. A foal had an initially normal CSF sample (collected by lumbosacral puncture), followed by a markedly abnormal sample 48 hours later (collected from the cisterna magna) [3]. Hypoglycorrhachia (defined as a CSF glucose concentration less than or equal to 50% of the serum glucose concentration) is a common finding in human patients with meningitis [26]. The usefulness of this test is unknown in horses. The CSF glucose concentration has been observed to be higher in newborn foals compared with adult horses (mean $\pm$ 1 standard deviation [SD]: 98.8 ± 12.0 mg/dL and 51.1 ± 2.5 mg/dL, respectively) [32]. If the clinical suspicion for bacterial meningitis is high, CSF sampling can be performed after the administration of the first dose of antimicrobials, because no changes in the ability to culture bacteria were observed for 1 to 2 hours after initiation of antimicrobial treatment [28,33]. CSF culture yields bacterial growth in a high percentage of human beings affected by bacterial meningitis [23,26], although it is frequently negative in horses [24,25]. In human medicine, to increase the chances of obtaining a causative diagnosis, a polymerase chain reaction (PCR) assay of CSF samples is frequently performed to test for the most common pathogens of infectious meningitis. This test is available for some of the common pathogens affecting horses (including *S equi* subsp *equi*, *Rhodococcus equi*, and *Salmonella* spp). Because of the relative frequency of *S equi* subsp *equi* infection in horses with meningitis and brain abscesses, an *S equi* PCR assay of a CSF sample may be helpful in evaluating a horse with a history of strangles, nasal discharge, and clinical and laboratory findings suggestive of meningitis. A CSF fluid PCR assay could also be performed in a neonatal foal with meningitis, when *Salmonella* spp bacteremia or enterocolitis is suspected.

In human patients with meningitis, there is a risk of high intracranial pressure (ICP) compared with normal, and performing a lumbar puncture may involve a risk of severe complications, such as cerebral herniation through the foramen magnum. For this reason, the sequence of diagnostic tests is somewhat controversial in human medicine [1,26,27], and cranial CT should be performed before lumbar puncture in human patients presenting with papilledema or focal neurologic signs [27,33]. This complication is rare in horses; however, cranial CT was successfully used to diagnose brain abscesses [14,15,22] and is recommended in horses with altered consciousness, focal neurologic deficits, and papilledema as well as historical, clinical, and laboratory findings indicating meningitis.

Management

Antimicrobial treatment

Antimicrobial drugs for the treatment of people [34] and horses [35,36] with bacterial meningitis have been reviewed recently. Only a brief overview is provided here, with a particular focus on antimicrobial-induced release of proinflammatory mediators and recent therapeutic guidelines suggested for people.

Factors affecting the effectiveness of antimicrobial drugs for the treatment of bacterial meningitis include the ability of the drug to penetrate into the CSF and nervous tissue, the activity in a purulent environment, and the pharmacodynamic relation between the CSF concentration of drugs and bactericidal activity [34].

The ability to penetrate the blood-CSF barrier is affected by the lipid or water solubility of the antimicrobial. Because of the presence of tight junctions, the transcellular pathway allows rapid diffusion of lipophilic drugs, such as fluoroquinolones, chloramphenicol, and rifampin. The paracellular pathway determines the delayed and poor penetration of hydrophilic drugs, such as β-lactams, through the intact barrier [34]. Fluoroquinolones and rifampin are also characterized by a low molecular weight, which enhances penetration [34,36]. Highly protein-bound agents (eg, ceftriaxone, a third-generation cephalosporin) have diminished CSF penetration [34], because only the free fraction is available for barrier crossing. β-lactams (and possibly aminoglycosides and fluoroquinolones) are pumped against a concentration gradient from the CSF into the serum by an active transport system operating in the choroid plexus, but meningeal inflammation impairs this mechanism and allows higher CSF concentrations [34,35].

The purulent environment of the CSF in bacterial meningitis may affect the penetration and activity of antimicrobials. The acidic CSF environment enhances the pH gradient between plasma and CSF and allows ion trapping of weak bases, such as aminoglycosides, macrolides, chloramphenicol, and trimethoprim [35,36]. In the absence of elevated CSF drug concentrations, however, the high ionization reduces drug activity; a poor clinical response to aminoglycosides and clarithromycin was observed in animal models of bacterial meningitis [33,34]. The high protein concentration in inflamed CSF may decrease the active fraction of highly protein-bound antimicrobials (eg, cephalosporins) after they cross the blood-CSF barrier [34]. Fever and high density of a bacterial population may decrease the rate of bacterial growth in the purulent CSF, affecting the efficiency of antimicrobials like β-lactams, which require active bacterial cell division for optimal bactericidal activity [33,34]. Some antimicrobial drugs are also metabolized in the CSF to compounds with decreased (eg, cephalothin) or increased (eg, cefotaxime) antibacterial activity [34] compared with the precursor parent compound.

Because early phagocytosis relies on complement-mediated opsonization, the negligible concentration of specific antibody and complement in the spinal fluid accounts for inefficient phagocytic activity in the initial phase of meningeal infection [37,38]. For this reason, the use of bactericidal rather than bacteriostatic antimicrobial agents has been recommended in the treatment of bacterial meningitis [33]. The concept of bactericidal or bacteriostatic activity of a specific drug is always related to a particular organism or strain against which the drug has been tested in vitro [39], however, and each antimicrobial drug may have different pathogen killing rates at different concentrations [37]. It has been suggested that high concentrations of an antimicrobial (up to 10 to 30 times the minimal bactericidal concentration against the organism in vitro) are required for optimal bactericidal activity in the CSF [33]. Experimental models of *Streptococcus pneumoniae* meningitis in laboratory animals have been used to demonstrate a significant correlation between CSF antimicrobial concentration and bacterial killing rate [33,37,40]. The dose choice is further complicated by the fact that bacterial killing may be affected by the "paradoxic effect": when the concentration of the drug is increased above an optimal threshold, the killing rate decreases [39]. The paradoxic effect has been described for penicillin, rifampin, and fluoroquinolones. For fluoroquinolones, higher drug concentrations paradoxically inhibit RNA and protein synthesis, thereby reducing the bactericidal activity [39].

Antimicrobial agents with good CNS penetration include fluoroquinolones, some third-generation cephalosporins, potentiated sulfonamides, doxycycline, chloramphenicol, rifampin, metronidazole, and macrolides [34,35,38]. Because of poor CSF penetration and the requirement of a log (growth) phase for optimal killing, penicillins are not considered drugs of choice for treatment of bacterial meningitis. Nevertheless, they have proven effectiveness against susceptible meningeal pathogens, because high systemic doses may achieve CSF concentrations well above the minimum inhibitory concentration (MIC) of sensitive isolates [34,41]. In the presence of antimicrobial resistance, newer β-lactams have been evaluated. Of the carbapenems, imipenem has been associated with a high incidence of seizure in children affected by meningitis, and its use is not recommended to treat children with bacterial meningitis [34]. Third-generation cephalosporins are drugs of choice for human patients for the treatment of meningitis, especially when the causative agent is a gram-negative bacterium [34,41]. Among this class of drugs, the pharmacokinetics of cefpodoxime, cefotaxime, ceftiofur, and ceftriaxone have been determined in adult horses [42–44] and neonatal foals [42,43,45–47]. Ceftriaxone was able to penetrate the CSF in horses [42], and cefotaxime has been successfully used to treat bacterial meningitis in a foal [3]. Ceftiofur was not detected in the CSF of healthy mares after repeated intramuscular injections at a dose of 2 mg/kg of body weight [44]. Because the CSF penetration of ceftiofur is poor [35], it is not recommended for treatment of horses with meningitis. Cefepime, a fourth-generation cephalosporin, was shown in experimental studies to have adequate CSF penetration and an in vivo bacterial killing rate superior to that of ceftriaxone [34]. Pharmacokinetic studies in horses revealed adequate serum concentrations after intravenous and intramuscular administration of cefepime but not after oral administration of cefepime [48]. The mode of administration may affect antibacterial activity; bolus dosing results in high peak concentrations but may not maintain drug levels above the minimum bactericidal concentration for a prolonged period versus continuous rate infusion, which produces lower peak but constant adequate concentrations [34]. The mode of administration may be particularly important for β-lactam antimicrobials, which have a time-dependent mechanism of action [34]. An experimental model of bacterial meningitis in rabbits demonstrated that maximal bacterial killing rates were only achieved when the CSF concentration of ceftriaxone was above the minimal bactericidal concentration for 95% to 100% of the dosing interval [34]. Treatment of meningitis using third-generation cephalosporins may be cost-prohibitive in adult horses but may be economically feasible in foals.

Chloramphenicol, because of its good penetration of the CNS (CSF and brain tissue concentrations reported as 0.5 and 9 times the plasma concentration, respectively) [36], may achieve bactericidal concentrations at high doses for most gram-positive meningeal pathogens [49]. Chloramphenicol is only bacteriostatic against enteric gram-negative bacilli, *S aureus*, and penicillin-resistant gram-positive bacteria, however [35,37]. A recent meta-analysis of 18 studies on the treatment of acute bacterial meningitis in human patients recommended that chloramphenicol should never be used alone because of its limited spectrum of action against bacteria causing meningeal infection. A combination of ampicillin and chloramphenicol, however, represents a broad-spectrum alternative to the more expensive third-generation cephalosporins [41]. Antagonism of action in the combination of chloramphenicol with penicillin, gentamicin, or fluoroquinolones has been reported [34–36]. Because of human health-related risks connected with handling of chloramphenicol, the utilization of this drug in equine medicine should be restricted and it should be used with caution.

Other bacteriostatic antibacterial agents that penetrate CSF efficiently and have been used successfully to treat gram-positive bacterial meningitis include tetracycline and potentiated sulfonamides [39]. Antagonism has been observed with the combination of ampicillin and oxytetracycline [36].

Intraventricular gentamicin administration has been proposed for treatment of human and equine neonates with enteric gram-negative meningitis [36]. A technique to access the cerebral ventricles in horses was described [50]; however, recent studies in infants have shown an increased risk of mortality with this technique compared with intravenous therapy alone [51].

Intrathecal administration of aminoglycosides did not yield adequate drug concentrations over the brain and ventricular system, and it may lead to arachnoiditis [38].

Antimicrobial treatment may lead to neuronal injury by causing bacterial lysis and the release of toxic bacterial products, particularly cell wall components. Lipopolysaccharides from gram-negative bacteria as well as teichoic acid, lipoteichoic acid, and peptidoglycan from gram-positive bacteria contribute to different extents to the propagation of the inflammatory cascade in the neuronal tissue. These bacterial products induce impairment of the barrier function of the vascular endothelium, stimulate synthesis of proinflammatory cytokines (particularly tumor necrosis factor-α [TNFα], interleukin [IL]-1β, and IL-6), upregulate expression of intercellular adhesion molecule (ICAM)-1 and nitric oxide synthesis, and promote release of matrix-metalloproteinase (MMP)-2 in cerebral endothelial cells [52–54]. Antimicrobial agents inducing cell wall lyses (β-lactams) may promote the liberation of proinflammatory bacterial cell wall components to a greater extent than agents inhibiting RNA or protein synthesis or DNA replication (eg, rifampin, macrolides, quinolones) [54]. A lower mortality rate and reduction of neuronal injury were observed in laboratory animals treated with these antimicrobials compared with β-lactams [53]. When the β-lactams are used against gram-negative bacteria, inhibition of bacterial penicillin-binding protein (PBP) 1A and 1B leads to bacterial cell lysis, inhibition of bacterial PBP-2 leads to cell wall–deficient round bacterial cells, and inhibition of PBP-3 leads to filament formation in bacteria. Filament formation leads to marked endotoxin release after cell lysis. When a PBP-3–specific agent (eg, ceftazidime) was compared with a PBP-2–specific agent (eg, imipenem), an increased amount of endotoxin was liberated [54]. When compared with ceftriaxone in a mouse model of pneumococcal meningitis, rifampin caused the release of less teichoic and lipoteichoic acid, which resulted in a lower mortality rate [34]. The use of rifampin as monotherapy is not indicated because of the high rate of bacterial resistance to this antimicrobial; however, treatment with rifampin before the administration of a third-generation cephalosporin has been recommended to reduce neuronal inflammation [34,54]. Despite their mechanism of action as protein synthesis inhibitors, aminoglycosides may also alter gram-negative cell surface lipids by interacting with anionic polysaccharides and may induce bacterial lysis, causing release of proinflammatory bacterial products [54]. Chloramphenicol induces the release of a lower amount of endotoxin compared with β-lactams in the early phase of treatment of gram-negative bacterial meningitis [54], possibly because of the lack of bactericidal activity of chloramphenicol against gram-negative meningeal pathogens.

Antimicrobials may affect the inflammatory cascade by a direct immunomodulatory effect. Immunosuppression and inhibition of T-cell activity was observed with rifampin therapy, and it was attributed to the binding of the drug to a glucocorticoid receptor [54]. In vitro, erythromycin and other macrolides inhibited cytokine (TNFα and IL-6) production [54].

Anti-inflammatory treatment
Dexamethasone. A logical step in the management of meningitis is the control of inflammation. The use of corticosteroids has been implemented and extensively discussed for this condition during the past 50 years. Corticosteroids exert their anti-inflammatory effects at different stages of the inflammatory cascade: they inhibit the expression of proinflammatory cytokine mRNA, the synthesis of arachidonic acid derivatives, and complement activation as well as the activity of inducible nitric oxide synthase. Thus, corticosteroids limit vasodilation, prevent increased endothelial permeability, and provide protection from the cytotoxic effects of neutrophil-mediated release of reactive oxygen species [55–57]. Dexamethasone is the corticosteroid of choice in the treatment of meningitis. Animal trials have demonstrated superior efficacy of this drug compared with methylprednisolone in the modulation of the inflammatory cascade in patients with meningitis [55].

Because of insufficient clinical and experimental studies on the use of corticosteroids for treatment of meningitis in the horse, it is not possible to formulate recommendations concerning their use. Dexamethasone was administered during the treatment of brain abscess in two horses [15], and its use was recommended for the management of cerebral edema [35,36].

By stabilizing the blood-CSF barrier (and thereby limiting the increase in permeability that accompanies meningitis), corticosteroids may actually impair the penetration of antimicrobial agents into the SAS [55]. In experimental animal models of meningitis, the percentage of CSF penetration of ampicillin, cefotaxime, and cefuroxime was not affected by treatment with dexamethasone; however, vancomycin entry into the SAS was reduced compared with untreated animals [55,58].

Innumerable experimental trials, clinical studies, and meta-analyses have evaluated the usefulness of dexamethasone treatment in bacterial meningitis. Evidence of beneficial effects in the management of *Haemophilus influenzae* in children was initially observed, but whether an improved outcome could be expected in the presence of different pathogens or in adult patients remains questionable [54,55]. The most recent information indicates that dexamethasone administration may improve the outcome in adults [57–60] and children with meningitis [56,60,61]. The use of corticosteroids should be avoided in infants younger than 6 weeks of age as well as in immunosuppressed patients, however [56,62]. The beneficial effect of treatment with corticosteroids is dependent on the pathogen. Improved clinical outcome and decreased markers of inflammation were observed when dexamethasone was used in human patients with meningitis caused by gram-positive bacteria [63,64], whereas a detrimental effect was reported when dexamethasone was administered to patients with gram-negative bacillary meningitis [56,57]. The recommended protocol for human patients (0.15 mg/kg administered every 6 hours) is based on the administration of dexamethasone before or at the same time as the first dose of antimicrobial drug so as to prevent the inflammatory events related to the release of toxic bacterial products secondary to bacteriolysis [56]. The administration of corticosteroids is not recommended if the patient has already received parenteral antimicrobials [57]. The recommended length of treatment with corticosteroids in human patients is 4 days [57].

Miscellaneous. Based on the physiopathology of neuronal injury, a number of adjunct anti-inflammatory treatments are currently undergoing experimental studies; however, the efficacy of these agents has not yet been proven in clinical trials. Experimental tests of MMP inhibitors, endothelin inhibitors, excitatory amino acid antagonists, antioxidants, and IL-1 inhibitors have so far produced encouraging results.

An inhibitor of MMPs and TNFα-converting enzyme decreased collagen degradation and showed neuroprotective effects in a neonatal rat model of meningitis [53,65]. A different MMP inhibitor administered intraperitoneally in rats with bacterial meningitis actually prevented brain damage [66]. Improved cerebral blood flow and the neuroprotective effect of the systemically administered endothelin inhibitor, bosentan (Tracleer; Actelion Pharmaceuticals, San Francisco, California), was noticed in laboratory animals [67]. High concentrations of glutamate were observed in the CSF of animal species and human patients during the course of meningitis; high concentrations of excitatory amino acids may induce membrane depolarization, Ca^{2+} influx, and energy failure [53]. Investigations of the glutamate antagonist kynurenic acid revealed a moderate neuroprotective effect [53]. Experimental studies on antioxidants, such as uric acid, N-acetyl-L-cysteine, tirilazad, and mannitol (possible hydroxyl radical scavenger), have so far yielded positive results, showing the beneficial effects of these agents in meningitis-associated cerebral ischemia, blood-CSF barrier permeability, and CSF pleocytosis [52,53,68]. Finally, systemic administration of IL-10 (especially when combined with dexamethasone) has produced encouraging results in animal models of bacterial meningitis [68]. IL-10 inhibits IL-1, IL-6, and TNFα production; enhances the synthesis of IL-1 receptor antagonist; decreases the release of reactive oxygen and nitrogen species; and downregulates leukocyte migration [68].

Conversely, contrasting results have emerged from experiments evaluating nitric oxide synthase inhibitors, leukocyte migration inhibitors, and pentoxifylline [68]. Inhibition of leukocyte migration into the SAS by antibodies against the CD18 epitope reduced neuronal damage in rabbits with meningitis [53]; however, the prevention of CSF leukocyte accumulation by the leukocyte blocker fucoidin increased the risk of bacteremia and fatal outcome in rats with experimental pneumococcal meningitis, suggesting that neutrophil blockage impairs the host's ability to control systemic infection [69]. Systemic pentoxifylline only showed mild anti-inflammatory effects and failed to reduce brain damage in a model of *E coli* meningitis in newborn pigs [70].

Treatment of high intracranial pressure

The occurrence of increased ICP compared with normal has not been documented in horses with meningitis; however, clinical signs suggestive of this condition (eg, altered mentation, papilledema, seizures) have been described [10,13–15,17,19–21,24,25]. Conversely, high ICP has been well described in human patients with meningitis [1] and is inversely associated with survival [71]. Three important pathogeneses of cerebral edema have been recognized in patients with meningitis: (1) vasogenic edema secondary to increased permeability of the blood-brain and blood-CSF barriers; (2) interstitial edema attributable to increased CSF outflow resistance, and (3) cytotoxic edema resulting from vasculitis and neuronal ischemia [53,56].

CSF pressure measurement in adult horses was performed in anesthetized and sedated standing horses by means of a 17-gauge subarachnoid catheter placed at the lumbosacral junction and connected by a heparinized line to a calibrated pressure transducer [72,73]. Under general anesthesia, CSF pressure measured at the lumbosacral space was closely correlated with pressure measured by lateral ventricle catheterization [72]. In healthy standing horses with the head aligned level with the thoracolumbar spine, the mean baseline lumbosacral CSF pressure was 23.7 mm Hg. Lumbosacral CSF pressure was not significantly affected by sedation with xylazine at a dose of 1.1 mg/kg; however, head positioning markedly changed the pressure recorded, and the authors recommended supporting the head at or above the thoracolumbar spine in horses at risk of high ICP [73]. In human patients, long-term ICP measurement devices are used to monitor the efficacy of therapy aimed at ICP reduction [71]. In equine medicine, lumbosacral catheterization maintained for 48 hours produced significant CSF pleocytosis (9360 ± 3878 white blood cells/µL), although there were no clinical signs or culture results suggestive of bacterial contamination [74].

Mannitol and dexamethasone are drugs commonly used to control ICP in human [75,76] and equine patients [35]. The use of dimethyl sulfoxide (DMSO) has also been advocated for equine patients for treatment of cerebral edema [35]. Alternative approaches used in human patients include an ICP-targeted therapy (the Lund concept based on the use of antihypertensive therapy) [77] and the administration of acetazolamide for chronically elevated ICP in fungal (*Cryptococcus neoformans* and *Coccidioides immitis*) meningitis [78].

Equine protozoal myeloencephalitis

EPM is a neurologic disease, first described 30 years ago, affecting horses on the North and South American continents. The parasite most commonly associated with the disease is *Sarcocystis neurona*; however, cases attributed to *Neospora hughesi* have also been reported [79]. Comprehensive reviews about EPM have been published recently [79,80], and the following discussion focuses on recent developments in EPM testing.

Antemortem diagnosis of EPM is difficult to establish, because there is diffuse exposure to the parasite among much of the horse population. A consensus statement published in 2002 by the American College of Veterinary Internal Medicine about the clinical diagnosis of EPM confirmed the diagnostic value of a positive result on immunoblot testing of an uncontaminated CSF sample (<50 red blood cells/μL) in a horse displaying neurologic signs suggestive of EPM (typically segmental, asymmetric, or multifocal) [81].

Recent studies, however, have raised doubts concerning the diagnostic utility of CSF testing [82–84]. The sensitivity and specificity of immunoblot testing of serum and CSF were evaluated in a postmortem study of 234 horses, including subjects with and without neurologic signs [82]. Although the study results reinforced the sensitivity of immunoblot testing, they indicated poor specificity (44%) of the CSF Western blot test in horses with neurologic abnormalities [82]. A weakness of the study was that, for the analysis, horses were classified as positive if lesions suggestive of *S neurona* infection were detected on histopathologic examination of the CNS. Because of the multifocal nature of the pathologic findings and the impracticality of examining the whole CNS, however, EPM may be difficult to diagnose even on postmortem examination. A cutoff of 100 red blood cells/mL was used in the definition of an uncontaminated CSF sample, and this degree of contamination may yield false-positive results [81,85].

The significance of a positive CSF immunoblot is questionable because of the presence of specific antibodies against *S neurona* in the serum. There is evidence that CSF antibody titers can be influenced by serum antibody titers. In healthy animals, CSF proteins are derived from the blood and are mainly composed of albumin, whereas globulin levels are negligible [86]. During CNS diseases, however, intrathecal production of immunoglobulin takes place. Intramuscular vaccination of healthy horses with ovalbumin induced rapid antibody production and measurable serum titers; positive CSF titers (markedly lower compared with the serum) were concurrently measured [83]. A high correlation was observed between serum and CSF titers [83]. The result of this experiment suggests that passive movement of antibodies across the blood-CSF barrier takes place and that CSF titers may be influenced by serum titers [83]. A similar result was demonstrated in a study evaluating serum and CSF Western blot results in horses after vaccination against *S neurona*: 77% of the horses that were negative on CSF immunoblot testing before vaccination were subsequently positive [84]. The horses in this study were potentially exposed to natural infection during the course of the experiment, however, and the criterion defining CSF blood contamination was 200 red blood cells/mL [84]. In contrast, another recent study testing the agreement of Western blot test results on 181 paired serum and CSF samples of naturally infected horses indicated only a moderate agreement, with approximately one third of the seropositive horses yielding negative CSF samples [87].

Additional information for the joint interpretation of serum- and CSF-specific antibody titers may be provided by the results of quantitative antibody tests. These tests are not available for clinical use, but are currently used in experimental models and are being evaluated for their possible application in the clinical diagnosis of the disease. A direct agglutination test provided 100% sensitivity and 90% specificity in a mouse model of experimental infection with *S neurona* [88]. Cross-reactions were not observed in mice fed sporocysts of different *Sarcocystis* spp. An indirect immunofluorescent antibody test (IFAT) was compared with the Western blot test for the diagnosis of EPM using serologic screening of 48 horses [89]. The horses were diagnosed, based on postmortem findings, as EPM-positive (histologic lesions compatible with EPM and positive immunostaining for *S neurona*) or EPM-negative (remaining horses) [89]. The overall accuracy of the IFAT was better than that of the Western blot test [89]. When the IFAT was evaluated in paired serum and CSF samples of naturally and experimentally infected horses as well as vaccinated horses, the test proved accurate and reliable [90]. Cross-reactivity with other Apicomplexan parasites, however, is a concern with the IFAT [91]. False-positive IFAT results were obtained after experimental administration of sporocysts of *Sarcocystis fayeri* to ponies testing negative for EPM on Western blot analysis [91]. When horses experimentally infected with *N hughesi* were tested with an *S neurona* IFAT, there was no cross-reactivity [90]. The study that evaluated the accuracy of the IFAT in naturally and experimentally infected horses as well as vaccinated horses reported an overall incidence of false-positive IFAT results of only 3%, suggesting that confounding factors attributable to cross-reactivity are minimal [90].

ELISAs for detection of *S neurona* surface antigens (SnSAGs) also have been evaluated [92]. The ELISA for detection of recombinant SnSAG2 showed a high sensitivity and specificity when compared with a Western blot test of serum samples, and cross-reactivity with *S fayeri* or *N hughesi* was not observed [92].

Although indexes that are not antigen specific (eg, albumin quotient, IgG index) have little diagnostic value and their use in EPM diagnosis is not recommended [81], the availability of quantitative serologic tests would allow the use of titer-specific ratios. The likelihood ratios (the likelihood that a certain serum titer is associated with a horse with EPM compared with the likelihood that the same serum titer is associated with a horse without EPM) or antigen-specific CSF-to-serum ratios, such as the C-value, which compares the antigen-specific antibody titer with the total IgG in CSF and serum, or the antibody index (Ab_{index}), which compares the antigen-specific antibody titer with the albumin in CSF and serum, may provide helpful information in the joint interpretation of CSF and serum tests [83,90].

Interpretation of a positive EPM immunoblot assay has been evaluated recently in foals [93,94]. Passive transfer of antibodies against *S neurona* with colostrum has been demonstrated by Western blot seroconversion in post-versus presuckle serum of foals born to seropositive mares [93]. All the foals became seronegative again by the age of 9 months, with a mean seroconversion time of 4.2 months [93]. A positive Western blot test result was also obtained from the CSF of neonatal foals born to seropositive mares up to 3 months after birth, indicating that CSF testing is not a suitable aid in the diagnosis of clinical disease in foals of this age [94]. A suspected case of EPM in a 2-month-old colt was recently reported [95]; the clinical signs were first noticed when the foal was 2 days of age, and in utero infection was hypothesized by the authors. Transplacental transmission of *S neurona* has never been documented in the equine species, however, and a study performed on 366 mares and their offspring (including aborted fetuses) did not support the possibility of in utero infection [96]. Presuckle serum IFAT titers were negative in all the foals, and no histologic evidence of the parasite was observed in aborted fetuses that were examined [96]. A large-scale study, including 484 horses in California whose serum was tested for *S neurona* using the IFAT, showed a low exposure in horses younger than 2.5 years of age and an increase in the prevalence of seropositivity with increasing age [96,97].

Recently, a vaccine constituted by killed merozoites (Fort Dodge Animal Health, Fort Dodge, Iowa) was introduced under a conditional US Department of Agriculture (USDA) license. When seronegative horses were vaccinated, a positive Western blot test result was observed 14 days after the booster vaccination in 89% of the horses [84]. No difference in Western blot testing was observed between vaccinated horses and a group of horses testing positive after natural exposure, indicating that a history of EPM vaccination may represent a confounding factor in diagnosing the clinical disease [84]. In a different study performed using the IFAT, the highest titers after EPM vaccination were observed between 14 and 28 days after the booster vaccination; however, by 112 days, the titers for all the vaccinated horses had decreased to values comparable to those of noninfected horses [90]. In addition to humoral immunity, stimulation of cellular immunity was demonstrated after administration of EPM vaccine [98]. Mononuclear cell proliferation in response to *S neurona* was demonstrated in vitro, and skin reactivity after intradermal inoculation of *S neurona* antigen in vaccinated horses was demonstrated in vivo [98]. Clinical performance of the vaccine and efficacy in disease prevention are currently being evaluated.

The drugs currently available for EPM treatment include folate-inhibiting drugs, triazines, and nitazoxanide, and they have been reviewed previously [79]. A recent study evaluated the efficacy of daily administration of pyrantel tartrate as a preventive agent against EPM based on promising results of in vitro studies [99]. The effectiveness of the drug was tested in vivo in 24 unexposed horses [99]; however, the administration of pyrantel tartrate at the labeled dose did not prevent infection after experimental challenge with *S neurona*.

Equine herpesvirus myeloencephalitis

Abortion caused by equine herpesvirus-1 (EHV-1) is recognized worldwide. Until recently, myeloencephalitis caused by the virus (EHM) was less often recognized. In the past few years, the neurologic form was more commonly documented, with reports of devastating outbreaks of EHV-1 in herds, on breeding farms, and on racetracks, with unusually high numbers of horses exhibiting the neurologic form of the disease. Recent reports suggest the emergence of an epidemiologic picture that resembles the well-known "abortion storms" caused by EHV-1 [100–104]; the possibility that there is an emerging hypervirulent form of EHV-1 evolving toward neuropathogenicity is a cause of concern. Outbreaks of the neurologic form highlight the fact that EHM is contagious; hence, barrier approaches to EHM cases, similar to those used in aborting mares, should help to reduce attack rates during outbreaks. Although EHV-1 and EHV-4 are able to induce the neurologic form of the disease, EHV-1 is much more commonly implicated [105–107].

Different outcomes of infections caused by EHV-1 and EHV-4 isolates were associated with varying cell tropisms in foals, and infection of vascular endothelial cells was a feature of high-virulence EHV-1 isolates. EHV-1 is more endotheliotropic than EHV-4, and the cell-associated viremia that characterizes EHV-1 infections permits systemic spread of the virus to additional sites of replication, including the endothelium of blood vessels in the endometrium and the CNS [108].

A recent comparative genomic study performed by scientists from the Maxwell Gluck Research Center in the United States and from the Animal Health Trust in the United Kingdom sequenced DNA on several key genes of the herpesvirus from 48 outbreaks of EHV-1 neurologic disease and 82 outbreaks of EHV-1 abortion without accompanying neurologic involvement [11,109]. A single-point mutation was identified, which was uniquely present in 83% of the neurologic cases and uniquely absent in 95% of EHV-1 abortion outbreaks [11,109]. The identified mutation was located in the catalytic subunit of the gene encoding the DNA polymerase, with the strategic positioning of this location providing evidence that the neuropathogenic EHV-1 virus may have enhanced replicative aggressiveness [11,109]. This finding was supported by studies in which foals inoculated with the paralytic strain of EHV-1 demonstrated a fivefold increase in magnitude and increased duration of leukocyte-associated viremia when compared with foals inoculated with abortigenic strains of EHV-1 [110].

Disease caused by EHV-1 and EHV-4 was reviewed recently [101]; hence, this discussion is confined to advances in diagnosis, treatment, and epidemiology as they pertain to control of a disease outbreak and immunoprophylaxis.

Diagnosis

History and clinical signs

A presumptive diagnosis of EHM often may be made on the basis of the typical clinical signs [101,111], especially if there is an epidemic and antecedent or concurrent respiratory tract disease. Ruling out differential diagnoses is helpful in supporting the diagnosis [101]. Establishment of an early definitive diagnosis is extremely important in managing an outbreak of EHV-1.

Cerebrospinal fluid analysis

CSF fluid from horses with EHM has a high total protein concentration, with little or no change in nucleated cell count compared with normal. Dissociation between albumin concentration and cytology, in conjunction with characteristic clinical signs, strongly supports the diagnosis of EHM; however, the magnitude of abnormalities in the CSF does not seem to correlate with clinical signs or prognosis [111,112]. The CSF frequently has a yellow discoloration (xanthochromia) associated with red blood cell breakdown. Cytologic evaluation of the CSF reveals primarily mononuclear cells [111,112]. A positive CSF antibody titer is of no value for diagnosis because it most likely reflects disruption of the blood-brain barrier as a result of vasculitis. Isolation of virus from the CSF is rare [101] in concordance with the pathophysiology of the disease, in which CNS damage is the result of hypoxic damage rather than direct neurologic insult by the virus. Damage to the blood-brain barrier as a result of vasculitis may allow circulating antibodies to *S neurona* to enter the CSF, which may lead to an incorrect diagnosis of EPM.

Serology

Retrospective serodiagnosis of EHV-1 infection can be accomplished by demonstrating a three- to fourfold increase in anti-EHV-1 neutralizing antibody or complement fixation titers between acute and convalescent phase serum samples taken 7 to 21 days apart; however, this delay in definitive diagnosis is a serious disadvantage in the early stages of an outbreak.

Serologic evidence for recent infection with EHV-1 can be obtained by examining a single serum sample by complement fixation [113] or by a recombinant glycoprotein G ELISA [114]; however, the results of these tests are not conclusive [115]. Measuring anti-EHV-1 neutralizing antibody titers in a single serum sample in the acute stages of the disease is not recommended, because the virus-neutralizing antibody titers increase more slowly than those of complement fixation and the recombinant glycoprotein G ELISA.

The confusion that arose previously because of the cross-reactivity of EHV-1 and EHV-4 antibodies in the complement fixation and virus-neutralizing antibody tests has been eliminated by the development of ELISAs that can differentiate between antibodies of the two viruses.

Type-specific epitopes located near the C-terminal of the glycoprotein gG of EHV-1 and EHV-4 have been described [114], and an ELISA has been developed in which the recombinant protein gG was used as antigen [114]. The ELISA can distinguish between the type-specific antibodies against EHV-1 and EHV-4 elicited by EHV infection [114]. A modified version of this ELISA was found to be useful for seroepizootiology and diagnosis, at first in unvaccinated horse populations [116] and later in vaccinated horse populations [117]. The ability to distinguish between antibodies elicited by vaccination and those elicited by infection is an added advantage of ELISA techniques over the complement fixation test. This ability is useful for serodiagnosis of EHV infection in the vaccinated horse population and for evaluation of the efficacy of EHV vaccination in the field. In summary, the use of ELISA techniques is a suitable alternative to the virus neutralization antibody test for screening large numbers of field sera and enables confirmatory EHV-1 serodiagnosis [118].

Detection of antigen

A definitive antemortem diagnosis of EHV-1 infection is achieved by laboratory isolation of the virus from samples of nasopharyngeal exudate collected on a Dacron-tipped swab or from the buffy coat of a blood sample. Given that EHV-1 was shown to be latent in leukocytes [119], the detection of EHV-1 nucleic acid in the buffy coat is not in itself of value in diagnosing an acute infection or recrudescence of an infection. Of greater significance is the identification of EHV-1 in nasal swabs of clinically affected mares and foals, combined with the increase in EHV-1–specific antibody titers compared with normal titers. Virus isolation is a time-consuming procedure, taking up to 4 weeks [120]; however, it is still important, because this is the only way to secure the isolate for further comparative analysis [121]. The diagnostic use of viral isolation has largely been superseded by the development of PCR techniques, which have increased the speed at which the viral antigen can be identified (same-day diagnosis) and, as such, may be used for rapid screening and detection of EHV-1 and EHV-4 isolates and clinical samples. Samples of nasopharyngeal exudate or whole blood are required for PCR analysis. Nasopharyngeal samples are preferred, because latency is established in the CD5 and CD8 leukocytes; hence, blood samples from animals with a latent infection may produce false-positive results [122–125]. Some PCR techniques are quantitative as well as qualitative and are of particular use in experimental work assessing the viral kinetics of EHV-1 and EHV-4 [126,127]. Recently, a PCR assay that permits quantification of the EHV-1 genome has been developed, allowing differentiation between latency and infection from blood samples [128]. The differentiation is based on copy number and on the assumption that there is probably more virus present in a lytic infection than in a latent infection [128].

The recent identification of a disease-conferring single-point mutation for the neuropathic form of EHV-1 [109] has provided a genetic marker that has allowed the development of a molecular diagnostic technique for antemortem detection of mutant EHV-1 DNA present in tissue biopsies from the submandibular lymph nodes of latently infected carrier horses, using sequence-capture nested PCR (nPCR) techniques [129]. The amplified polymorphic region of the latent EHV-1 DNA undergoes subsequent DNA sequencing [109,129]. Biopsy collection was performed on anesthetized horses [130] but could be performed on adequately sedated standing horses. Comparison of the sequence-capture nPCR technique in this study with conventional nPCR and real-time PCR techniques showed it to have a much higher sensitivity for detection of the EHV-1 virus [129]. The presence of EHV-1 virus was not detected in the peripheral blood mononuclear cells of carrier horses in this study; hence, utilization of this technique on the buffy coat of blood samples collected from suspected carriers would not be useful [129].

Postmortem diagnosis

Histologic evaluation of nervous tissue shows classic vasculitis changes with ischemic damage to contiguous nervous tissue [131]. Immunohistochemical studies may be used to detect the presence of EHV-1 antigen, but results may be equivocal, with the antigen only rarely being detected in CNS endothelial cells from field cases (ie, false-negative results are common) [104,132]. This may be because EHV-1 may be complexed with antibody if there is an immunologic component of the disease. The positive detection of EHV-1 antigen may be dependent on the stage of the disease and on the temporal class of viral protein recognized by the antibody.

Failure to isolate EHV-1 in cell culture from CNS tissues is typical of EHV-1 myeloencephalopathy [133] and is attributed to high levels of circulating neutralizing antibodies; however, high levels of circulating antibody were not found to be present in a recent EHV-1 outbreak in which the virus could not be cultured from CNS tissues [104]. PCR techniques may be more sensitive for detection of viral antigen in tissues, but special preparation techniques may be required. In the outbreak described previously [104], the PCR assay did not detect viral antigen in crude homogenates, but viral antigen was detected after phenol chloroform extraction of DNA from these homogenates; this occurred because the phenol chloroform step removes many impurities and inhibitors of Taq polymerase (a heat-stable DNA polymerase isolated from the bacterium *Thermus aquaticus* used in the PCR assay).

An ongoing study at the Livestock Disease Diagnostic Center of Kentucky University using PCR techniques based on the point mutation found in the neuropathotypic EHV-1 strains [109,129,130] involves testing submandibular lymph nodes collected from horses submitted for postmortem examination for the presence of the neuropathotypic strains of EHV-1 [109]. This is part of a new epidemiology initiative to provide real-time surveillance of the prevalence and distribution of neuropathotypic strains of EHV-1 as latent viral DNA in the Kentucky Thoroughbred population [109].

Management

Any horse with suspected EHV-1 infection should be isolated until the diagnosis is ruled out, because that animal may be contagious. The horse should be kept in an environment that minimizes injuries resulting from ataxia. A sling may be required to raise and support paralyzed horses. For horses with bladder paralysis, aseptic evacuation of the bladder may be required. Bladder evacuation can be performed using an indwelling Foley catheter with an extension to avoid perineal urine scalding. In stallions, the Foley catheter may be placed via a perineal incision. Prophylactic antimicrobials are useful for preventing urinary infections and infections of decubital ulcers in a recumbent horse [101]. The horse should be monitored to ensure adequate intake of food and water. The use of DMSO at a rate of 0.9 g/kg as a 10% solution once daily for 3 days and then once every other day for three to four additional treatments has been advocated on the basis of its free radical scavenging properties and, theoretically, may slow down propagation of membrane degeneration [101,111]. The efficacy of treatment with DMSO has not been evaluated scientifically.

Anti-inflammatory drugs, most notably corticosteroids (dexamethasone, 0.05–0.1 mg/kg, administered every 12 hours the first day and thereafter in diminishing doses and lengthening intervals depending on the response to treatment and the prednisolone dosing regimen), have been advocated in the treatment of EHM, purportedly for treatment of the supposed immune-mediated component of the disease process [101]. Administration of corticosteroids may be associated with some risk, because exogenous steroid administration has been shown to reactivate presumed latent infection in horses [134] and may increase the quantity and duration of virus shedding. Moreover, the viremia in the treated horse may be prolonged, which possibly means propagation of endothelial infection throughout the entire vasculature of the CNS [113]. Additionally, corticosteroid use in horses has been anecdotally associated with an increased risk of laminitis. Currently, however, corticosteroid therapy is routinely used to treat horses with EHM [101,111].

Acyclovir, an antiviral drug, has been advocated for treatment of EHV [135]. It is an acyclic nucleoside analogue that has high activity and selectivity for herpesviruses, particularly herpes simplex viruses types 1 and 2 and varicella zoster virus [136]. The drug is initially activated by phosphorylation by a herpesvirus-specified thymidine kinase [137]. This results in acyclovir monophosphate being converted to a triphosphate that is a more potent inhibitor of herpesvirus DNA polymerases than of cellular DNA polymerases [137]. The drug, no longer under patent and therefore potentially more affordable, is available in oral and intravenous preparations. If treatment is effective, the cost of the drug may be offset by lower mortality and fewer requirements for intensive management compared with untreated clinically affected horses [137]. Animal model studies have demonstrated that EHV-1 is sensitive to inhibition by acyclovir in vivo [138–140], and the drug is reported to inhibit replication of EHV-1 in vitro. It should be stressed, however, that there are no controlled studies reporting on the efficacy of acyclovir in the treatment or prevention of EHM.

There have been reports describing the use of acyclovir in the management of EHM [140,141]. Treatment of horses in these cases was empiric, because pharmacokinetic studies of acyclovir in horses had not been performed. In the recent outbreak of EHM in Findlay, Ohio, two dose rates of acyclovir and two dosing intervals were used prophylactically and therapeutically in managing the outbreak [142]. Horses were initially treated with 20 mg/kg administered orally at 8-hour intervals. Treatment was later changed to 10 mg/kg administered five times daily, which is the recommended human dose rate and administration interval [100]. Horses did develop EHM after acyclovir treatment was initiated, but neurologic signs seemed to be less severe [100]. There were no problems identified in any patient receiving acyclovir that were attributed to administration of the drug [100,142]. Preliminary data suggested that reasonable plasma levels are achievable and that multiple isolates of EHV-1 are sensitive to the drug, although sensitivity seems to vary with the isolate [142]. Recently, pharmacokinetic studies of acyclovir have been performed in horses [143,144]. These studies demonstrated poor bioavailability of orally administered acyclovir, even when administered at the higher dose rate of 20 mg/kg [143,144]. Poor oral bioavailability is a problem of acyclovir in all species. In human beings, there has been considerable research into developing prodrugs with a higher bioavailability that would make oral dosing a practical and successful option. The results of these investigations are not supportive of a therapeutic benefit when acyclovir is administered orally to adult horses at dosages as high as 20 mg/kg. It is therefore difficult to explain the reported beneficial effects of oral acyclovir administration in the outbreak in Findlay, Ohio. It has been suggested that multiple dosing may allow sufficient plasma accumulation because of the prolonged half-life of the drug [143]. Acyclovir was detected in the plasma of five horses with confirmed EHM treated with acyclovir at a dose of 10 mg/kg orally five times daily for 3 to 4 days before blood sampling [142]; however, the concentrations were significantly lower than the therapeutic dose range suggested by in vitro studies. Intravenous administration of an acyclovir infusion (10 mg/kg infused over 1 hour in crystalloid solution [1 L]) resulted in peak plasma concentrations of 13.7 ± 5.9 µg/mL [143]. Adverse effects were noted in one horse administered intravenous acyclovir, characterized by sweating, colic, and generalized muscle tremors [144]. Therefore, intravenous administration of the drug at a dose of 10 mg/kg would seem to result in a plasma concentration above the therapeutic range. Additional pharmacokinetic and safety studies are necessary to support the use of intravenously administered acyclovir in adult horses and foals. There are no reported serious complications associated with administration of acyclovir; however, monitoring of renal function is recommended.

Studies testing the efficacy of other nucleoside analogues have been performed. EHV-1 was sensitive to penciclovir, a compound related to acyclovir, when tested in tissue culture [145]. 9-[[2-Hydroxy-1-(hydroxymethyl)-ethoxy]methyl]guanine (BIOLF-62) showed high antiviral potency and low cell toxicity in tissue cultures and a mouse model [146]. These and other antiviral medications with improved oral bioavailability, such as valacyclovir, may become affordable for use in the horse in the future and may be more effective than acyclovir.

Prevention and control

The strategies for containing and managing an outbreak of EHV-1 have been reviewed recently [115]. The emphasis is on minimizing exposure of susceptible animals to the three main sources of virus: actively infected horses, placental membranes and fluids from an EHV-1 abortion, and recrudescence of infection in a latently infected carrier horse [115]. Preventative strategies include subdivision and maintenance of the herd into smaller, physically separated, and epidemiologically isolated subgroups. Horses should be subdivided into like groups if possible. Use of PCR and ELISA techniques helps with management of groupings. Stringent hygiene is essential, and disinfection of contaminated housing should be performed promptly using 1 part sodium hypochlorite to 10 parts water. Minimizing the risks of endogenous introduction of virus into each subgroup as well as into the herd as a whole can be achieved by the use of space barriers between paddocks and 21-day isolation of new or reintroduced horses. The likelihood of stress-induced reactivation of virus in latently infected horses should be reduced by avoiding overcrowding, transport, high parasite burdens, and poor nutrition. The new neuropathotype carrier identification procedure [109,129] described previously provides the option of an additional test and segregate approach for minimizing the risk of outbreaks of EHV-1 neurologic virus reactivation in carrier horses [109,130].

Routine vaccination should be practiced to maintain an effective level of immune protection against EHV throughout the whole herd. The aim of EHV vaccination is not individual protection against disease, which is not realistic with presently available vaccines, but the herd-wide goal of reduction in contact transmission.

Prevention of EHV-1 infection has been attempted by the use of vaccines, none of which are specifically labeled for use to prevent the neurologic form of the disease. After it was realized that EHV-1 and EHV-4 are distinct viruses, newer inactivated vaccines include both virus types [147]. Currently, there are at least 12 multivalent EHV-1 and EHV-4 multidose inactivated,

2 EHV-1 only multidose inactivated, and 2 multidose live EHV-1 vaccines marketed for parenteral use only [121]. Most manufacturers only claim protection against respiratory disease caused by EHV-1 and EHV-4. Frequent revaccination at 60- to 90-day intervals has been recommended to reduce viral shedding [101]. Although frequent vaccination does not prevent infection, it clearly reduces clinical symptoms, duration of virus shedding, and quantity of virus shed, and it significantly reduces the risk of abortions and outbreaks of respiratory disease caused by circulating field viruses [147].

Vaccination is controversial in the face of an outbreak of EHM. Killed vaccines take too long to generate immunity to be of any use in limiting disease spread. Vaccination has even been proposed by some to result in an increased risk of development of EHM [115]. The underlying concern is that the vasculitis is immune mediated; hence, vaccination may aggravate the situation by generating anti-EHV1 antibodies. There is no convincing evidence to support this, however. The efficacy of current-generation vaccines in reducing the losses from EHV-1 abortigenic disease is not mirrored in prevention of neurologic outbreaks, perhaps because the enhanced replicative vigor of the mutant neuropathotype EHV-1 strains allows them to overcome the level of immune responses induced by such vaccines [109]. Prevention of additional cases once an outbreak has been established and identified as caused by EHV-1 has been attempted by using corticosteroids and acyclovir [100], but the efficacy of this approach is questionable and may not be financially feasible in many cases.

Immunoprophylaxis against EHV-1 and EHV-4 infections has, until recently, been hampered by the difficulty in demonstrating protective immune responses after natural infection [148]. Prechallenge levels of circulating complement-fixing and virus-neutralizing antibodies do not correlate fully with protection [149]. A recent study has shown that preinfection frequencies of EHV-1–specific cytotoxic T lymphocytes correlate with protection against abortion after experimental infection of pregnant mares [150]. Cytotoxic T-lymphocyte precursor (CTLp) frequencies are the best correlate of protection identified so far, and thus may be useful as a marker in assessing protective response to vaccination and in the development of more effective vaccines.

Vaccine research trends

Much effort has gone into the development of live deletion mutant vaccines, mostly using EHV-1 strains, largely encouraged by successes with other alphavirus vaccines, such as bovine herpesvirus-1 [151] and pseudorabies virus [152]. Despite these efforts, no suitable live deletion mutant vaccine candidate for EHV-1 or EHV-4 has been identified so far [153–155]. A possible downside in the development of a live EHV-1 vaccine is reported in a recent study [156], which concluded that attenuated EHV-1 vaccines are likely to induce major histocompatibility complex class 1 downregulation and result in incomplete protection. It is not known whether this applies to all EHV-1 strains; however, the advantage conferred by a live virus (the ability to generate antigen-specific cytotoxic T lymphocytes) may outweigh these more subtle immunosuppressive effects of infection.

Glycoproteins play an important role in the biology of herpes viruses, particularly in the pathogenicity (virus adsorption, cell penetration, and cell-to-cell spread) and as immunologic targets by virtue of their expression on the surface of host infected cells [121,157]. The envelope glycoprotein D of EHV was found to evoke comparable neutralizing antibody responses in horses to those of a whole-virus vaccine, indicating that it may be a promising candidate for inclusion in subunit vaccines against EHV-1 [158].

Different routes of vaccine administration, such as the intranasal route, which elicits locally produced antibody or immune cells, may provide superior protection [159,160]. A clone of EHV-1 isolated after classic mutagenesis in vitro and having a temperature-sensitive and host range phenotype typically found in EHV-4 strains significantly protected pregnant mares from EHV-1 for up to 6 months against febrile respiratory disease, virus shedding in nasal mucus, and abortions after a single intranasal administration [159]. A live EHV-1 vaccine significantly cross-protected adult horses against EHV-4 [160] and also afforded virologic and clinical protection against EHV-1 to sucking foals with maternally derived neutralizing antibody [161]. Because sucking foals are now considered an important reservoir in the transmission of EHV-1 [162–164], it was suggested that sucking foals with maternal antibodies ought to be the target for immunoprophylaxis so as to eliminate or reduce EHV-1 in the field eventually [165]. This vaccine could therefore be useful in minimizing the reservoir of infection. Serologic evidence indicates that multidose inactivated vaccines are unlikely to be effective in protecting sucking foals with maternally derived antibodies; hence, the use of temperature-sensitive live intranasal vaccines may afford the best level of protection and might prevent establishment of viremia and consequent spread to the vascular endothelium of target organs [166,167].

The activation of cytotoxic T lymphocytes should be considered a cornerstone of successful vaccination. A multifactorial approach to the induction of immunity that involves mucosal antibodies, serum virus-neutralizing antibodies, and cytotoxic T lymphocytes should be used.

West Nile virus encephalitis

West Nile virus (WNV) belongs to the Japanese encephalitis virus complex, genus *Flavivirus*, family Flaviviridae [168]. The natural cycle of the virus includes birds as amplifying hosts because of their significant levels of viremia and ornithophilic mosquitos, especially but not limited to *Culex* spp, as transmitting vectors [168]. Mammalians, including the equine and human species, are considered dead-end hosts because they rarely reach the high levels of viremia required to infect mosquitoes [168,169].

Clinical signs described in horses include ataxia, weakness, muscle fasciculations, fever, abnormal mentation, hyperesthesia, facial nerve paralysis, dysphagia, and tongue paresis [168,170–174]. The mechanism of neuronal damage has not yet been clarified, and although the presence of neuronal apoptosis without associated inflammatory cells may indicate direct virus-induced cellular damage, an immune-mediated pathologic component has also been suggested based on inflammatory changes accompanied by scarce viral antigen [168]. Typical pathologic lesions consist of a nonsuppurative polioencephalomyelitis, and they are observed most commonly in the lower brain stem and ventral horns of the spinal cord rather than in the cerebral or cerebellar cortex [168].

Diagnosis

An antemortem diagnosis is mainly based on epidemiologic considerations (eg, geographic location; time of the year; presence of potential vectors in the area; previously reported cases in birds, horses, or people), evaluation of clinical signs, and serologic test results. The results of CSF analysis are abnormal in most affected horses. In a study of CSF analysis in 30 horses diagnosed with WNV based on the IgM antibody-capture (MAC) ELISA, 73% of the horses had abnormal results [175]. The cytologic findings are not pathognomonic for the disease, and the most common abnormalities consist of mononuclear pleocytosis with lymphocytic predominance [175]. In a limited number of cases (27% of 22 abnormal CSF samples), the only abnormality was a high protein concentration, whereas the nucleated cell count was within the normal reference range [175]. A significantly higher protein concentration was observed in samples collected from the lumbosacral space compared with the cisterna magna; this difference doubled that of normal healthy horses, and the authors suggested that it may be secondary to spinal cord inflammation caused by WNV [175].

Serologic tests are currently the most helpful tool in antemortem diagnosis of the disease. Detection of IgG by ELISA has been used in surveillance studies, based on the persistence of IgG in the bloodstream for up to 15 months after infection [168]. Vaccination also induces measurable IgG titers [172,176]. Recent infection is diagnosed based on a fourfold (or greater) increase in IgG titer on analysis of paired samples collected 14 days apart [168]. The plaque reduction virus neutralization test (PRNT) measures virus-neutralizing antibodies, and it is more specific for WNV than the IgG ELISA, which may cross-react with antibodies against other flaviviruses [168,169]. Although a single vaccination with killed WNV vaccine (Fort Dodge Laboratories, Fort Dodge, Iowa) does not consistently yield measurable PRNT titers [172], after a second vaccination, a substantial increase in neutralizing antibodies was observed, which lasted for 5 to 7 months [176].

IgM antibodies indicate acute exposure [168]. They appear in the bloodstream 6 to 7 days after infection and persist for less than 3 months

[168,169]. A positive result of the MAC-ELISA and a concomitantly positive single PRNT titer are considered confirmatory of a diagnosis of WNV [177]. If the clinical signs have been present for less than 21 days and the PRNT is negative, a positive MAC-ELISA in the presence of clinical signs suggestive of WNV encephalomyelitis is a strong diagnostic indicator if the presence of the virus has been documented in the area in a mosquito, bird, horse, or human being [177].

In people, intrathecal production of IgM antibodies against WNV takes place during WNV encephalitis, and in approximately 30% of the patients, IgM is present in the CSF earlier than in the serum [178]. The diagnostic value of measuring CSF IgM was evaluated in naturally infected horses [178]. All the horses that were positive for IgM in the CSF were also positive in the serum, suggesting that CSF IgM is present concomitantly with serum IgM in horses [178]. The albumin quotient measured in the same horses was within the normal reference range for healthy horses, indicating no evidence of blood-brain barrier damage [178]. The IgG index, conversely, was increased compared with normal in horses with WNV encephalomyelitis in samples collected from the lumbosacral space [178]. The joint interpretation of the albumin quotient and IgG index in these horses was suggestive of intrathecal immunoglobulin synthesis [178]. The same study also evaluated the IgM antibody response to vaccination in serum and CSF [178]. Three of 28 vaccinated horses were positive with the serum MAC-ELISA 3 to 4 weeks after the initial vaccination [178]. Thus, in a small number of vaccinated horses, vaccination may induce positive MAC-ELISA results.

An additional test in the serodiagnosis of WNV is a recombinant envelope protein–based ELISA [179]. The envelope protein E contains three antigenic domains and is responsible for many viral biologic features, such as tropism, cell binding, virulence, and antigenicity [168]. The ELISA test recognizes IgM and IgG against a purified recombinant envelope protein E. The assay yielded encouraging results when tested on horses with confirmed WNV infection [179].

Detection of viral genomic material in blood of suspected positive horses by a reverse transcriptase (RT) nPCR assay was also investigated as an antemortem test for WNV in the equine species [180]. The diagnostic sensitivity of the RT-nPCR assay performed on whole blood of clinically affected horses was low: of 140 clinically affected horses, only 18 were positive on the RT-nPCR assay [180]. Interestingly, when the test was run in normal herd mates, it was consistent in detecting subclinically affected horses [168]. Positive results were also obtained in samples collected from experimentally infected horses during the 6 days after inoculation [168]. The RT-nPCR assay can be used to detect viremia before immunoglobulin production, and the limitation of the test is the short duration and low titers of the viremia [180]; the virus is unlikely to be present in the blood by the time the clinical signs are manifest.

Postmortem diagnosis is based on detection of WNV by a PCR assay, virus isolation, or immunohistochemistry in the CNS [181].

Treatment

Treatment of WNV encephalomyelitis is mainly supportive and symptomatic and is aimed at reducing inflammation in the CNS. The survival rate of horses with WNV infection is high; in many cases, horses seem to show signs of recovery between 3 and 5 days after the onset of clinical signs [181]. It is thus difficult to assess the effects of any pharmacologic intervention in the face of resolving clinical signs [181]. To date, no controlled trials have studied the use of corticosteroids, anticonvulsants, or osmotic agents for the treatment of neurologic disease caused by WNV in human beings or horses. Therapy has thus been empiric and based on the same rationale as that used for other viral causes of myeloencephalitis. Commonly used therapies in horses include nonsteroidal anti-inflammatory drugs (eg, flunixin meglumine, phenylbutazone), osmotic and antioxidant agents (eg, DMSO, mannitol), and corticosteroids (eg, dexamethasone, prednisolone) in an attempt to limit inflammation in the CNS [169, 171–174,182]. In a cross-sectional study evaluating factors associated with outcome in 484 equids with a confirmed diagnosis of WNV infection, treatment with corticosteroids did not seem to affect disease severity or outcome [183]. In human patients, treatment of viral encephalitis with corticosteroids is limited because of the concern about immunosuppressive effects that may lead to virus replication and spread of the infection [184]. The use of high-dose corticosteroids, however, has been reported for the management of acute flaccid paralysis attributable to WNV infection in a man [184].

Ribavirin, a synthetic nucleoside analogue with immunomodulatory properties, has in vitro antiviral activity against WNV; its efficacy, however, has not been documented in animal models or clinical trials [185]. The lack of in vivo effectiveness has been attributed to incomplete penetration of the blood-brain barrier [185].

Manifestation of WNV clinical disease is linked to host factors, particularly the innate immune response, such as type I interferon (IFN)-α or IFNβ [168]. IFNα is an immunotherapic used in viral diseases [185]. It inhibits intracellular viral replication and participates in antigen presentation and activation of cytotoxic T-cell responses. IFNα inhibited in vitro WNV-induced cytotoxicity; its in vivo efficacy has not yet been evaluated, however [185]. IFN has been used successfully in some equine cases at a dose of 3×10^6 U administered subcutaneously once daily [182].

Intravenous fluid therapy is required in horses that are not drinking adequately. Deep bedding, regular turning, and use of slings are indicated in recumbent cases. Affected horses are often excitable and unpredictable. Acepromazine has been recommended for its anxiolytic properties (0.02 mg/kg administered intravenously or 0.05 mg/kg administered intramuscularly) [181]. Detomidine (0.02–0.04 mg/kg) intravenously or intramuscularly is often used when more profound sedation is required [181].

Hyperimmune plasma (Lake Immunogenics, Ontario, New York) and serum (Novartis Animal Health US, Greensboro, North Carolina) products are available and have been used in clinical cases to provide a state of immediate immunity. Their effects have not been fully evaluated; however, there is some evidence to support the use of these products on the basis of in vivo studies in murine models [186–188]. Mice received full protection from WNV infection when treated with pooled plasma or intravenous immunoglobulin containing WNV-specific antibodies [186]. Beneficial effects were not seen when plasma or intravenous immunoglobulin that did not contain the specific antibodies was administered. These results indicate that antibodies play a major role in protection and recovery from WNV infection. A linear correlation was found between the level of protection and the amount of plasma product containing a specific antibody that was given, and an inverse correlation was found between virus load and the protective efficacy of passive transfer [186]. Treatment of WNV-infected pregnant mice with reactive immunoglobulin seemed to offer protection to the dam and fetus [187]. The recommended dose of the WNV equine antibody plasma is 2.2 mL/kg (1 mL/lb). This dose resulted in a WNV PRNT titer of 1:30 based on tests performed by a commercial company (Lakeimmunogenics, Rochester, New York), which is four times higher than the level that the USDA considers protective after vaccination. These higher doses of antibody would theoretically seem to be advantageous on the basis of the dose-related benefits demonstrated by the murine model [186]. Although the administration of specific antibody-containing products is best performed as early as possible in the disease process, laboratory animal models have shown that clinical outcome is improved by passive transfer of immune antibody even after WNV has disseminated into the CNS [188]. Dissemination into the CNS occurred several days before clinical signs of disease, and administration of immunoglobulin only had a therapeutic effect when it was given before the development of clinical neurologic disease [188]. In summary, there is not yet any experimental evidence that therapy with immunoglobulin can improve survival or neurologic outcome when this therapy is initiated after the development of clinical neurologic disease [185]. Results are not available from controlled studies critically evaluating the use of hyperimmune products in equine WNV cases. As such, any protective affects in the horse are as yet unproven, and optimal dosages and frequency of administration are unknown. If there is an autoimmune pathologic component to the CNS damage caused by WNV, it may conceivably be exacerbated by administration of hyperimmune products.

Prevention

WNV infection is best prevented by a combination of environmental control and vaccination. Management procedures to minimize or prevent the risk of spread and transmission of WNV from infected mosquitoes include elimination of standing or stagnant water, keeping horses in barns from dawn until dusk, and removing organic debris promptly. Mosquito traps, topical antimosquito repellent agents approved for use in the horse, and fans to increase air movement are also recommended.

There are two commercially available vaccines, and a third, a DNA vaccine, is expected to be on the market in 2006. The risk of infection is reduced by use of these vaccines, but clinical disease is not fully prevented [183]. The first vaccine to be developed was a formalin-killed WNV vaccine (Fort Dodge Animal Health, Overland Park, Kansas) that has been available to equine practitioners since 2001. A trial performed using this killed vaccine in horses demonstrated significant protection (94% of preventable fraction) against viremia [189]. The protective effect of this vaccine was further supported by the fact that fewer clinical cases of WNV were recognized in fully vaccinated horses and that unvaccinated equids were twice as likely to die as vaccinated equids in a retrospective clinical study [183]. An observational study showed that some horses responded poorly to the killed WNV vaccine, with antibody levels waning significantly by 6 months [176]. Therefore, current guidelines for WNV vaccination include a high frequency of vaccination given at strategic times in high-risk areas (this may be semiannually or more frequently). Annual revaccination is best completed in the spring, before the onset of peak insect vector season. A retrospective study reviewing the records of 595 mares showed no evidence that the killed vaccine compromised pregnancy in any of the horses [190]. It would thus seem that although the killed vaccine is not labeled for use in pregnant mares, the benefits of its use in mares located in areas where the disease is endemic outweigh the possible risks.

The second vaccine is a live canarypox vector vaccine (Merial Limited, Athens, Georgia) which came on the market in 2004. This vaccine expresses the premembrane and envelope genes of WNV, which results in presentation of antigens in a manner analogous to that of the wild-type infection [191]. A primary course of two doses of vaccine 5 weeks apart resulted in protection of horses against a WNV mosquito challenge 2 weeks after the second vaccination and seemed to confer long-lasting protection (12 months) [191]. Only 1 of 10 horses challenged at 1 year developed detectable viremia as opposed to 8 of 10 in the control group [191].

A study using WNV-naive horses vaccinated with the live canarypox vector vaccine found that the vaccine generated a protective response 26 days after administration of a single dose and that administration of two doses of the vaccine resulted in protection from viremia at day 14 [192]. The canarypox vector vaccine is able to produce a substantial anamnestic response sufficient to provide a protective immune response against WNV infection in horses previously vaccinated with the killed WNV vaccine; hence, this vaccine can be used interchangeably with the killed vaccine [193]. This study, however, did not evaluate the duration of immunity. The safety of the recombinant vaccine in pregnant mares has not yet been established.

In July 2005, the USDA granted a license for a DNA vaccine (Fort Dodge Animal Health, Overland Park, Kansas), and it is anticipated that the product should reach the market in the early part of 2006.

Acknowledgments

The authors acknowledge Dr. John Schumacher and Dr. Josh Slater for critical reading of the manuscript and Dr. George Allen for allowing inclusion of information not yet published at the time of submission of this manuscript.

References

[1] Snyder RD. Bacterial meningitis: diagnosis and treatment. Curr Neurol Neurosci Rep 2003;3:461–9.
[2] Santschi EM, Foreman JH. Equine bacterial meningitis—part I. Compend Contin Educ Pract Vet 1989;11:479–83.
[3] Morris DD, Rutkowski J. Therapy in two cases of neonatal foal septicaemia and meningitis with cefotaxime sodium. Equine Vet J 1987;19:151–4.
[4] Platt H. Septicaemia in the foal. A review of 61 cases. Br Vet J 1973;129:221–9.
[5] Stuart BP, Martin BR, Williams LP Jr, et al. Salmonella-induced meningoencephalitis in a foal. J Am Vet Med Assoc 1973;162:211–3.
[6] Rush Moore B. Bacterial meningitis in foals. Compend Contin Educ Pract Vet 1995;17: 1417–20.
[7] Tyler CM, Davis RE, Begg AP, et al. A survey of neurological diseases in horses. Aust Vet J 1993;70:445–9.
[8] Adams R, Mayhew IG. Neurologic diseases. Vet Clin North Am Equine Pract 1985;1: 209–34.
[9] Barklay WP, deLahunta A. Cryptococcal meningitis in a horse. J Am Vet Med Assoc 1979; 174:1236–8.
[10] Steckel RR, Adams SB, Long GG, et al. Antemortem diagnosis and treatment of cryptococcal meningitis in a horse. J Am Vet Med Assoc 1982;180:1085–9.
[11] Barton MD, Knight I. Cryptococcal meningitis of a horse. Aust Vet J 1972;48:534.
[12] Smith JJ, Provost PJ, Paradis MR. Bacterial meningitis and brain abscesses secondary to infectious disease processes involving the head in horses: seven cases (1980–2001). J Am Vet Med Assoc 2004;224:739–42.
[13] Ford J, Lokai MD. Complications of *Streptococcus equi* infection. Equine Pract 1980;2: 41–4.
[14] Allen JR, Barbee DD, Boulton CR, et al. Brain abscess in a horse: diagnosis by computed tomography and successful surgical treatment. Equine Vet J 1987;19:552–5.
[15] Cornelisse CJ, Schott HC II, Lowrie CT, et al. Successful treatment of intracranial abscesses in 2 horses. J Vet Intern Med 2001;15:494–500.
[16] Foreman JH, Santschi EM. Equine bacterial meningitis—part II. Compend Contin Educ Pract Vet 1989;11:640–4.
[17] Raphael CF. Brain abscess in three horses. J Am Vet Med Assoc 1973;180:874–7.
[18] Devriese LA, Sustronck B, Maenhout T, et al. *Streptococcus suis* meningitis in a horse. Vet Rec 1990;21:68.
[19] Rumbaugh GE. Disseminated meningitis in a mare. J Am Vet Med Assoc 1977;171:452–4.
[20] Timoney PJ, McArdle JF, Bryne MJ. Abortion and meningitis in a Thoroughbred mare associated with *Klebsiella pneumoniae*, type 1. Equine Vet J 1983;15:64–5.

[21] Reilly L, Habecker P, Beech J, et al. Pituitary abscess and basilar empyema in 4 horses. Equine Vet J 1994;26:424–6.
[22] Tietje S, Becker M, Bockenhoff G. Computed tomographic evaluation of head diseases in the horse: 15 cases. Equine Vet J 1996;28:98–105.
[23] Brass DA. Pathophysiology and neuroimmunology of bacterial meningitis. Compend Contin Educ Pract Vet 1994;16:45–53.
[24] Newton SA. Suspected bacterial meningoencephalitis in two adult horses. Vet Rec 1998; 142:665–9.
[25] Pellegrini-Masini A, Bentz AI, Johns IC, et al. Common variable immunodeficiency in three horses with presumptive bacterial meningitis. J Am Vet Med Assoc 2005;227:114–22.
[26] Hussein AS, Shafran SD. Acute bacterial meningitis in adults: a 12-year review. Medicine (Baltimore) 2000;79:360–8.
[27] Tunbridge A, Read RC. Management of meningitis. Clin Med 2004;4:499–505.
[28] Coant PN, Kornberg AE, Duffy LC, et al. Blood culture results as determinants in the organism identification of bacterial meningitis. Pediatr Emerg Care 1992;8:200–5.
[29] Seehusen DA, Reeves MM, Fomin DA. Cerebrospinal fluid analysis. Am Fam Physician 2003;68:1103–8.
[30] Araj GF, Hamati AI, Sinno DD, et al. Bacterial meningitis with normal cerebrospinal fluid findings. Report of a case and review of the literature. J Med Liban 1993;41:86–9.
[31] Rebeu-Dartiguelongue I, Laurent JP, Clarac A, et al. Early lumbar puncture and cutaneous rash: a clear CSF is not always a normal CSF. Med Mal Infect 2005;35:422–4.
[32] Furr MO, Bender H. Cerebrospinal fluid variables in clinically normal foals from birth to 42 days of age. Am J Vet Res 1994;55:781–4.
[33] Quagliarello VJ, Scheld WM. Treatment of bacterial meningitis. N Engl J Med 1997;336: 708–16.
[34] Sinner SW, Tunkel AR. Antimicrobial agents in the treatment of bacterial meningitis. Infect Dis Clin North Am 2004;18:581–602.
[35] Dowling PM. Clinical pharmacology of nervous system diseases. Vet Clin North Am Equine Pract 1999;15:575–88.
[36] Brewer BD. Therapeutic strategies involving antimicrobial treatment of the central nervous system in large animals. J Am Vet Med Assoc 1984;185:1217–21.
[37] Rahal JJ, Simberkoff MS. Bactericidal and bacteriostatic action of chloramphenicol against meningeal pathogens. Antimicrob Agents Chemother 1979;16:13–8.
[38] Garvey G. Current concepts of bacterial infections of the central nervous system. J Neurosurg 1983;59:735–44.
[39] Pankey GA, Sabath LD. Clinical relevance of bacteriostatic versus bactericidal mechanisms of action in the treatment of gram-positive bacterial infections. Clin Infect Dis 2004;38:864–70.
[40] Tauber MG, Doroshow CA, Hackbarth CJ, et al. Antibacterial activity of beta-lactam antibiotics in experimental meningitis due to Streptococcus pneumoniae. J Infect Dis 1984; 149:568–74.
[41] Prasad K, Singhal T, Jain N, et al. Third generation cephalosporins versus conventional antibiotics for treating acute bacterial meningitis. Cochrane Database Syst Rev 2004;2: CD001832.
[42] Ringger NC, Pearson EG, Gronwall R, et al. Pharmacokinetics of ceftriaxone in healthy horses. Equine Vet J 1996;28:476–9.
[43] Carrillo NA, Giguere S, Gronwall RR, et al. Disposition of orally administered cefpodoxime proxetil in foals and adult horses and minimum inhibitory concentration of the drug against common bacterial pathogens of horses. Am J Vet Res 2005;66:30–5.
[44] Cervantes CC, Brown MP, Gronwall R, et al. Pharmacokinetics and concentrations of ceftiofur sodium in body fluids and endometrium after repeated intramuscular injections in mares. Am J Vet Res 1993;54:573–5.

[45] Ringger NC, Browns MP, Kohlepp SJ, et al. Pharmacokinetics of ceftriaxone in neonatal foals. Equine Vet J 1998;30:163–5.
[46] Gardner SY, Sweeney RW, Divers TJ. Pharmacokinetics of cefotaxime in neonatal pony foals. Am J Vet Res 1993;54:576–9.
[47] Meyer JC, Brown MP, Gronwall RR, et al. Pharmacokinetics of ceftiofur sodium in neonatal foals after intramuscular injection. Equine Vet J 1992;24:485–6.
[48] Guglick MA, MacAllister CG, Clarke CR, et al. Pharmacokinetics of cefepime and comparison with those of ceftiofur in horses. Am J Vet Res 1998;59:458–63.
[49] Scheld WM, Sande MA. Bactericidal versus bacteriostatic antibiotic therapy of experimental pneumococcal meningitis in rabbits. J Clin Invest 1983;71:411–9.
[50] Regodon S, Franco A, Lignereux Y, et al. A new technique for accessing the cerebral ventricles of the horse. Res Vet Sci 1993;55:389–91.
[51] Shah S, Ohlsson A, Shah V. Intraventricular antibiotics for bacterial meningitis in neonates. Cochrane Database Syst Rev 2004;4:CD004496.
[52] Scheld WM, Koedel U, Nathan B, et al. Pathophysiology of bacterial meningitis: mechanism(s) of neuronal injury. J Infect Dis 2002;186(Suppl):S225–33.
[53] Nau R, Bruck W. Neuronal injury in bacterial meningitis: mechanisms and implications for therapy. Trends Neurosci 2002;25:38–45.
[54] Nau R, Eiffert H. Modulation of release of proinflammatory bacterial compounds by antibacterials: potential impact on course of inflammation and outcome in sepsis and meningitis. Clin Microbiol Rev 2002;15:95–110.
[55] Townsend GC, Scheld WM. The use of corticosteroids in the management of bacterial meningitis in adults. J Antimicrob Chemother 1996;37:1051–61.
[56] Chaudhuri A. Adjunctive dexamethasone treatment in acute bacterial meningitis. Lancet Neurol 2004;3:54–62.
[57] van de Beek D, de Gans J, McIntyre P, et al. Steroids in adults with acute bacterial meningitis: a systematic review. Lancet Infect Dis 2004;4:139–43.
[58] Gomes JA, Stevens RD, Lewin JJ III, et al. Glucocorticoid therapy in neurologic critical care. Crit Care Med 2005;33:1214–24.
[59] Pile JC, Longworth DL. Should adults with suspected acute bacterial meningitis get adjunctive corticosteroids? Cleve Clin J Med 2005;72:67–70.
[60] van de Beek D, de Gans J, McIntyre P, et al. Review: adjuvant corticosteroid therapy reduces death, hearing loss, and neurological sequelae in bacterial meningitis. Cochrane Database Syst Rev 2003;3:CD004305.
[61] Bonadio WA. Adjunctive dexamethasone therapy for pediatric bacterial meningitis. J Emerg Med 1996;14:165–72.
[62] Feigin RD. Use of corticosteroids in bacterial meningitis. Pediatr Infect Dis J 2004;23: 355–7.
[63] Irazuzta J, Pretzlaff RK, deCourten-Myers G. Dexamethasone decreases neurological sequelae and caspase activity. Intensive Care Med 2005;31:146–50.
[64] Gupta S, Tuladhar AB. Does early administration of dexamethasone improve neurological outcome in children with meningococcal meningitis? Arch Dis Chil 2004;89: 82–3.
[65] Meli DN, Loeffler JM, Baumann P, et al. In pneumococcal meningitis a novel water-soluble inhibitor of matrix metalloproteinases and TNF-alpha converting enzyme attenuates seizures and injury of the cerebral cortex. J Neuroimmunol 2004;151:6–11.
[66] Leib SL, Leppert D, Clements J, et al. Matrix metalloproteinases contribute to brain damage in experimental pneumococcal meningitis. Infect Immun 2000;68:615–20.
[67] Pfister LA, Tureen JH, Shaw S, et al. Endothelin inhibition improves cerebral blood flow and is neuroprotective in pneumococcal meninigitis. Ann Neurol 2000;47:329–35.
[68] Pfister HW, Scheld WM. Brain injury in bacterial meningitis: therapeutic implications. Curr Opin Neurol 1997;10:254–9.

[69] Brandt CT, Lundgren JD, Frimodt-Moller N, et al. Blocking of leukocyte accumulation in the cerebrospinal fluid augments bacteremia and increases lethality in experimental pneumococcal meningitis. J Neuroimmunol 2005;166:126–31.
[70] Park WS, Chang YS, Lee M. The efficacy of pentoxifylline as an anti-inflammatory agent in experimental Escherichia coli meningitis in the newborn piglet. Biol Neonate 2000;77:236–42.
[71] Lindvall P, Ahlm C, Ericsson M, et al. Reducing intracranial pressure may increase survival among patients with bacterial meningitis. Clin Infect Dis 2004;38:384–90.
[72] Moore RM, Trims CM. Effect of xylazine on intracranial pressure in conscious horses [abstract]. Vet Surg 1991;20:155–6.
[73] Moore RM, Trims CM. Effect of xylazine on cerebrospinal fluid pressure in conscious horses. Am J Vet Res 1992;53:1558–61.
[74] Natalini CC, Robinson EP. Effects of lumbosacral subarachnoid catheterization in horses. Vet Surg 1999;28:525–8.
[75] Lorenzl S, Koedel U, Pfister HW. Mannitol, but not allopurinol, modulates changes in cerebral blood flow, intracranial pressure, and brain water content during pneumococcal meningitis in the rat. Crit Care Med 1996;24:1874–80.
[76] Murthy JM. Management of intracranial pressure in tuberculous meningitis. Neurocrit Care 2005;2:306–12.
[77] Grande PO, Myhre EB, Nordstrom CH, et al. Treatment of intracranial hypertension and aspects on lumbar dural puncture in severe bacterial meningitis. Acta Anaesthesiol Scand 2002;46:264–70.
[78] Patel S, Lederman E, Wallace M. Acetazolamide therapy and intracranial pressure. Clin Infect Dis 2003;36:538.
[79] MacKay RJ, Granstrom DE, Saville WJ, et al. Equine protozoal myeloencephalitis. Vet Clin North Am Equine Pract 2000;16:405–25.
[80] Dubey JP, Lindsay DS, Saville WJ, et al. A review of *Sarcocystis neurona* and equine protozoal myeloencephalitis (EPM). Vet Parasitol 2001;95:89–131.
[81] Furr M, MacKay R, Granstrom D, et al. Clinical diagnosis of equine protozoal myeloencephalitis (EPM). J Vet Intern Med 2002;16:618–21.
[82] Daft BM, Barr BC, Gardner IA, et al. Sensitivity and specificity of Western blot testing of cerebrospinal fluid and serum for diagnosis of equine protozoal myeloencephalitis in horses with and without neurologic abnormalities. J Am Vet Med Assoc 2002;221:1007–13.
[83] Furr M. Antigen-specific antibodies in cerebrospinal fluid after intramuscular injection of ovalbumin in a horse. J Vet Intern Med 2002;16:588–92.
[84] Witonsky S, Morrow JK, Leger C, et al. *Sarcocystis neurona*-specific immunoglobulin G in the serum and cerebrospinal fluid of horses administered *S neurona* vaccine. J Vet Intern Med 2004;18:98–103.
[85] Miller MM, Sweeney CR, Russel GE, et al. Effects of blood contamination of cerebrospinal fluid on Western blot analysis for detection of antibodies against Sarcocystis neurona and on albumin quotient and immunoglobulin G index in horses. J Am Vet Med Assoc 1999;215:67–71.
[86] Tipold A. Cerebrospinal fluid. In: Braund KG, editor. Clinical neurology in small animals: localization, diagnosis and treatment. Ithaca (NY): International Veterinary Information Service; 2003. B0235.0803. Available at: www.ivis.org.
[87] Rossano MG, Kaneene JB, Schott HC II, et al. Assessing the agreement of Western blot test results for paired serum and cerebrospinal fluid samples from horses tested for antibodies to *Sarcocystis neurona*. Vet Parasitol 2003;115:233–8.
[88] Lindsay DS, Dubey JP. Direct agglutination test for the detection of antibodies to *Sarcocystis neurona* in experimentally infected animals. Vet Parasitol 2001;95:179–86.
[89] Duarte PC, Daft BM, Conrad PA, et al. Comparison of a serum indirect fluorescent antibody test with two Western blot tests for the diagnosis of equine protozoal myeloencephalitis. J Vet Diagn Invest 2003;15:8–13.

[90] Duarte PC, Daft BM, Conrad PA, et al. Evaluation and comparison of an indirect fluorescent antibody test for detection of antibodies to *Sarcocystis neurona*, using serum and cerebrospinal fluid of naturally and experimentally infected, and vaccinated horses. J Parasitol 2004;90:379–86.
[91] Saville WJ, Dubey JP, Oglesbee MJ, et al. Experimental infection of ponies with Sarcocystis fayeri and differentiation from Sarcocystis neurona infections in horses. J Parasitol 2004;90: 1487–91.
[92] Hoane JS, Morrow JK, Saville WJ, et al. Enzyme-linked immunosorbent assays for detection of equine antibodies specific to Sarcocystis neurona surface antigens. Clin Diagn Lab Immunol 2005;12:1050–6.
[93] Cook AG, Buechner-Maxwell V, Morrow JK, et al. Interpretation of the detection of *Sarcocystis neurona* antibodies in the serum of young horses. Vet Parasitol 2001;95:187–95.
[94] Cook AG, Buechner-Maxwell V, Donaldson LL, et al. Detection of antibodies against *Sarcocystis neurona* in cerebrospinal fluid from clinically normal neonatal foals. J Am Vet Med Assoc 2002;220:208–11.
[95] Gray LC, Magdesian KG, Sturges BK, et al. Suspected protozoal myeloencephalitis in a two-month-old colt. Vet Rec 2001;149:269–73.
[96] Duarte PC, Conrad PA, Barr BC, et al. Risk of transplacental transmission of *Sarcocystis neurona* and *Neospora hughesi* in California horses. J Parasitol 2004;90:1345–51.
[97] Duarte PC, Conrad PA, Wilson WD, et al. Risk of postnatal exposure to *Sarcocystis neurona* and *Neospora hughesi* in horses. Am J Vet Res 2004;65:1047–52.
[98] Marsh AE, Lakritz J, Johnson PJ, et al. Evaluation of immune responses in horses immunized using a killed *Sarcocystis neurona* vaccine. Vet Ther 2004;5:34–42.
[99] Rossano MG, Schott HC III, Kaneene JB, et al. Effect of daily administration of pyrantel tartrate in preventing infection in horses experimentally challenged with *Sarcocystis neurona*. J Am Vet Med Assoc 2005;66:846–52.
[100] Henninger R. Epidemic neurologic disease due to equine herpesvirus 1: the University of Findlay English Equestrian Center. In: Proceedings of the Ninth International Veterinary Emergency and Critical Care Symposium. New Orleans (LA); 2003. p. 621–4.
[101] Reed S, Toribio R. Equine herpes virus 1 and 4. Vet Clin North Am Equine Pract 2004;20: 631–42.
[102] Friday P, Scarratt W, Elvinger F, et al. Ataxia and paresis with equine herpes type 1 infection in a herd of riding school horses. J Vet Intern Med 2000;14:197–201.
[103] Van Maanen C, Sloet van Oldruitenborgh-Oosterbaan MM, Damen EA, et al. Neurological disease associated with EHV-1 infection in a riding school: clinical and virological characteristics. Equine Vet J 2001;33:191–6.
[104] Studdert MJ, Hartley CA, Dynon K, et al. Outbreak of equine herpesvirus type 1 myeloencephalitis: new insights from virus identification by PCR and the application of an EHV-1-specific antibody detection ELISA. Vet Rec 2003;153:417–23.
[105] Ostlund EN. The equine herpesviruses. Vet Clin North Am Equine Pract 1993;9:283–94.
[106] Wilson WD. Equine herpesvirus 1 myeloencephalopathy. Vet Clin North Am Equine Pract 1997;13:53–72.
[107] O'Callaghan DJ, Osterrieder N. Equine herpes viruses. In: Webster RG, Granoff A, editors. Encyclopedia of virology. San Diego (CA): Harcourt Brace & Company; 1999. p. 508–15.
[108] Patel JR, Edington N, Mumford JA. Variation in cellular tropism between isolates of equine herpes virus-1 in foals. Arch Virol 1982;7:41–51.
[109] Allen G. New insights into equine herpesvirus-1 (EHV-1) neurological disease. Equine Dis Q 200;15(1):2–3.
[110] Allen GP, Breathnach CC. Quantification by real-time PCR of the magnitude and duration of leukocyte-associated viraemia in horses infected with neuropathogenic versus non-neuropathogenic strains of Equid herpesvirus-1. Equine Vet J 2006;38:252–7.
[111] Donaldson MT, Sweeney CR. Equine herpes myeloencephalopathy. Compend Contin Educ Pract Vet 1997;19:864–71.

[112] Donaldson MT, Sweeney CR. Herpesvirus myeloencephalopathy in horses: 11 cases (1982–1996). J Am Vet Med Assoc 1998;213:671–5.
[113] McCartan CG, Russell MM, Wood JL, et al. Clinical, serological and virological characteristics of an outbreak of paresis and neonatal foal disease due to equine herpesvirus-1 on a stud farm. Vet Rec 1995;136:7–12.
[114] Crabb BS, Studdert MJ. Epitopes of glycoprotein G of equine herpesviruses 4 and 1 located near the C termini elicit type-specific antibody responses in the natural host. J Virol 1993;67:6332–8.
[115] Allen GP. Epidemic disease caused by Equine herpesvirus-1: recommendations for prevention and control. Equine Vet Educ 2002;14:136–42.
[116] Yasunaga S, Maeda K, Matsumura T, et al. Diagnosis and sero-epizootiology of equine herpesvirus type 1 and type 4 infections in Japan using a type-specific ELISA. J Vet Med Sci 1998;60:1133–7.
[117] Yasunaga S, Maeda K, Matsumura T, et al. Application of a type-specific enzyme-linked immunosorbent assay for equine herpesvirus types 1 and 4 (EHV-1 and -4) to horse populations inoculated with inactivated EHV-1 vaccine. J Vet Med Sci 2000;62:687–91.
[118] Singh BK, Ahuja S, Gulati BR. Development of a neutralizing monoclonal antibody-based blocking ELISA for detection of equine herpesvirus 1 antibodies. Vet Res Commun 2004;28:437–46.
[119] Smith DJ, Iqbal J, Purewal A, et al. In vitro reactivation of latent equid herpesvirus-1 from CD5+/CD8+ leukocytes indirectly by IL-2 or chorionic gonadotrophin. J Gen Virol 1998;79:2997–3004.
[120] Mumford JA. The development of diagnostic techniques for equine viral diseases. Vet Ann 1984;24:182–9.
[121] Patel JR, Heldens J. Equine herpesviruses 1 (EHV-1) and 4 (EHV-4)—epidemiology, disease and immunoprophylaxis: a brief review. Vet J 2005;170:14–23.
[122] Carvalho R, Passos LM, Martins AS. Development of a differential multiplex PCR assay for equine herpesvirus 1 and 4 as a diagnostic tool. J Vet Med B Infect Dis Vet Public Health 2000;47:351–9.
[123] Lawrence GL, Gilkerson J, Love DN, et al. Rapid, single-step differentiation of equid herpesviruses 1 and 4 from clinical material using the polymerase chain reaction and virus-specific primers. J Virol Methods 1994;47:59–72.
[124] Daly P, Doyle S. The development of a competitive PCR-ELISA for the detection of equine herpesvirus-1. J Virol Methods 2003;107:237–44.
[125] Varrasso A, Dynon K, Ficorilli N, et al. Identification of equine herpesviruses 1 and 4 by polymerase chain reaction. Aust Vet J 2001;79:563–9.
[126] Pusterla N, Leutenegger CM, Wilson WD, et al. Equine herpesvirus 4 infection in foals: quantitation of viral DNA in nasal secretions and peripheral blood leukocytes during an outbreak using the real-time Taqman® PCR. In: Proceedings of the 21st Annual American College of Veterinary Internal Medicine Forum. Charlotte (NC); 2003. p. 33.
[127] Goehring LS. Equine herpes virus type 1 myeloencephalopathy: a quantitative approach. In: Proceedings of the 22nd Annual American College of Veterinary Internal Medicine Forum. Minneapolis (MN); 2004. p. 168–9.
[128] Pronost S, Gouarin S, Leon A, et al. The development of a real time PCR assay for differentiation of EHV-1 infection or latent states in tissues. In: Proceedings of the 11th Societa Italiana Veterinari per Equini National Congress. Pisa (Italy); 2005. p. 204.
[129] Allen GP. Antemortem detection of horses latently infected with neuropathogenic strains of equine herpesvirus-1. Am J Vet Res 2006, accepted for publication.
[130] Nugent J, Birch-Machin I, Smith KC, et al. Analysis of equine herpes-virus type 1 strain variation reveals a point mutation of the DNA polymerase strongly associated with neuropathogenic versus non-neuropathogenic disease outbreaks. J Virol 2006;80:4047–60.
[131] Bryans JT, Allen GP. Herpesviral diseases of the horse. In: Wittmann G, editor. Herpesviral diseases of cattle, horses and pigs. Boston (MA): Kluwer; 1989. p. 176–229.

[132] Whitwell KE, Blunden AS. Pathological findings in horses dying during an outbreak of the paralytic form of Equid herpesvirus type 1 (EHV-1) infection. Equine Vet J 1992;24:13–9.
[133] Platt H, Singh H, Whitwell KE. Pathological observations on an outbreak of paralysis in broodmares. Equine Vet J 1980;12:118–26.
[134] Slater JD, Borchers K, Thackery AM, et al. The trigeminal ganglion is a location for equine herpesvirus 1 latency and reactivation in the horse. J Gen Virol 1994;75:2007–16.
[135] Collins P. The spectrum of antiviral activities of acyclovir in vitro and in vivo. J Antimicrob Chemother 1983;12:19–27.
[136] Schaeffer HJ. Acyclovir chemistry and spectrum of activity. Am J Med 1982;73:4–6.
[137] Wilkins PA. Controversies in EHV-1 myeloencephalopathy. In: Proceedings of the Ninth International Veterinary Emergency and Critical Care Symposium. New Orleans (LA); 2003. p. 669–70.
[138] Collins P. The spectrum of antiviral activities of acyclovir in vitro and in vivo. J Antimicrob Chemother 1983;12:19–27.
[139] Rollinson EA, White G. Relative activities of acyclovir and BW759 against Aujeszky's disease and equine rhinopneumonitis viruses. Antimicrob Agents Chemother 1983;24:221–6.
[140] Wilkins PA, Del Piero F, de Lahunta A, et al. Paralytic equine herpes virus: 1978–1997. In: Proceedings of the Eighth International Conference on Equine Infectious Diseases. Dubai (United Arab Emirates); 1998. p. 596–7.
[141] Friday PA, Scarratt WK, Elvinger F, et al. Ataxia and paresis with equine herpesvirus type 1 infection in a herd of riding school horses. J Vet Intern Med 2000;14:197–201.
[142] Wilkins PA, Henninger R, Reed SM, et al. Acyclovir as treatment for EHV-1 myeloencephalopathy. In: Proceedings of the 49th Annual Convention of the American Association of Equine Practitioners. New Orleans (LA); 2003. p. 394–6.
[143] Wikins P, Papich M, Sweeney RW. Acyclovir pharmacokinetics in the horse. In: Proceedings of the American College of Veterinary Internal Medicine Forum. Baltimore (MD); 2005. p. 945.
[144] Bentz BG, Maxwell LK, Clarke CR, et al. The pharmacokinetics of acyclovir in adult horses following single intravenous and intragastric dosing. In: Proceedings of the American College of Veterinary Internal Medicine Forum. Baltimore (MD); 2005. p. 945–6.
[145] de la Fuente R, Awan AR, Field HJ. The acyclic nucleoside analogue penciclovir is a potent inhibitor of equine herpesvirus type 1 (EHV-1) in tissue culture and in a murine model. Antiviral Res 1992;18:77–89.
[146] Smith KO, Galloway KS, Hodges SL, et al. Sensitivity of equine herpesviruses 1 and 3 in vitro to a new nucleoside analogue, 9-[[2-hydroxy-1-(hydroxymethyl) ethoxy] methyl] guanine. Am J Vet Res 1983;44:1032–5.
[147] Heldens JGM, Hannant D, Cullinane AA, et al. Clinical evaluation of the efficacy of an inactivated EH-1 and EH-4 whole virus vaccine (Duvaxyn EHV1, 4). Vaccination/challenge experiments in foals and pregnant mares. Vaccine 2001;19:4307–17.
[148] Slater J, Hannant D. Equine immunity to viruses. Vet Clin North Am Equine Pract 2000; 16:49–68.
[149] Mumford JA, Hannant DA, Jessett DM, et al. Abortigenic and neurological disease caused by infection with equid herpesvirus-1. In: Proceedings of the Seventh International Conference of Equine Infectious Diseases. Newmarket (England); 1995. p. 261–75.
[150] Kydd JH, Wattrang E, Hannant D. Pre-infection frequencies of equine herpesvirus-1 specific cytotoxic lymphocytes correlate with protection against abortion following experimental infection of pregnant mares. Vet Immunol Immunopathol 2003;96:207–17.
[151] Kaashoek MJ, Moerman A, Madic J, et al. A conventionally attenuated glycoprotein E-negative strain of bovine herpesvirus type 1 is an efficacious and safe vaccine. Vaccine 1994;12:439–44.
[152] Mettenleiter TC, Klupp BG, Weiland F, et al. Characterization of a quadruple glycoprotein-deleted pseudorabies virus mutant for use as a biologically safe live virus vaccine. J Gen Virol 1994;75:1723–33.

[153] Matsumura T, O'Callaghan DJ, Kondo T, et al. Lack of virulence of the murine fibroblast adopted strain, Kentucky A (KyA) of equine herpesvirus type 1 (EHV-1) in young horses. Vet Microbiol 1996;48:353–65.

[154] Cornick J, Martens J, Crandell R, et al. Safety and efficacy of a thymidine kinase negative equine herpesvirus-1 vaccine in young horses. Can J Vet Res 1990;54:260–6.

[155] Matsumara T, Kondo T, Sugita S, et al. An equine herpesvirus type 1 recombinant with a deletion in the gE and gI genes is avirulent in young horses. Virology 1998;242:68–79.

[156] Rappocciolo G, Birch J, Ellis SA. Down-regulation of MHC class 1 expression by equine herpesvirus-1. J Gen Virol 2003;84:293–300.

[157] Spear P. Glycoproteins specified by herpes simplex virus. In: Roizman B, editor. The herpesviruses. New York: Plenum Press; 1984. p. 315–56.

[158] Foote CE, Love DN, Gilkerson JR, et al. Serum antibody responses to equine herpes virus 1 glycoprotein D in horses, pregnant mares and young foals. Vet Immunol Immunopathol 2005;105:47–57.

[159] Patel JR, Bateman H, Williams J, et al. Derivation and characterisation of a live equid herpesvirus-1 (EHV-1) vaccine to protect against abortion and respiratory disease due to EHV-1. Vet Microbiol 2003;91:23–39.

[160] Patel JR, Foldi J, Bateman H, et al. Equid herpesvirus (EHV-1) live vaccine strain C147: efficacy against respiratory diseases following EHV types 1 and 4 challenges. Vet Microbiol 2003;92:1–17.

[161] Patel JR, Didlick S, Bateman H. Efficacy of a live equine herpesvirus-1 (EHV-1) strain C147 vaccine in foals with maternally derived antibody. Protection against EHV-1 infection. Equine Vet J 2004;36:447–51.

[162] Gilkerson JR, Love DN, Whalley JM. Incidence of equine herpesvirus 1 infection in Thoroughbred weanlings on two stud farms. Aust Vet J 2000;78:277–8.

[163] Gilkerson JR, Whalley JM, Drummer HE, et al. Epidemiological studies of equine herpesvirus 1 (EHV-1) in Thoroughbred foals: a review of studies conducted in the Hunter Valley of New South Wales between 1995 and 1997. Vet Microbiol 1999;68:15–25.

[164] Gilkerson JR, Whalley JM, Drummer HE, et al. Epidemiology of EHV-1 and EHV-4 in the mare and foal populations on a Hunter Valley stud farm: are mares the source of EHV-1 for unweaned foals. Vet Microbiol 1999;68:27–34.

[165] Foote CE, Love DN, Gilkerson JR, et al. Serological responses of mares and weanlings following vaccination with an inactivated whole virus equine herpesvirus-1 and equine herpesvirus 4 vaccine. Vet Microbiol 2002;88:13–25.

[166] Wilson W, Rossdale PD. Effect of age on the serological responses of Thoroughbred foals to vaccination with an inactivated EHV-1/EHV-4 vaccine. In: Proceedings of the Eighth International Conference on Equine Infectious Diseases. Newmarket (England); 1999. p. 428.

[167] Breathnach CC, Allen GP, Holland RE, et al. Problems associated with vaccination of foals against equine herpesvirus-4 and the role of EHV-4 maternal antibodies. In: Proceedings of the Eighth International Conference on Equine Infectious Diseases. Newmarket (England); 1999. p. 418–9.

[168] Castillo-Olivares J, Wood J. West Nile virus infection of horses. Vet Res 2004;35:467–83.

[169] Ostlund EN, Andresen JE, Andresen M. West Nile encephalitis. Vet Clin North Am Equine Pract 2000;16:427–41.

[170] Long MT, Porter MB. West Nile virus—clinical presentation, differentiation from other encephalitides, and management. In: Proceedings of the 20th Annual American College of Veterinary Internal Medicine Forum. Dallas (TX); 2002. p. 151–3.

[171] Ward MP, Levy M, Thacker HL, et al. Investigation of an outbreak of encephalomyelitis caused by West Nile virus in 136 horses. J Am Vet Med Assoc 2004;225:84–9.

[172] Porter MB, Long MT, Getman LM, et al. West Nile Virus encephalomyelitis in horses: 46 cases (2001). J Am Vet Med Assoc 2003;222:1241–7.

[173] Snook CS, Hyman SS, Del Piero F, et al. West Nile virus encephalomyelitis in eight horses. J Am Vet Med Assoc 2001;218:1576–9.

[174] Schuler LA, Khaitsa ML, Dyer NW, et al. Evaluation of an outbreak of West Nile virus infection in horses: 569 cases (2002). J Am Vet Med Assoc 2004;225:1084–8.
[175] Wamsley HL, Alleman AR, Porter MB, et al. Findings in cerebrospinal fluids of horses infected with West Nile virus: 30 cases (2001). J Am Vet Med Assoc 2002;221:1303–5.
[176] Davidson AH, Traub-Dargatz JL, Rodeheaver RM, et al. Immunologic responses to West Nile virus in vaccinated and clinically affected horses. J Am Vet Med Assoc 2005;226: 240–5.
[177] Ostlund EN, Crom RL, Pederson DD, et al. Equine West Nile encephalitis, United States. Emerg Infect Dis 2001;7:665–9.
[178] Porter MB, Long M, Gosche DG, et al. Immunoglobulin M-capture enzyme-linked immunosorbent assay testing of cerebrospinal fluid and serum from horses exposed to West Nile virus by vaccination or natural infection. J Vet Intern Med 2004;18:866–70.
[179] Wang T, Magnarelli LA, Anderson JF, et al. A recombinant envelope protein-based enzyme-linked immunosorbent assay for West Nile virus serodiagnosis. Vector Borne Zoonotic Dis 2002;2:105–9.
[180] Kleiboeker SB, Loiacono CM, Rottinghaus A, et al. Diagnosis of west Nile virus infection in horses. J Vet Diagn Invest 2004;16:2–10.
[181] Long MT, Ostlund EN, Porter MB, et al. Equine West Nile encephalitis: epidemiological and clinical review for practitioners. In: Proceedings of the 48th American Association of Equine Practitioners. Orlando (FL); 2002. p. 1–6.
[182] Wilkins PA, Del Piero F. West Nile virus: lessons from the 21st century. J Vet Emerg Crit Care 2004;14:2–14.
[183] Salazar P, Traub-Dargatz JL, Morley PS, et al. Outcome of equids with clinical signs of West Nile virus infection and factors associated with death. J Am Vet Med Assoc 2004; 225:267–74.
[184] Pyrgos V, Younus F. High-dose steroids in the management of acute flaccid paralysis due to West Nile virus infection. Scand J Infect Dis 2004;36:509–12.
[185] Jackson AC. Therapy of West Nile virus infection. Can J Neurol Sci 2004;31:131–4.
[186] Ben-Nathan D, Lustig S, Tam G, et al. Prophylactic and therapeutic efficacy of human intravenous immunoglobulin in treating West Nile virus infection in mice. J Infect Dis 2003; 188:5–12.
[187] Julander JG, Winger QA, Olsen AL, et al. Treatment of West Nile virus-infected mice with reactive immunoglobulin reduces fetal titers and increases dam survival. Antiviral Res 2005;65:79–85.
[188] Engle MJ, Diamond MS. Antibody prophylaxis and therapy against West Nile virus infection in wild-type and immunodeficient mice. J Virol 2003;77:12941–9.
[189] Ng T, Hathaway D, Jennings N, et al. Equine vaccine for West Nile virus. Dev Biol (Basel) 2003;114:221–7.
[190] Vest DJ, Cohen ND, Berezoski CJ, et al. Evaluation of administration of West Nile virus vaccine to pregnant broodmares. J Am Vet Med Assoc 2004;225:1894–7.
[191] Minke JM, Siger L, Karaca K, et al. Recombinant canarypoxvirus vaccine carrying the prM/E genes of West Nile virus protects horses against a West Nile virus-mosquito challenge. Arch Virol Suppl 2004;18:221–30.
[192] Siger L, Bowen RA, Karaca K, et al. Assessment of the efficacy of a single dose of a recombinant vaccine against West Nile virus in response to a natural challenge with West Nile virus-infected mosquitoes in horses. Am J Vet Res 2004;65:1459–62.
[193] Grosenbaugh DA, Backus CS, Karaca K, et al. The anamnestic serologic response to vaccination with a canarypox virus-vectored recombinant West Nile virus (WNV) vaccine in horses previously vaccinated with an inactivated WNV vaccine. Vet Ther 2004; 5:251–7.

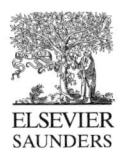

Infections of the Head and Ocular Structures in the Horse

Mathew P. Gerard, BVSc, PhD[a],*,
Kathryn L. Wotman, DVM[b],
András M. Komáromy, Dr Med Vet, PhD[c]

[a]*Department of Clinical Sciences, College of Veterinary Medicine, North Carolina State University, 4700 Hillsborough Street, Raleigh, NC 27606, USA*
[b]*New Bolton Center, School of Veterinary Medicine, University of Pennsylvania, 382 West Street Road, Kennett Square, PA 19348, USA*
[c]*Department of Clinical Studies, School of Veterinary Medicine, University of Pennsylvania, 3900 Delancey Street, Philadelphia, PA 19104-6010, USA*

The horse is prone to infections of the head. Commensal normal flora of the upper airway and oral cavity has the potential to become pathogenic and cause disease when the host-organism relation is disrupted [1]. The extensive nasal passages and paranasal sinuses are also readily exposed to inhaled contaminants and infectious organisms that may colonize and result in primary rhinitis or sinusitis. The roots of the upper three caudal cheek teeth (modified Triadan numbers 109–111 and 209–211) in the mature horse occupy the floor of the maxillary sinuses; therefore, infection in the paranasal sinuses secondary to dental disease is a common condition. The guttural pouches (diverticula of the Eustachian tubes) are susceptible to being contaminated directly or indirectly and developing subsequent infection.

Anamnesis and physical examination findings provide a high index of suspicion of an infectious condition of the head. Radiography and endoscopy are currently the most commonly used imaging modalities to aid in the diagnosis of disease. CT and MRI represent advances in diagnostic imaging that are becoming more accessible for the equine patient.

For any cavity type infection, the general principles of treatment are to ensure effective lavage and drainage. This approach is instrumental for the management of many infections of the equine head. The scope of this article is directed at bacterial and fungal infections, with an emphasis on

* Corresponding author.
 E-mail address: mat_gerard@ncsu.edu (M.P. Gerard).

disease conditions in which new approaches to diagnosis and management have been developed or consolidated in recent years.

The equine eye is susceptible to injury because of its lateral position and the horse's fractious nature. Bacteria and fungi inherent to the ocular surface and the environment of the horse can become serious pathogens. Although infections can occur in any part of the equine eye and its adnexa, recent advances in the management of such infectious diseases have mostly been made for corneal diseases and equine recurrent uveitis (ERU). New medical and surgical treatment options have improved the prognosis for vision in horses with infectious corneal disease. With ERU, multiple advances in techniques for determining possible infectious inciting causes as well as potential vision-sparing treatments have recently been developed and are addressed in this article.

Paranasal sinusitis

Infectious sinusitis is a relatively common clinical condition in the horse, typically affecting the conchofrontal (combined frontal and dorsal conchal), maxillary, and ventral conchal sinuses [2]. Sinusitis is classified as primary or secondary according to the inciting cause. Primary sinusitis with a single bacterial, viral, or fungal cause is considered less common than sinusitis secondary to another disease [3]. Bacteria cultured in primary sinusitis include *Streptococcus equi* subsp *equi* (strangles agent) and *S equi* subsp *zooepidemicus* [4]; however, polymicrobial cultures are possible [5]. Fungal etiologies include *Aspergillus* spp [6,7] and, less commonly, cryptococcal organisms [8,9]. *Aspergillus* spp are a common cause of paranasal and nasal passage fungal infection in human beings and dogs, whereas cryptococcal organisms are most frequently isolated from cats [10,11]. Secondary sinusitis is most commonly caused by dental disease or may be associated with space-occupying obstructive or destructive masses (eg, cysts, neoplasia) or trauma [2,6,12–15].

Diagnosis

The approach to diagnosis of paranasal sinusitis is generally straightforward [3,12,16,17]. Nasal discharge may be absent in chronic sinusitis if the nasomaxillary aperture is obstructed by accumulated exudate, tissue inflammation, or a mass. A malodorous breath often accompanies sinusitis secondary to dental disease or tissue necrosis within the sinus and can also be a feature of primary sinusitis. A thorough oral and dental examination is imperative to assess possible dental disease as a cause of the sinus infection.

Sinocentesis or sinus trephination and sinoscopy can confirm sinus empyema and likely provide a definitive cause for the sinusitis [12,18–21]. These procedures are often performed after other imaging techniques have indicated that the paranasal sinuses are the site of exudative accumulation. Rhinoscopy is used to evaluate the source of nasal discharge and to detect any abnormalities or extension of sinus disease into the nasal passage.

In the mid-1980s, radiography was reported to be the most useful diagnostic procedure for diseases of the nasal passage and paranasal sinuses [13], and this probably remains true today in most cases, despite the availability of more advanced imaging techniques. Radiography continues to be the most accessible and widely used imaging modality available to veterinarians, and diagnostic head radiographs are obtainable with portable units [22]. Careful review of the standard paranasal sinus projections usually allows detection of fluid accumulation and the presence of masses (Fig. 1). Accurate interpretation and exact anatomic locations of disease can be difficult to determine on radiographs, however, because of multiple tissue superimpositions. Contrast sinusography is not commonly used but can enhance visualization of a mass when compared with plain radiographs [23,24]. Ultrasonography is also not commonly used to assess the paranasal sinuses because of the bony casing and air interface. If there is facial distortion with a protruding mass, ultrasonography may help to define the nature of the mass, for example, an expanding fluid-filled structure or a soft tissue mass (Fig. 2).

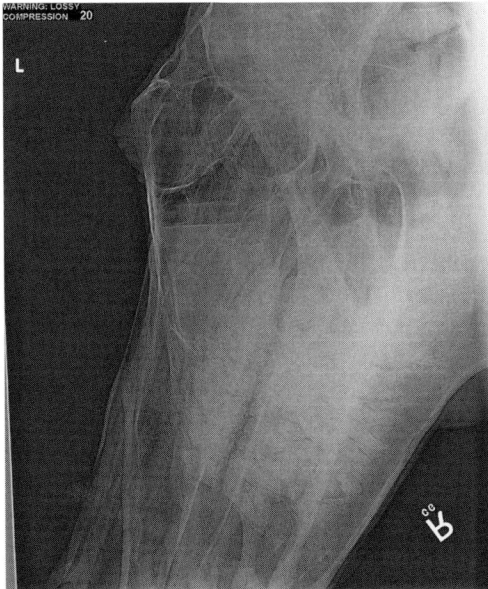

Fig. 1. Oblique radiographic projection of the left paranasal sinuses shows two horizontal air and soft tissue density interfaces consistent with fluid accumulation in the maxillary sinus.

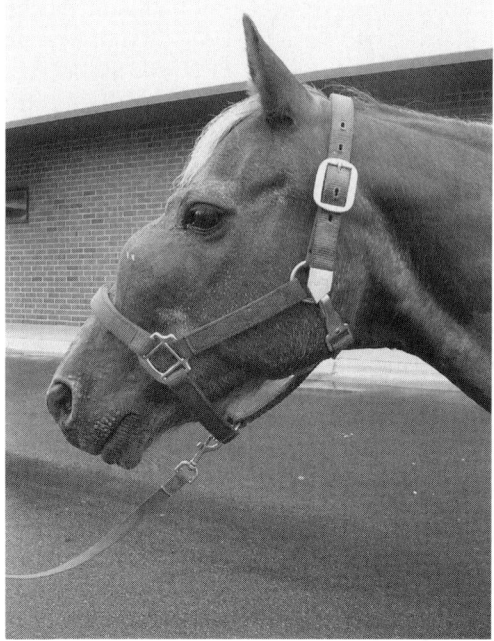

Fig. 2. Left-sided facial mass that can be imaged using ultrasonography to help determine the nature of the mass.

Nuclear scintigraphy remains a possibly underused imaging modality for the equine head [25]. Its primary indication for use is in the evaluation of suspected dental disease as a cause of secondary sinusitis, and it allows differentiation of this disease process from primary sinusitis conditions [26]. Frontal sinus trephination performed up to 7 days before scintigraphic examination of the head has no significant effect on local uptake of the radiopharmaceutic agent [27].

When available, CT is often the imaging procedure of choice for the paranasal sinuses and associated structures [28,29]. The advantage of CT compared with radiography is excellent cross-sectional imaging of the head with no superimposition of structures (Fig. 3A). Dental structures, bone, and soft tissues are clearly evaluated and can provide definitive evidence of disease when radiographs have led to equivocal findings [28,30]. Excessive thickening of the respiratory epithelium and maxillary bone reaction are CT features in horses with chronic sinusitis (see Fig. 3B) [31]. Exact localization of accumulated exudate is confirmed with a CT scan and can allow more appropriate surgical management of cases by defining what cavities need to be specifically explored to access the exudate (see Fig. 3B). MRI provides superior soft tissue anatomic and physiologic detail compared with CT, but improvements in osseous and dental structure evaluation are less significant

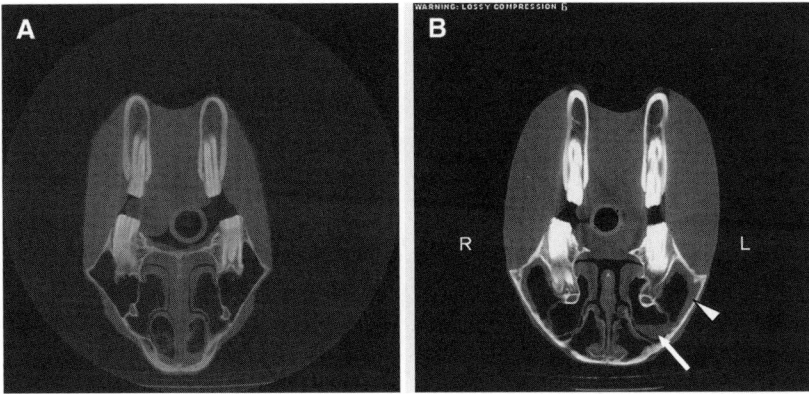

Fig. 3. (A) Cross-sectional CT scan of a normal mature equine head in dorsal recumbency. (B) Cross-sectional CT scan of an equine head in dorsal recumbency shows dependent mild accumulation of fluid in the left ventral conchal bulla (arrow) and increased thickness of the left maxillary sinus epithelium (arrowhead) compared with the right side.

[28,32]. In the authors' opinion, the current advantages of performing MRI versus CT for evaluating the equine head in most cases of sinusitis may be too minimal or nonexistent to justify the greater expense of MRI.

In refractory cases of sinusitis or when a mass is present, it is appropriate to obtain specimens of mucosa or the mass for histopathologic examination as well as culture and sensitivity testing. Sinus mucosa is preferably obtained from the lateral wall of the caudal maxillary sinus because of its accessibility and ease of identification of the site during sinoscopy and sinusotomy [6]. Fungal elements accompanied by a severe neutrophilic infiltration were observed in cases of mycotic sinusitis. Mucosa from chronic sinusitis cases revealed the presence of granulation tissue underlying the epithelium, which, to varying degrees, was replaced by immature or mature fibrous tissue. The transition from acute to chronic sinusitis is manifested histologically by the presence of progressively increasing mucosal fibroplasia [6]. The appearance is similar to that of the mucosa in human patients with chronic sinusitis [33]. Chronic and irreversible changes in the mucosa may contribute to unsatisfactory treatment responses.

Management

Acute cases of primary sinusitis, accurately diagnosed, may respond to medical management, including appropriate antimicrobials (ideally based on culture and sensitivity testing), nonsteroidal anti-inflammatory drugs (NSAIDs), steam inhalations, mucolytics, and continued exercise at light intensity [34]. The effective use of a nasal irrigation solution containing antimicrobials and pancreatic dornase in chronic cases of sinusitis with catarrhal discharge has been described for the horse [35]. Nasal irrigation with hypertonic saline solution is considered an important adjunctive therapy in the management of acute sinusitis in human beings, with a significant reduction in the need for antimicrobials being one key benefit [36].

Surgical procedures are reserved for chronic cases of primary sinusitis that do not respond to medical therapy and for sinus infections secondary to dental disease or space-occupying masses [12,34]. An early return to exercise is advocated after sinus surgery to encourage forced nasal ventilation and subsequent evaporation of postoperative secretions [34]. Frontal or maxillary sinus trephination (using a 2–4-mm Steinmann pin or Michele trephine up to a 0.5-in diameter Galt trephine) to allow access for direct lavage with copious volumes of preferably warm sterile physiologic saline is common practice. This technique is performed in cases of primary sinusitis that persists or recurs after a course of antimicrobials and before a more invasive procedure might need to be considered [12]. Inspissated material can collect in the ventral conchal sinus and requires vigorous lavage via the trephination hole to achieve its removal [5,37,38].

The greatest surgical exposure and access to the paranasal sinuses is achieved by a conchofrontal or maxillary sinus bone flap technique [8,9,12,34]. The conchofrontal bone flap allows access to most regions of the paranasal sinuses and is the favored approach in most cases. Maxillary sinusotomy is reserved for direct access to dental structures or masses, particularly those in the rostral cavity. Often, the nasomaxillary aperture would be enlarged or a new ostium through a conchal wall would be made into the nasal passage, ostensibly to facilitate postoperative sinus drainage. The benefit of doing this is now being questioned because of an apparent failure to improve disease resolution when a patent nasomaxillary aperture is present [38]. Altered mucociliary clearance mechanisms and paranasal sinus nitric oxide concentrations may be important in the pathogenesis of various sinusitis conditions in human beings [39] and might be affected by a surgically created ostium. If a functioning nasomaxillary aperture exists, the possible long-term adverse effects on paranasal sinus physiology of creating an extra hole for drainage into the nasal passage need to be considered and further researched.

Standing sinusotomy in the horse has been described and is becoming more routine with careful patient selection and an accurate understanding of the disease process being managed [38,40]. Horses tolerate the procedure well, and hemorrhage is noticeably less compared with a similar procedure performed with the horse anesthetized and in lateral recumbency. Recently, for standing sinus surgery, use of a trephined hole 5 cm in diameter has been described as a modification of the standard conchofrontal sinusotomy [41]. The center of the hole is located 5 cm axial to the nasolacrimal duct pathway, 4 cm lateral to the nasal midline, and 2 cm below the horizontal line joining the medial canthi [41]. Despite the need to discard the disk of bone, the cosmetic outcome was satisfactory to excellent for owners in 86% of horses [41]. Exposure of the sinuses was considered sufficient, and successful treatment of various conditions was possible (ethmoid hematoma, primary empyema, mycotic sinusitis, sinus cyst, and neoplasia) [41].

For nasal and paranasal sinus surgery performed under general anesthesia, the potential for massive hemorrhage remains a concern. Temporary bilateral carotid artery occlusion can reduce blood flow to the head [42,43], but the clinical effectiveness of this procedure is unpredictable [12]. A rapid surgical procedure and firm packing of the sinus spaces with gauze are currently the best intraoperative techniques to minimize the volume of blood loss. Future options for replenishing an anticipated large reduction in blood volume may include the use of preoperative autologous donation (PAD) programs and intraoperative autotransfusion techniques (V. Cook, VetMB, MA, MS, personal communication, 2005) [44]. The potential for a prolonged lifespan for transfused autologous red blood cells (ie, longer than the 2–4 days associated with homologous transfusions) and the minimal risk of transfusion reactions and disease transmission are clear advantages of such techniques. Equine whole blood can be adequately preserved for up to 5 weeks when stored in plastic bags containing citrate-phosphate-dextrose with supplemental adenine [44]. Further refining of protocols for storage of blood and for intraoperative autologous transfusions is required.

Infection of the teeth and supporting structures

Advances in dental imaging, treatment for periodontal disease, and endodontic therapy for apically infected cheek teeth are areas of intense clinical study in the horse [45]. Apical and periapical infections of teeth refer to disease of the apex or root portion of the tooth and adjacent tissues. Infection can be primary (probably caused by anachoresis [ie, hematogenous or lymphatic-borne bacterial localization]) or secondary to other conditions, including periodontal disease, infundibular decay, dental overgrowths and wear abnormalities, dental trauma, idiopathic dental fractures, supernumerary and displaced cheek teeth, and diastemata [46–50]. Sinusitis secondary to periapical infection of the caudal three upper cheek teeth is a common head infection in horses, because the roots of teeth 09 through 11 extend into the maxillary sinus. Incisors and canines and the third mandibular molars (number 311 or 411) are rarely affected [51,52]; however, the incidence of infection of these teeth may increase with the surge in equine dentistry care and the consequent possible overaggressive reduction of teeth leading to exposed vital pulp [52].

Diagnosis

Diagnosis of dental infection is based on a thorough physical examination, including a detailed oral examination and, often, multiple ancillary imaging modalities. Clinical signs of dental disease encompass a variety of findings that may include abnormal head carriage, abnormal eating and riding habits, ptyalism, halitosis, purulent nasal discharge, an external painful bony swelling, draining tracts, and, rarely, anorexia [53,54]. One of the most significant advances in the diagnosis of dental disease is the recognition of the critical importance of a thorough oral examination and the right instruments to perform it. Comprehensive oral examination in the horse is greatly facilitated by adequate chemical restraint of the patient, a full-mouth speculum, a bright light source, and dental mirrors and picks and probes to explore occlusal surfaces and gingival margins. Advances in equipment design in recent years have allowed the detection of more dental pathologic findings than previously realized [47,50,54,55].

Radiographs remain useful in evaluating dental pathologic findings; however, limitations with interpretation or accurate diagnosis are apparent. Radiographically, infected tooth apices develop lytic changes, manifested as a loss of sharp projections in mature teeth, causing a rounded (clubbing) appearance and a generalized radiolucency of the apex area surrounded by a rim of sclerotic bone [56]. This can also be characteristic of recently erupted permanent cheek teeth; thus, caution is needed in interpretation of findings, particularly in the young horse (Fig. 4) [56,57]. Needle aspiration through the thin cortex under sterile conditions can be useful to confirm the presence of purulent exudate over the apices of suspicious teeth on radiographs [46,57]. Other findings include disruption of the lamina dura denta, widening of the periodontal space, pearls of excessive cementum (produced in the presence of chronic infection), densities in periapical

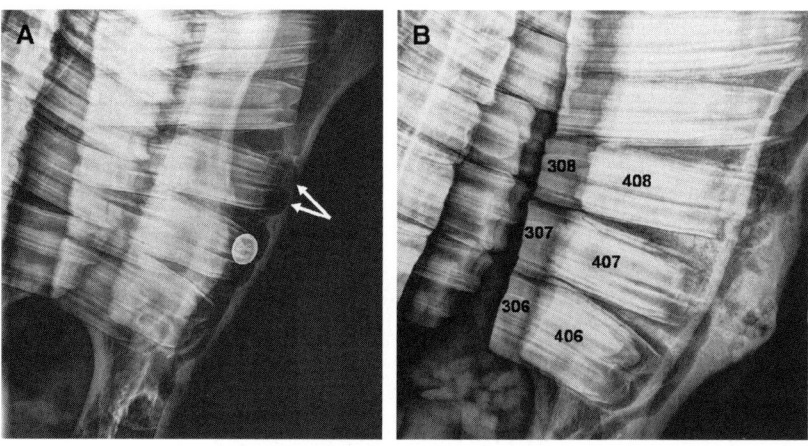

Fig. 4. (*A*) Oblique radiographic projection of the left mandible of a 3-year-old horse shows normal periapical smooth-bordered lucencies with sclerotic margins (*arrows*) consistent with eruption cysts. The coin marks a draining tract on the opposite mandible. (*B*) Right mandibular oblique radiographic projection in the same horse. Punctate lucency and irregular sclerotic margins adjacent to the roots of third cheek tooth (number 408) are consistent with periapical disease. There is also a lytic tract extending through the thickened mandibular cortex to tooth 407. Tooth 406 is normal.

tissues, lytic tracts through bone, and metaplastic calcification of nasal concha ("coral" formation) [56,58]. In some cases, a rounded soft tissue mass representing a granuloma or, later, an encapsulated abscess may be apparent over the apices of an affected tooth. This can resemble a maxillary cyst [57].

Superimposition of multiple tissue densities makes accurate radiographic interpretation difficult. Open-mouth oblique views separate occlusal surfaces of teeth and allow better visualization of the interproximal space and tooth roots (Fig. 5) [59,60]. Intraoral radiography is valuable for the incisors and canines, and techniques have also been described for the cheek teeth [56,61]. Fistulography should be considered when external draining tracts are present. Placing a metallic bead at the skin surface of a draining tract or putting a metal probe into the tract can be helpful in correlating radiographic findings in deeper tissues with those present on the surface. In many cases of early periapical disease, it is difficult to obtain any conclusive evidence of disease on radiographs alone, even for experienced clinicians and radiologists.

Ultrasonography allows examination of cortical bone surfaces and surrounding soft tissues and can be sensitive for detecting cortical defects and fluid accumulation associated with or without draining tracts in horses with periapical tooth infections. Ultrasonography was the most specific imaging modality used in the diagnosis of third mandibular molar abscessation in four of five horses [52], and its routine use in the diagnosis of dental disease with associated clinical signs of external swelling or draining tracts is recommended.

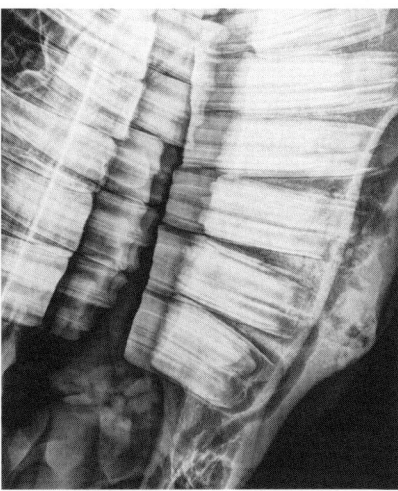

Fig. 5. Right mandibular open-mouth oblique radiograph of the same horse as in Fig. 4. Increased visualization of the interproximal spaces and occlusal surfaces with less superimposition is achieved when the mouth is wedged open.

Nuclear scintigraphy may be helpful in the diagnostic workup of horses with dental disease with suspected infection [26,62,63]. In three horses, nuclear scintigraphy was considered invaluable in supporting or discounting a diagnosis of periapical cheek tooth infection after radiographs, nasal endoscopy, and oral examination were inconclusive [64]. In one case, a lack of increased radiopharmaceutic uptake over tooth roots of suspicion on radiographs averted the clinician's consideration for a sinusotomy under general anesthesia; the case was successfully managed with exploratory standing sinoscopy, lavage, and drainage [64]. Other authors also support the use of scintigraphic examination of the equine head in cases of suspected dental disease when radiographs are inconclusive, particularly in terms of localizing the affected tooth [65]. In a comparison of radiography and scintigraphy for the diagnosis of dental disease in the horse, it was found that scintigraphy using ^{99m}Tc-methylene diphosphonate was approximately 95% sensitive but only 86% specific, whereas radiography had 52% sensitivity and 95% specificity [66]. It was recommended that when radiographic evidence of dental disease is equivocal but still suspected, scintigraphy should be performed. Radiography and scintigraphy are highly complementary, increasing the likelihood of an accurate diagnosis compared with when either is performed alone. Scintigraphy with ^{99m}Tc-labeled leukocytes was considered ineffective in diagnosing dental disease because of diffuse distribution of the marker cells, resulting in a lack of detail to determine the affected tooth or teeth [66].

CT is the current state-of-the-art imaging tool for dental structures and surrounding tissues and has proven to be an excellent diagnostic aid when available (Fig. 6) [28–30]. MRI may gain in popularity as it becomes more available and economic; however, in the authors' opinion, the

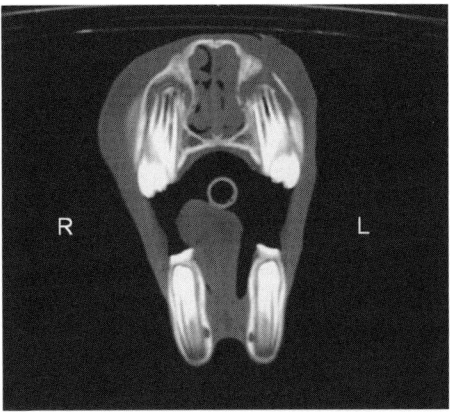

Fig. 6. Cross-sectional CT scan of an immature Miniature Horse with a draining sinus on the left side of its face. A direct communication between the external surface and the periapical region of a cheek tooth is apparent that was not visible on radiographs.

advantages of MRI over CT for dental imaging are not recognized to be sufficiently significant at this time to justify the increased expense.

Management

In early primary apical and periapical abscessation, an intensive long-term course of antimicrobials may be effective in resolving the condition, particularly in younger horses that have wider apical pulp canals and a generous blood supply. Combination therapy with trimethoprim-sulfonamide and metronidazole antimicrobials for a minimum of 6 to 8 weeks, and possibly for 12 to 16 weeks, is recommended [53]. Recurrent clinical signs after medical treatment indicate a need for tooth extraction or tooth restoration techniques. Tooth removal currently remains the most common definitive management approach to unresolved apical and periapical abscessation of equine cheek teeth. This is accomplished by repulsion [52,67–70], a lateral buccotomy, and sectioning of the tooth [68,70,71] or by oral extraction [46,68,70,72–75]. Apical curettage of infected mandibular cheek teeth with the objective of salvaging the tooth is an appropriate alternative to tooth removal in some cases [76]. Repulsion of cheek teeth has up to a 47% incidence of complications (fractured mandible or alveolus, damage to neighboring teeth, removal of the wrong tooth, loss of bone flap, sinusitis, draining tracts, loss of dental packing, retention of dental packing, damage to surrounding neurovascular structures and salivary and lacrimal ducts, dental and alveolar bone sequestration, oroantral fistula formation, and osteomyelitis) and should be reserved for patients only when oral extraction, lateral buccotomy, apical curettage, or restoration techniques are not possible [46,69]. Oral extraction is now the favored technique for tooth removal, and there are few cases in which it is not applicable. The reduced patient morbidity, postoperative complications, and expense associated with oral extraction are distinct advantages over repulsion and lateral buccotomy techniques. Advances in instrument design are being marketed regularly, increasing the versatility of oral extraction methods. For example, three-pronged arcade-specific molar forceps, narrow-profiled fragment forceps, and reverse fulcrum molar forceps have facilitated grasping of low-profile clinical crowns, root fragments, and rostral premolars, respectively. A renewed interest in local anesthesia techniques of the equine head using selective nerve blocks (maxillary, infraorbital, mandibular, and mental nerves) has also greatly facilitated standing tooth extractions in the horse [77]. In particular, the mandibular and maxillary nerve blocks are now routinely performed for extractions of cheek teeth in their respective arcades [77].

What to pack dental sockets with after tooth removal remains an area of controversy and personal preference. Plaster of Paris, dental wax, cold-curing polymethylmethacrylate bone cement, silicone, and gauze sponges have been used [70,72,73,75,78]. Antimicrobial-impregnated plaster of Paris has the advantage of being biodegradable, and thus does not need to be removed. In a series of eight horses managed with plaster of Paris, only one horse required repacking at the time of surgery and all eight horses healed without complication [78]. A longer curing time makes plaster of Paris less advantageous, particularly in standing sedated patients that have had an oral extraction.

Regardless of the method of tooth removal, for this procedure to be successful, the diseased tooth must be accurately identified. Removal of the whole tooth and damage to nothing but this tooth must then be foremost in the clinician's mind [48].

Endodontic procedures for management of periapical cheek teeth infections and occlusal surface restoration techniques for infundibular decay and exposed vital pulp tissue are being applied to equine patients with increasing frequency [50,79–81]. Endodontic treatment is most suitable for the first through third mandibular cheek teeth and for the first and second maxillary cheek teeth [68]. Its use should be restricted to horses with early periapical abscessation that have no gross occlusal surface defects or widespread periodontal disease and no gross osteomyelitis of the supporting bones [68,79,80]. It has been suggested that endodontic treatment is usually ineffective in horses with affected immature teeth because of intercommunicating pulp cavities and that a permanent tooth should have been erupted for at least 3 years to be a good candidate for treatment [82,83]. Others have found that horses with affected immature teeth respond satisfactorily [79]. The objective of endodontic treatment is to extirpate necrotic pulp and then to plug the pulp canal system so that no communication exists between the oral cavity and the periradicular tissues. Postoperative antimicrobials are used routinely, and follow-up clinical and radiographic examination is needed to assess tooth viability. The affected tooth continues to erupt normally after successful endodontic treatment. The advantages of endodontic procedures are the avoidance of considerable postoperative complications and the prevention of long-term abnormalities of wear and eruption (eg, step mouth, diastemata formation) that may follow a tooth removal procedure [68]. The disadvantages of endodontics are that the procedure is slower, necessitates general anesthesia, and requires additional specialized equipment and skills [80]. Teeth that do not maintain viability can be removed at a later date. In one study, short-term success (up to 12 months) was achieved in 60% of horses with treated teeth and long-term success (at least 24 months) was achieved in 44% of horses with treated teeth, with a slightly better outcome for mandibular cheek teeth than for maxillary cheek teeth in both time frames [79]. A lack of recognition of occlusal surface disease may have accounted for the high failure rate and poor outcome (compared with other species) after restorative apical surgery [79]. More recently, success rates up to 80% were suggested with careful case selection [79]. Periodontitis is considered incurable in its advanced stages unless the affected tooth is removed. Prevention is highly desirable. Regular oral examinations and appropriate correction of dental wear abnormalities that may initiate periodontal disease are the keys to prevention [50,84,85]. If early disease is recognized, attempts should be made to halt the process before tooth loss occurs. High-pressure irrigation of pockets (using water mixed with baking soda) can assist in cleaning, and antimicrobial preparations may then be packed into the cavity, with the area protected by impression materials [50,84]. Periodontitis that is associated with valved or closed diastema formation may be managed by physically widening the diastema to encourage easy exiting of feed material that enters the space [86].

Guttural pouch empyema and mycosis

The auditory tube diverticula (guttural pouches) present a unique challenge when infected because of their intricate anatomic relations with vital neurovascular structures and their relative inaccessibility. It is fortunate that fungal infections of the guttural pouches are less common than bacterial empyemas because they can result in rapid fatality if not diagnosed and managed in a timely manner.

Diagnosis

Physical examination findings in cases of established guttural pouch infection invariably include nasal discharge (mucopurulent to acute epistaxis) that can be bilateral, even with unilateral disease. Empyema cases may also present with painful retropharyngeal swelling, cough, inappetence or anorexia, fever, respiratory noise, dyspnea, and dysphagia [87]. Horses with mycotic infections are presented with various neurologic disorders (eg, dysphagia, Horner's syndrome, laryngeal hemiplegia); however, in the early stages of the disease, a mild greenish yellow discharge may be the first external clinical sign noted [88].

Imaging of the guttural pouches is critical in obtaining an accurate diagnosis, and for any infectious process, the use of endoscopy and radiography remains the minimal standard. In advanced disease, it may be difficult or impossible to access the pouch if the ostium is obstructed by a mass or accumulated exudate, and in cases of mycosis with acute hemorrhage, visibility is often limited by the presence of blood.

Radiography complements endoscopy, especially when endoscopy is limited by a lack of visibility. Portable machines are adequate to obtain lateral images from both sides. For unilateral disease, fluid lines and other pathologic findings should be more sharply defined when the affected side is closer to the cassette; however, this can be difficult to assess. A dorsoventral view is possible and may help to differentiate unilateral from bilateral disease. Alternatively, caudal-to-cranial oblique views from either side can separate the pouches enough to distinguish unilateral from bilateral disease [87].

Diagnosis and treatment of guttural pouch disease may also be aided by a parotid sialogram [89], carotid angiography [90,91], and ultrasonography.

Carotid angiography allows accurate evaluation of the vasculature that may be affected by mycotic infections. Ultrasonography of the retropharyngeal region may be helpful to distinguish the source and nature of space-occupying masses or swellings in that region but is not often used if endoscopy and radiology have confirmed primary guttural pouch disease. Advanced imaging with CT or MRI is used infrequently for guttural pouch infections.

Culturing of sampled exudate is required for definitive diagnosis of the causative agent in infectious guttural pouch disease. Samples are best obtained directly from the pouch via endoscopic guidance using guarded swabs or by performing a guttural pouch wash using sterile technique [87]. If access to the pouch is not possible transendoscopically, nasopharyngeal swabs may be obtained or a percutaneous guttural pouch wash can be performed [92]. Percutaneous guttural pouch lavages from clinically normal horses indicated 59% positive cultures of mostly transient flora and no fungal organisms [93]. When horses were prevented from lowering their heads for 12 or 24 hours, there was an increasing frequency of positive bacterial cultures (50%) in the 24-hour group but no fungal growth [94]. *S equi* subsp *equi* and *S equi* subsp *zooepidemicus* account for most primary bacterial infections of the guttural pouch, but other isolates include *Escherichia coli, Klebsiella* spp, *Corynebacterium* spp, *Bordetella* spp, and *Salmonella* spp [95]. Approximately one third of horses with empyema cultured positive for *S equi* subsp *equi* [95], and the predominant locale for *S equi* subsp *equi* in persistent and asymptomatic carriers is the guttural pouch [96,97]. Therefore, it is critical that any horse suspected of guttural pouch empyema be handled as an isolated infectious patient until a culture indicates the primary pathogen involved. *Aspergillus* spp (particularly *Aspergillus fumigatus*) is the most common fungus isolated from guttural pouch mycoses [98]. *Scopulariopsis* spp and *Mucor* spp were found rarely, and their pathogenic importance is not clear [98]. Emphasis on methods of establishing an early diagnosis of guttural pouch mycosis is needed to reduce the incidence of fatal hemorrhage or permanent neurologic damage [99]. Detection of antibodies to *A fumigatus* by molecular techniques has been investigated [100]. Serum antibody titers were similar on ELISA analysis for normal and infected horses; however, immunoblot analysis detected antigens specific to sera from infected horses.

Management

Empyema

Medical treatment is effective in many cases of empyema, particularly when instituted early in the disease process. Systemic anti-inflammatory drugs and culture- and sensitivity-defined antimicrobials should be administered as adjunctive therapies to lavage and drainage procedures. Endoscopic-assisted lavage or lavage via indwelling catheters (eg, Foley) can be used to get fluid into the guttural pouch [87,101,102]. With experience, catheterization of the guttural pouch can be performed without endoscopic guidance. The addition of antimicrobials or antiseptics to the lavage solution is controversial and generally not recommended because of the potential to irritate sensitive mucosa and neurovascular structures [87,95,103]. Instillation of acetylcysteine into the guttural pouch to break down mucoproteins and facilitate drainage of exudate has been used successfully [104] but not consistently [96]. When performing high-volume lavage of the guttural pouch, caution should be taken to ensure that there is appropriate outflow to match the inflow rate of the fluid being instilled. Inflamed pouches secondary to chronic empyema may rupture with increased pressure from inflowing fluids when the outflow tract is partially or completely obstructed by accumulated exudate, especially inspissated material. If wall rupture occurs, surgical exploration and drainage of the pouch are recommended to evacuate the debris that has tracked into surrounding retropharyngeal tissue planes.

Surgical access to the guttural pouch to remove large amounts of inspissated purulent material and to establish drainage is frequently considered as a last resort because of the apparent high risk of adverse side effects associated with surgical trauma to the cranial nerves. In chronic cases of empyema with significant accumulation of exudate (particularly chondroids), however, it may be more economic and effective to perform a surgical procedure early in the management plan. The favored external surgical approach to the guttural pouch is the modified Whitehouse incision, with the horse in dorsal recumbency [105]. Access through Viborg's triangle can be accomplished in the standing horse but does not provide the most dependent ventral drainage. Once all the major debris has been extracted, a balloon-tipped Foley catheter can be passed through the surgical incision into the pouch and sutured to the skin to facilitate standing lavage of the pouch after surgery. Excellent ventral drainage is achieved using a modified Whitehouse approach, and once the pouch appears clean on endoscopic examination, the catheter can be removed and the surgical wound allowed to heal by second intention.

A less invasive surgical approach to create a permanent or temporary drainage route is laser-assisted fistulation of the guttural pouch via transendoscopic guidance [106]. This procedure is similar to that used for management of guttural pouch tympany [107] and is relatively economic to perform in the standing sedated horse. The fistula is made in the dorsocaudal pharyngeal wall adjacent the normal salpingopharyngeal orifice and allows for passive drainage of the pouch when the horse lowers its head to eat or drink. Alternatively, laser-assisted fenestration of the guttural pouch median septum can be performed from the normal side to access an infected guttural pouch if the salpingopharyngeal orifice is obstructed on the diseased side [108]. There are isolated case reports of successful removal of chondroids via endoscopy from the guttural pouches without the need for surgery [109,110]. These cases involved relatively small chondroids up to 3 cm in diameter that were easily sectioned and snared for retrieval or that eventually dissolved with long-term lavaging [109,110].

Mycosis

The current need for medical treatment of guttural pouch mycosis remains questionable [111]. The use of antifungal agents in the horse is limited by expense, difficult effective topical application in the guttural pouch, and lack of known efficacy after topical or systemic administration. There are real risks of advancing disease causing a fatal epistatic event or permanent neurologic dysfunction if medical treatment alone is chosen [112,113]. Isolated case reports of successful medical treatment exist, however, and various antifungal agents (eg, iconazole, itraconazole, enilconazole) have been used [114]. Mechanical removal of the plaque and cryosurgery are not recommended treatment options because of the high risk of epistaxis and damage to adjacent vital neurovascular structures.

Innovative surgical approaches to the treatment of guttural pouch mycosis have been directed at reducing the risk of fatal hemorrhage by occluding vessels that have already been compromised by fungal invasion or that may be susceptible to fungal invasion in the near future. For reasons that are not clear, after surgical thrombosis of adjacent vessels has occurred, it is common for fungal plaques to retract and disappear on their own accord without further medical intervention [88,111]. Fungal plaque regression may take 8 to 16 weeks before there is no visible endoscopic evidence of disease [88,111,115]. Most frequently, hemorrhage occurs from the internal carotid artery (ICA), but the external carotid and maxillary arteries may also be affected [116–119]. Classically, the simplest way to induce thrombosis of the ICA was to ligate it just distal to its origin on the common carotid artery. This approach has been quite effective and may be a reasonable (and more economic) treatment option in cases of early diagnosis of mycosis in which hemorrhage does not seem to be an imminent threat [120–122]. Often, the occipital artery is ligated at the same time, because the vascular anatomy can be variable, and without intraoperative angiography, it may be difficult to definitively differentiate the ICA from the occipital vessel [120]. Ligation of the ICA near its origin does not alter blood pressure distal to the ligature (at least for 3 days), however, indicating significant retrograde blood flow from the circle of Willis [123]. Therefore, ligation of the ICA at its origin alone does not prevent hemorrhage from fungal invasion of an arterial wall more distally until the vessel has thrombosed to the level of the lesion. This potential problem was addressed by balloon-tipped catheter embolization of affected arteries so that arterial flow could be occluded on the proximal (cardiac) side and distal (cerebral) side of the fungal plaque and compromised segment of vessel [118,124]. Results with this technique have been favorable [116]. Catheters may also be inserted into the maxillary artery and into the external carotid artery to eliminate normograde and retrograde flow in those vessels if they are affected by the fungal plaque [117]. Complications of the balloon-tipped catheterization technique include failure of cuff inflation, premature cuff leakage, protrusion of the catheter through the vessel wall defect (Fig. 7), infection at catheter insertion sites,

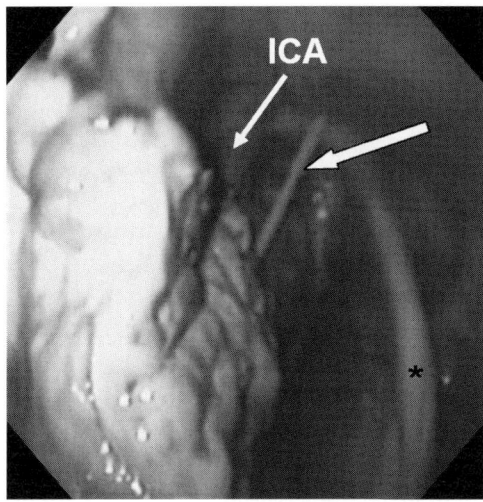

Fig. 7. Endoscopic view of balloon-tipped catheter (balloon has deflated, *arrow*) protruding through a defect in the left internal carotid artery (ICA) created by an eroding fungal plaque (present in left foreground). The stylohyoid bone is indicated by an asterisk.

breakage of the catheter, cosmetic blemish with the buried subcutaneous catheter at the ICA site, the need for multiple catheter insertion sites in some cases, and the need for catheter removal [116–118]. Blindness secondary to optic ischemia has been reported as a complication when the external carotid artery and its branches have been occluded during a single operation [119,125]. It is proposed that a significant reduction in blood flow to the eye is the result of a "steal phenomenon," whereby collateral flow into the external ophthalmic artery is preferentially drawn into the larger maxillary and major palatine arterial trees [126]. The risk of blindness may be related to the method of normograde and retrograde occlusion of the arterial supply in the external carotid and maxillary arteries [126]. Aberrant vascular anatomy can result in unsuccessful catheter occlusion and death of the horse secondary to hemorrhage [127,128], and carotid angiography is an excellent imaging method to assess vascular supply before surgery is undertaken to occlude a vessel [90,129].

The most recent advance in vessel thrombosis techniques for the horse uses intraoperative angiography to facilitate transarterial coil embolization [130,131] or detachable latex balloon occlusion [129,132] of affected arteries. One coil embolization technique is performed via a common carotid arteriotomy in the proximal neck and has the desirable qualities of being minimally invasive, safe, quick, and effective. Management of guttural pouch mycosis with this approach has been described in 31 horses with excellent long-term results [115]. Unfortunately, the need for fluoroscopy and a custom-designed Plexiglas head and neck table to enable its use may currently limit the practicality of this technique in many surgical practices. Latex balloons were inserted via an ICA arteriotomy after a modified hyovertebrotomy approach. This technique is more amenable to radiographic angiography and is also safe and effective. Regardless of the vessel thrombosis technique, intraoperative angiography should be strongly considered in all cases to reduce the risk of life-threatening complications associated with a failure to identify and correctly occlude all affected arteries.

Ocular structures

Infectious corneal diseases

The equine cornea is composed of five layers: stratified squamous epithelium, epithelial basement membrane, stroma, Descemet's membrane, and the corneal endothelium from the outer to inner layers. The eyelids, preocular tear film, resident flora, and corneal epithelium form an effective barrier that prevents entry and colonization of the collagen-rich avascular corneal stroma by microorganisms [133–136]. Fungi and gram-positive bacteria (gram-negative bacteria make up a small portion) are part of the normal resident flora of the equine cornea and conjunctiva resulting from their environment [137]. Predictably, ocular flora varies based on the geographic location of the horse and weather conditions [138].

Etiologies and diagnosis

Most microorganisms do not invade the cornea easily but require trauma, tissue devitalization, or immunologic compromise for infection [139]. Infectious corneal diseases are often suspected based on clinical signs, such as blepharospasm, epiphora, and corneal edema, as well as on miosis attributable to secondary uveitis. The diagnosis of a corneal ulcer is made with positive fluorescein stain uptake by the exposed stroma (Fig. 8). In cases with corneal stromal abscesses, the cornea is often fluorescein-negative;

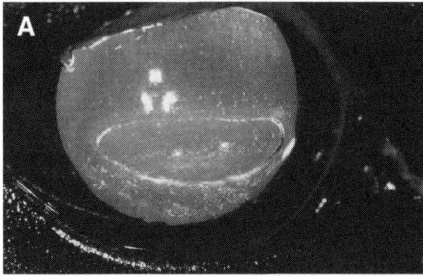
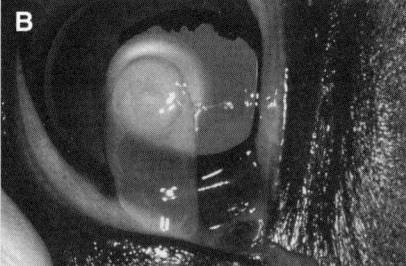

Fig. 8. Corneal ulceration. (*A*) Uncomplicated superficial corneal ulcer without stromal loss. The pupil is dilated because of treatment with topical atropine sulfate. (*B*) Melting corneal ulcer with severe keratomalacia. The exposed corneal stroma appears fluorescein-positive.

the infectious nature of the disease has to be suspected based on the clinical appearance, because the lesion is not accessible by the usual sampling techniques.

Fungi and bacteria can pose a serious problem to the corneal stroma if the defense mechanisms of the epithelium are overwhelmed or dysfunctional [140]. Once in the stroma, bacteria are able to spread through the collagen lamellae, whereas fungi generally burrow deep in the stroma toward Descemet's membrane [140]. Corneal stromal abscesses then form if the bacteria or fungi are sealed into the stroma when epithelial cells close the epithelial defect that originally allowed the infectious organisms to enter the stroma [140–143]. The diagnosis of stromal abscesses is generally based on their appearance of a white-yellow stromal infiltrate with variable amounts of corneal edema, neovascularization, and iridocyclitis (Fig. 9) [141–143]. The differential diagnosis for stromal abscesses includes other nonulcerative corneal diseases, such as immune-mediated keratitis [144,145].

In the case of ulcerative keratitis, the potentially involved infectious agent can be identified by aerobic and fungal culture as well as by cytologic examination of a corneal scraping (eg, Gram stain). Although *Staphylococcus* spp, *Streptococcus* spp, and *Pseudomonas* spp are the most commonly isolated bacteria [146], *Aspergillus* spp and *Fusarium* spp are the most commonly isolated fungi in infectious keratopathies [147]. Geographic location and the associated change in climate result in varied fungal etiologies as well as frequency of ocular disease. A retrospective study performed at the College of Veterinary Medicine of the University of Georgia suggests that the frequency of equine fungal keratitis may increase during or after periods of draft and warm temperature [148]. A retrospective evaluation of the most common fungi isolated from horses with fungal keratitis at the New Bolton Center of the University of Pennsylvania in 2004 included *Aspergillus flavus*, *A fumigatus*, and *Fusarium* spp.

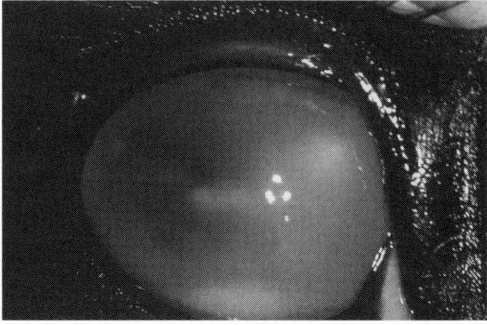

Fig. 9. A yellow-white stromal abscess is visible dorsomedially in the cornea. Corneal vascularization is present along the entire limbus. In this patient, the abscess is associated with severe anterior uveitis recognizable by the generalized corneal edema, hypopyon, and miotic pupil.

Fungal keratitis can be a diagnostic and management challenge, because, as opposed to bacterial keratitis, culture can take several days to weeks. Cytology complements culturing because it may reveal septate or branching fungal hyphae on the day of the initial presentation. Special stains, including Gomori methenamine silver, periodic acid–Schiff, Wright's, and Giemsa, are helpful in their identification. A polymerase chain reaction (PCR) assay is more timely than fungal culture results and may lead to more appropriate treatment [149]. A PCR assay is less specific than fungal culture; therefore, the possibility of false-positive results with PCR needs to be considered [149]. Real-time PCR is currently being studied at the Ohio State University to aid in the identification of fungal elements from horses with infectious keratitis [150]. It may prove to be a quick and effective diagnostic tool [150].

Equine herpesvirus (EHV) type 2 has been recognized as an infectious etiologic agent with equine keratitis and keratoconjunctivitis. Horses affected are usually presented with multifocal, diffuse, punctate opacities that may or may not retain fluorescein dye but are often positive with rose bengal dye [151]. EHV-2 may also manifest as a cornea with more diffuse superficial opacification or with more sparse lacy opacities that are variable in stain retention (Fig. 10) [152]. Diagnosis is usually based on clinical signs and response to therapy. Virus isolation or faster and more sensitive techniques, such as nested PCR analysis on citrated blood or ocular and nasal swabs (with ocular swabs being the most important sample), can aid in cases with suspected viral keratitis [153,154]. Detection of a viral etiology may be difficult, bearing in mind that clinically normal horses may also test positive for EHV-2 [155].

Medical therapy

In general, medical therapy is aimed at treating the inciting infectious cause that has been identified by cytology or culture. Antimicrobial choices should be based on susceptibility testing, although for fungal organisms, this

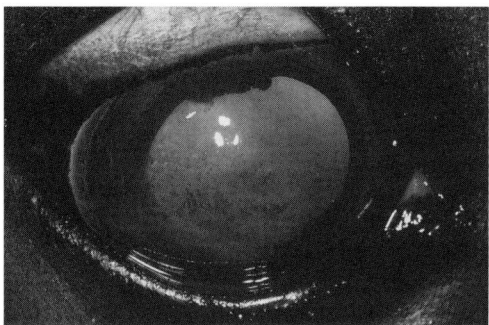

Fig. 10. Superficial keratitis recognizable by the irregular corneal surface. The cornea is fluorescein-negative, but there is diffuse multifocal rose bengal stain uptake, which could indicate a viral or early fungal infection. Corneal culture and cytology are indicated.

information may not be obtainable within the critical time frame for the treatment of a case. In cases with keratomalacia (stromal and melting ulcers), antiproteases are also used. The secondary anterior uveitis is addressed with topical atropine sulfate and systemic NSAIDs to effect. Systemic antimicrobials may be indicated for deep corneal infections and are definitely indicated in any case with corneal perforation. Medications that are commonly used for suspected viral keratitis include antiviral agents and topical (diclofenac 0.1% or flurbiprofen 0.03%) as well as systemic anti-inflammatory agents (flunixin meglumine, 1.1 mg/kg) [151]. Some recommendations have been made to use glucocorticoids (dexamethasone or prednisolone acetate) as anti-inflammatory and potential immunosuppressive agents [153,156]. The use of these drugs is cautioned, however, because the diagnosis of viral keratitis can be difficult to make. Topical NSAIDs may prove to be a safer choice and may be used in combination with antivirals.

Antimicrobial agents

First-choice topical antimicrobials include triple antibiotics (neomycin-polymyxin B-bacitracin or neomycin-polymyxin B-gramicidin) and chloramphenicol. Most other topical antimicrobials should be used only if there is a strong suggestion of infection with certain microorganisms based on clinical appearance, cytology, or culture and sensitivity testing. These antimicrobials include ciprofloxacin, amikacin, oxytetracycline, and cefazolin [147]. The authors routinely use the antimicrobial combination of tobramycin and cefazolin in cases with severe keratomalacia that may be infected by *Pseudomonas* spp or β-hemolytic *Streptococcus* spp [137]. Increasing resistance of isolates from the equine cornea to ophthalmic antimicrobials has been reported, including resistance of *S equi* subsp *zooepidemicus* to gentamicin or *Pseudomonas aeruginosa* to tobramycin [146]. Ciprofloxacin 0.3% was shown in normal equine eyes to reach mean tear concentrations after topical application greater than the minimal inhibitory concentration (MIC) for common equine bacteria isolates (*S equi* subsp *zooepidemicus*, *Staphylococcus* spp, and *P aeruginosa*) for 6 hours after administration [157]. The pharmacokinetics of ciprofloxacin and many ocular drugs in the ulcerated equine cornea have yet to be studied and may indeed be different from those in the normal equine eye.

The in vitro effect of topical antimicrobials on canine corneal epithelial cells has recently been studied [158]. Antimicrobials used included ciprofloxacin, cefazolin, neomycin-polymyxin B-gramicidin, gentamicin sulfate, tobramycin, and chloramphenicol. Ciprofloxacin and cefazolin were most detrimental to epithelial morphology and caused rounding and shrinkage, with detachment of the cells from the plate. Gentamicin had greater cytopathologic effects and slowed cell migration when compared with tobramycin. Neomycin-polymyxin B-gramicidin had intermediate effects on the epithelial cells and cell migration. Chloramphenicol and tobramycin were least detrimental on the epithelial cells [158]. This study, although on canine corneal epithelial cells, illustrates what we often observe anecdotally in many ulcerative keratitis cases in horses. Noninfected superficial corneal ulcers seem to heal faster once dosing frequency decreases, which may be attributable to the cytotoxic effects of routinely used drugs.

Antifungal agents

Antifungal agents that have been used topically in horses are the polyenes (eg, amphotericin-B 0.15%, natamycin 5%), imidazoles (eg, miconazole 1%, ketoconazole 1%, fluconazole 2%, itraconazole 1%), iodides, and silver sulfadiazine (SSD). In general, these drugs penetrate the cornea poorly, which makes the treatment of deep fungal keratitis difficult [149]. Recent formulations of topical 1% itraconazole have included dimethyl sulfoxide (DMSO) 30% for better corneal penetration [159].

Over the past 15 to 20 years, the following sensitivities of fungal isolates were determined at the University of Pennsylvania: *Fusarium* spp isolates were only sensitive to natamycin and nystatin, and *Aspergillus* spp isolates had a wider spectrum of drug sensitivities, including clotrimazole, ketoconazole, itraconazole, amphotericin-B, and nystatin. The *Aspergillus* spp isolates were most consistently sensitive to itraconazole. These sensitivity patterns may be useful when treating horses with keratomycosis in the mid-Atlantic region. Similarly, fungal sensitivities were evaluated at the University of Florida. *Aspergillus* spp and *Fusarium* spp were the most commonly isolated fungi (16 of 22 cases of ulcerative keratomycosis), and susceptibilities against the following were found in decreasing order: natamycin and miconazole equally, itraconazole, and ketoconazole, with no significant difference among drugs [160]. Fluconazole was found to be significantly less effective compared with the other drugs against fungi, however [160].

A study from Cornell University demonstrated itraconazole 1%–DMSO 30% to be effective against most fungal agents responsible for keratitis in the northeastern United States [159]. SSD has been used in the past as a topical treatment for equine fungal keratitis. In vitro studies comparing SSD versus natamycin against 17 filamentous fungal isolates (13 of the 17 included *Fusarium* spp and *Aspergillus* spp) showed SSD to be fungistatic and fungicidal against all the fungal isolates [161]. Natamycin was fungistatic and fungicidal only to some of the equine fungal isolates at the drug doses used in the study [161]. SSD may provide another form of effective topical medical treatment that should be revisited in cases of equine keratomycosis.

Oral administration of antifungal agents has been used in conjunction with topical treatment in more severe and deep fungal keratitis. Systemic administration is limited by the cost of treatment in the horse as well as by questionable absorption of the antifungal agent and concentrations reached in the cornea and potential systemic side effects. In normal horses, the maximum plasma concentration and terminal half-life of fluconazole after intravenous and oral dosing were similar when used at 10 mg/kg [162]. Fluconazole also reached concentrations greater than the MIC (8.0 mg/mL) for fungus in plasma, cerebrospinal fluid (CSF), synovial fluid, aqueous humor, and urine after long-term oral administration (14-mg/kg loading dose, followed by 5 mg/kg every 24 hours for 10 days) [162]. Pharmacokinetic analysis of systemically administered itraconazole has recently been performed [163]. Normal horses were given two types of oral formulations (solution and capsule) at a dose of 5 mg/kg as well as intravenous itraconazole at dose of 1.5 mg/kg [163]. The itraconazole solution reached plasma concentrations that would be effective against most fungal pathogens in horses, especially *Aspergillus* spp, and may be more economically feasible than the intravenous form, which was also shown to reach therapeutic concentrations against *Aspergillus* spp [163]. However, this may not be clinically relevant as the blood-aqueous barrier is broken down with anterior uveitis. Systemic itraconazole did not reach significant aqueous humor concentrations in the normal horses studied [163]. A newer antifungal, voriconazole, has been evaluated topically and orally in the normal horse in terms of the aqueous humor concentration reached [164]. Topical voriconazole at three different concentrations (0.5%, 1.0%, and 3.0%) was given every 4 hours for a total of seven treatments, and aqueous humor levels were then measured 1 hour after the last dose [164]. Signs of ocular toxicity (eg, blepharospasm, epiphora, chemosis) were seen using the 3% voriconazole; however, the 1% and 3% voriconazole concentrations reached significantly higher levels in the aqueous humor compared with the 0.5% solution [164]. The antifungal agent was detectable in the plasma after the final dose at each concentration [164]. Two and a half hours after a single dose of oral voriconazole, aqueous humor concentrations were found that would likely be therapeutic based on reported MICs of fungi [164]. Further studies to evaluate voriconazole in ulcerated and inflamed equine eyes likely need to be performed, because drug effectiveness may differ in the diseased eye.

Antiviral agents

The most commonly used topical antiviral agents are idoxuridine 0.1% and trifluridine 1%. Initially, they should be used at more frequent intervals (4–12 times per day) and can then be decreased to 3 to 6 times per day when the cornea shows improvement (usually in 3–5 days) [151]. L-lysine is being used in cats to aid in decreasing virus replication and controlling keratoconjunctivitis caused by feline herpesvirus-1 [165,166]. Commercial supplements are also widely available for horses, and the suggested dosage varies from 10 to 30 g/d for potentially long-term treatment [151]. To the best of our knowledge, no studies have been performed regarding the effectiveness of L-lysine in the treatment of herpesvirus infection in horses.

Other agents

The cornea relies on certain inherent substances for protection and healing, including peptide growth factors locally and systemically as well as matrix metalloproteinases (MMPs) in the precorneal tear film [167,168]. The MMP proteolytic activity is generally held in check by protease inhibitors so as to prevent destruction of normal corneal tissue [169]. It has been shown that MMP2, MMP9, and neutrophil elastase are increased in the tear film with ulcerative keratitis, indicating increased proteolytic activity [170,171]. *P aeruginosa* and *Aspergillus* spp have been determined to produce MMPs directly, whereas other pathogens may induce endogenous corneal proteases or cytokines (from corneal epithelium and inflammatory cells) during ulceration [140,169,172–176]. Treatments aimed at decreasing MMP activity have included autogenous serum (contains α_2-macroglobulin), 0.2% ethylenediaminetetraacetic acid (EDTA), 0.1% doxycycline, ilomostat (solution of modified dipeptide that contains hydroxamic acid), and 10% *N*-acetylcysteine [169]. Several treatments have different mechanisms of action against MMPs, and thus have been suggested for use in combination for maximum effect [169]. Serum has been shown to have the broadest spectrum against proteases likely attributable to α_2-macroglobulin, which is a nonspecific protease inhibitor, and EDTA and ilomostat had the highest inhibitory action on MMPs in the equine tear film in vitro [169]. These substances generally have few adverse affects and should potentially be used in cases of ulcerative keratitis to decrease the digestion of the cornea by proteolytic enzymes [169].

Different types of growth factors have been evaluated that potentially speed corneal healing and include epidermal growth factor (EGF) [177]. In horses the beneficial effects of topical EGF application on the corneal healing were outweighed by the intensity of the associated inflammatory response [178]. In the future, growth factors may provide a valuable therapy in corneal ulceration.

Surgical therapy

Surgical treatment should be considered in conjunction with medical treatment of infectious corneal disease if the ulcer is deeper than one third of the corneal stroma, keratomalacia is present, or the lesion fails to respond to medical treatment alone [179]. Surgical treatment options include keratectomy to remove the diseased cornea and placement of a conjunctival graft to provide mechanical support as well as a blood supply with healing factors and systemic antimicrobials [180,181]. Corneal transplantation in horses is generally indicated if conjunctival grafts alone cannot provide sufficient mechanical support (tectonic graft) [182]. Generally, fresh or frozen corneal tissue from a donor horse is implanted. The graft is usually invaded by blood vessels; therefore, it does not remain clear [140,182–184].

A variety of surgical options have been described to remove corneal stromal abscesses, including penetrating keratoplasty (PK), posterior lamellar keratoplasty (PLK), deep lamellar endothelial keratoplasty (DLEK), keratectomy with a conjunctival flap, and corneal conjunctival transposition [179,181,185]. PLK and DLEK may be more appropriate surgical options for deep (posterior) stromal abscesses. The advantage of PLK is that it preserves the corneal epithelium and anterior stroma, which seems to allow for faster corneal neovascularization and subsequent healing [184]. DLEK resulted in faster healing times in four of six horses with deep limbal stromal abscesses [185]. From excised stromal abscesses in horses in which a PLK was performed, cultures were positive for infectious agents in only 50% of patients; however, histopathologic examination was used to detect an infectious etiology in 62.5% [184]. This demonstrates that histopathologic examination is likely to be a more sensitive diagnostic technique and aids in directing therapy after surgery.

PK has been used primarily in full-thickness corneal stromal abscesses [181]. The corneal epithelium and anterior stroma are not preserved; therefore, a pedicle conjunctival graft may need to be placed over the corneal graft for mechanical support and an improved blood supply [181]. More complications are reported with larger diameter (>6–8 mm) compared with smaller diameter (<6 mm) abscesses with PK and PLK [182,184].

Other natural and synthetic grafting materials have been proposed in the human and veterinary literature for corneal repair. Porcine small intestinal submucosa (SIS) has been used in dogs, cats, and horses with full-thickness corneal defects [186]. The SIS grafts were sutured to the equine cornea to cover the defect, and a conjunctival flap was placed over the graft for additional mechanical support and blood supply [186].

Harvested and frozen equine amniotic membrane has been used in cases of corneal ulceration and keratomalacia that were refractory to appropriate medical therapy [187]. Three horses that were treated at the College of Veterinary Medicine of the University of Florida have recently been described [187]. Each horse had severe keratomalacia that covered 50% or more of the cornea and was nonresponsive to medical therapy [187]. An amniotic membrane transplant (AMT) was sutured onto the cornea so that the corneal ulcers were covered; no conjunctival graft was placed [187]. Each horse had vision, although limited, after treatment and returned to their previous function [187]. AMTs may provide an alternative to conjunctival grafts, which often result in large corneal scars and decreased vision compared with normal. AMTs seem to have improved ability to survive in the face of proteases that may digest conjunctival grafts [187]. Studies in murine viral stromal keratitis treated with AMTs showed actual reduced expression and activity of MMP-8 and MMP-9 and increased expression of certain tissue inhibitors of MMPs compared with normal [188]. In human patients, AMTs are being used in conjunction with fibrin glue for corneal perforations secondary to ulceration with good success [189].

Biosynthetic corneas have been developed as alternatives to cornea grafts and AMTs because they may be more readily available and easier to store.

They could offer a low rejection rate, and thus an improved visual outcome [190]. One such biosynthetic cornea has recently been used in normal dogs [190]. It consisted of glutaraldehyde cross-linked collagen and copolymers of collagen and poly (*N*-isopropylacryamide-co-acrylic acid-co-acryloxysuccinimide) [190]. The corneal implants were quickly covered by corneal epithelium, with no rejection of the implant noted, and resulted in minimal corneal haze [190].

Other biomaterials being studied in human ophthalmology include corneal prosthetics made partially of hexaethyleneglycolmethacrylate and butylmethacrylate, with promising results for surgical corneal repair [191]. Human corneal epithelial stem cells in a cross-linked fibrin gel have shown potential as a stable and compatible corneal tissue replacement that may provide possibilities for the equine eye [149].

Equine recurrent uveitis

Etiologies and diagnosis

ERU is the leading cause of blindness in horses in the United States [192–195]. Recent developments in the treatment of ERU have improved the veterinarian's ability to achieve a better visual outcome, however. Also known as moon blindness, iridocyclitis, and periodic ophthalmia, ERU is an immune-mediated panuveitis typically seen in horses older than 4 years of age [192–195]. The inciting cause of the initial uveitis event, and subsequent ERU, is often unknown, but many infectious causes have been discussed, including bacterial (eg, *Leptospira* spp, *Brucella* spp, *Rhodococcus equi*, *Borrelia burgdorferi*), viral (eg, equine influenza, equine viral arteritis, parainfluenza type 3, EHV-1 and EHV-2), and parasitic (eg, *Onchocerca* spp, *Strongylus* spp, *Toxoplasma* spp) agents [196].

ERU can be classified based on anatomic location (ie, anterior uveitis involving the iris, ciliary body, and anterior chamber versus posterior uveitis with inflammation in the vitreous, retina, and choroid) [196]. Panuveitis is inflammation of the anterior and posterior segments of the eye [196]. Further classification of uveitis includes the type: "classic ERU" and "insidious ERU" [196]. Classic ERU is the most common form and is recognized by an acute active inflammatory phase (manifested as a painful eye, with corneal edema, miosis, and conjunctival hyperemia) involving primarily anterior segments, followed by variable periods of dormancy (Fig. 11) [196]. Uveitis bouts recur and are generally more severe each time; they eventually lead to visual deficits or blindness if left untreated [196]. Insidious ERU is generally less severe and chronic and affects draft breeds and Appaloosas [196]. When evaluating a horse presenting with uveitis, it is important to determine whether there is an obvious underlying problem, such as corneal or systemic disease. Tools to aid in the diagnosis of uveitis include thorough physical and ophthalmic examination, hematology and serum chemistry, and serum titers for various infectious diseases depending on the geographic region.

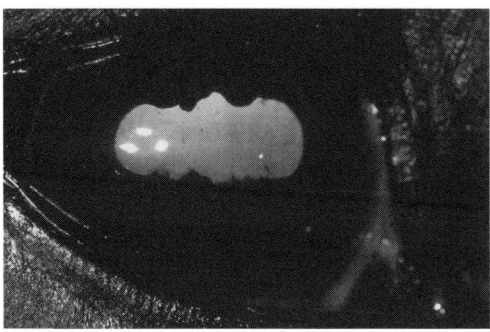

Fig. 11. Classic form of ERU with signs of anterior uveitis. Posterior synechiae with focal cataract formation and dark discoloration of the iris are indications of the chronicity of the disease. The yellowish reflection through the pupil is caused by inflammatory debris accumulating in the vitreous.

Many studies have investigated how an episode of uveitis develops into ERU, and it is thought that at least a portion of the disease process is immune mediated. Questions still remain, however, regarding the role of infectious agents in recurrent uveitis episodes [197]. Models demonstrating the autoimmune component of the disease have recently included determination of the type of inflammation and humoral and T-cell–mediated immune responses to retinal antigens [197–199]. Equine leukocyte antigen (ELA) typing has been used to determine whether the patient is susceptible to developing ERU [200,201]. Links between ERU and leptospirosis have been made with serologic and ocular fluid agglutinin, indicating the role of leptospirosis in ERU in many cases around the world [196,202]. It has already been determined that the equine cornea and *Leptospira* spp share some antigenic identity, supporting the fact that ERU is at least partially an organ-specific autoimmune disease [196,203–205].

The question remains as to what is the inciting cause for the likely autoimmunity. *Leptospira interrogans* serovar *pomona* has been implicated as the infectious cause of the autoimmune reaction. The prevalence of seropositive horses in affected populations has been shown to be high, with up to 56% of ERU cases positive for *L interrogans* serovar *pomona* in a New York river valley [206]. Conclusions from these studies suggest that a high positive titer (ie, ≥1:400) for *L interrogans* serovar *pomona* is a contributing factor for horses that may develop ERU [207]. Recent studies have shown, however, that serovars other than *pomona* also contain a DNA sequence with antigen sequences similar to the equine cornea; therefore, other serovars and strains are likely pathogenic [205]. The difficulty in diagnosis includes the fact that the uveitis episode usually occurs months to years after horses have been naturally or experimentally infected and serologic testing may not be indicative of the current disease state [202,208–211]. Serum leptospiral titers may persist for longer than 7 years [212]. Studies have found that higher antibody titers in the aqueous humor, or vitreous, to leptospiral serovars are suggestive of a causative role when compared with serum antibody titers [213,214]. Most of our equine patients from the mid-Atlantic region that underwent sampling of aqueous humor or vitreous are PCR-negative for *Leptospira* spp despite positive serum antibody titers. This finding is supported by Faber and colleagues [202], who found that positive serologic results were not predicative of aqueous PCR status. In addition, they found that horses with positive PCR assay results and culture from the aqueous were serologically negative [202]. It is difficult to grow leptospiral organisms in culture, and studies have shown that PCR is a more dependable tool for detecting leptospires [202].

The role of Lyme disease, *B burgdorferi*, has also been questioned in relation to ERU. Several horses affected by ERU and seen at the University of Pennsylvania in 2005 have had extremely high serum titers for Lyme disease. One study conducted several years ago showed no significant correlation between clinical signs of ERU and increased serum antibody titers against *B burgdorferi*, however [215]. The highest serum titers were noted 1 month later than the activity of the transmitting tick (*Ixodes ricinus*) in May and November [215]. It is likely still valuable to run serum titers and a Western blot analysis for Lyme disease on horses presented with uveitis [196].

Treatment of equine recurrent uveitis

Once the diagnosis of ERU has been made, clients should be educated as to its insidious nature, long-term care requirements, and financial commitments. Treatment is aimed at reducing ocular inflammation and is often symptomatic, because there is no cure for ERU. In general, mydriatics, and anti-inflammatory drugs (systemic and topical) have been the mainstay of treatment. Treatment should be tapered once clinical signs show improvement, because most medical therapies may result in adverse side effects in the horse, including gastric or colonic ulceration, nephrotoxicity, and laminitis.

Vaccination against leptospirosis has recently been evaluated for decreasing the recurrence of ERU [216]. Forty-one horses diagnosed with ERU were included in the study, and half received a vaccine containing six serovars of *L interrogans* serovars *bratislava, canicola, hardjo, icterohemorragica,* and *pomona* and *L kershneri* serovar *grippotyphosa*). Blood samples were drawn for antibody titers and ophthalmic examinations were performed several times over a 12-month period [216]. Results showed that the vaccinated horses had significantly increased days to recurrence (median of 126 days in experimental groups after second vaccination versus median of 86 days in control groups) [216]. Vaccination did not protect against progression of the disease; therefore, its use is not advocated at this time [216].

Systemic antimicrobials aimed at treating suspected infectious causes of ERU have also been used. Doxycycline (10 mg/kg administered every 12 hours for 28 days) has been used to treat horses with suspected or confirmed *Leptospira* spp infections (B.C. Gilger, DVM, MS, unpublished data, 2004). Lyme disease, also suspected to trigger ERU in the horse, has traditionally been treated with oral doxycycline. Recent studies have shown that intravenous tetracycline treatments are most effective at eliminating persistent infection with *B burgdorferi* in horses and ponies, and thus may be useful in ERU medical management [217].

Inroads have been made in the management of ERU via surgical techniques. One surgical approach to controlling ERU is pars plana vitrectomy (PPV). In one European report, 38 eyes with ERU underwent this procedure, and cessation of uveitis was seen in 85% of affected eyes [218]. The goals of PPV are to improve vision and to decrease the recurrence rate and severity of uveitis by removing inflammatory debris, potential immune mediators, and antigens (eg, leptospiral organisms) [218–221]. During the procedure, the vitreal cavity was irrigated with a balanced saline solution containing gentamicin at a dose of 0.2 mg/mL [218]. The gentamicin may have played a role in attenuating inflammation and eliminating residual organisms. Complications of PPV included cataract development or progression and vision loss [218]. More than 1200 affected eyes have undergone PPV at the University of Munich, and a success rate of 98% was reported, with no recurrence of ERU in horses that had minimal or no ocular inflammation at the time of surgery [222]. PPV has seen more success in Europe (mostly in warmbloods) than in the United States (mostly in Appaloosas and the Quarter Horses) [223]. It is possible that the disease recognized in Europe differs in that it has a primary posterior segment presentation that may be more responsive to PPV [223].

Another management option for ERU includes the use of intravitreal injections of gentamicin at a dose of 4 mg [224]. Eighteen eyes were included in one study that had follow-up ranging from 62 to 781 days [224]. Seventeen of the 18 eyes had no recurrence of uveitis episodes; however, a small number of eyes lost vision after injection [224]. The suspected mechanism is gentamicin's antimicrobial effect, although only 3 of 12 eyes tested via PCR assay were positive for *Leptospira* spp [224]. Intravitreal gentamicin may offer another option in terms of decreasing the frequency of uveitis bouts, and thus decreasing the costs associated with managing a horse with ERU.

Cyclosporin A (CsA) is a peptide capable of inhibiting the transcription of intraocular interleukin (IL)-2, which is found in high concentrations in horses with chronic ERU, and in decreasing T-cell activation, which is likely partially responsible for uveitis recurrence [225]. Topically applied CsA does not penetrate the intact equine cornea and sclera effectively [226,227]. Therefore, intravitreal and, more recently, suprachoroidal matrix reservoir devices have been developed that slowly release CsA over years. In horses with experimental uveitis, the chronic intravitreal release of CsA led to decreases in the severity and duration of uveitis episodes, number of T lymphocytes present, and IL-2 concentration in the eye [225]. Histologically, the eyes showed fewer pathologic changes resulting from inflammation, and there were no complications associated with the implant device [225]. Long-term follow-up (12 months) by this group showed the CsA implant to be well tolerated [228].

A recent prospective multicentric study tested the suprachoroidal bioerodible cyclosporine device in 63 eyes with ERU [229]. Except for 6 eyes that displayed blindness, 57 eyes had a clinically important decrease in the recurrence of uveitis flares, with no reported postoperative complications [229]. The use of the sustained release cyclosporine device in the suprachoroidal space holds promise for decreasing episodes and progression of ERU.

Ocular manifestation of systemic diseases

Certain systemic diseases have been increasingly recognized in the horse over the past 10 to 15 years, and their effect on the equine eye has been explored. Such diseases are generally recognized as causing various neurologic deficits in an affected horse. In general, any horse presented for systemic disease should have an ophthalmic examination.

Equine protozoal myeloencephalitis (EPM) has not yet been described in association with ocular changes [230]; however, it is likely that many horses are diagnosed in the field by clinical signs (eg, asymmetric hind limb ataxia, weakness) and that full ophthalmic examinations are not performed. Cerebral or brain stem lesions caused by EPM may lead to vision loss [231], and it is advisable to perform an ophthalmic examination on any horse suspected of having EPM.

The viral encephalitides have gained attention in recent years. Togaviruses (including Eastern, Western, and Venezuelan equine encephalomyelitis) cause progressive neurologic signs, including cerebral, cerebrocortical, and cranial nerve deficits, that manifest as blindness, facial nerve paralysis, ataxia, paresis, and proprioceptive deficits [232–234].

West Nile virus, a flavivirus, causes encephalitis and often manifests as fever, hind limb ataxia, recumbency, and muscle fasciculations [235,236]. Ocular changes that have been identified include unilateral or bilateral facial nerve paralysis and associated consequences to the globe [230]. Other reports have included loss of menace [235] and blindness possibly secondary to encephalitis [230].

Summary

Diagnostic and treatment advances in recent years for infections of the equine head have included improvements in imaging techniques and equipment as well as the development of less invasive and less traumatic surgical procedures. These advances have resulted in more accurate case diagnoses and less morbidity for our patients. Future investigations into the pathogenesis of the conditions discussed in this article should further enhance our ability to make a timely diagnosis and perhaps to reduce the frequency of complications associated with advanced disease. In addition, advances in diagnosis as well as medical and surgical techniques have improved the visual outcome of horses affected by infectious corneal disease and ERU. We also now recognize the importance of an ophthalmic evaluation and treatment of ocular disease when faced with a horse with systemic disease.

References

[1] Long MT. Mechanisms of establishment and spread of bacterial and fungal infections. In: Reed SM, Bayly WM, Sellon DC, editors. Equine internal medicine. 2nd edition. Philadelphia: WB Saunders; 2004. p. 59–74.
[2] Tremaine WH, Dixon PM. A long-term study of 277 cases of equine sinonasal disease. Part 1: details of horses, historical, clinical and ancillary diagnostic findings. Equine Vet J 2001; 33:274–82.
[3] Honnas CM, Pascoe JR. Diseases of the paranasal sinuses: sinusitis. In: Smith BP, editor. Large animal internal medicine. 3rd edition. St Louis (MO): Mosby; 2002. p. 537–9.
[4] Laverty S, Pascoe JR. Sinusitis. In: Robinson NE, editor. Current therapy in equine medicine 4. Philadelphia: WB Saunders; 1997. p. 419–21.
[5] Schumacher J, Honnas C, Smith B. Paranasal sinusitis complicated by inspissated exudate in the ventral conchal sinus. Vet Surg 1987;16:373–7.
[6] Tremaine WH, Clarke CJ, Dixon PM. Histopathological findings in equine sinonasal disorders. Equine Vet J 1999;31:296–303.
[7] Arnauld des Lions J, Guillot J, Legrand E, et al. Aspergillosis involving the frontal sinus in a horse. Equine Vet Educ 2000;12:248–50.
[8] Freeman DE, Orsini PG, Ross MW, et al. A large frontonasal bone flap for sinus surgery in the horse. Vet Surg 1990;19:122–30.
[9] Blackford JT, Goble DO, Henry RW, et al. Triangulated flap technique for nasofrontal surgery: results in five horses. Vet Surg 1985;14:287–94.
[10] Chakrabarti A, Sharma SC. Paranasal sinus mycoses. Indian J Chest Dis Allied Sci 2000;42: 293–304.
[11] Wolf AM. Fungal diseases of the nasal cavity of the dog and cat. Vet Clin North Am Small Anim Pract 1992;22:1119–32.
[12] Freeman DE. Sinus disease. Vet Clin North Am Equine Pract 2003;19:209–43.
[13] Boulton CH. Equine nasal cavity and paranasal sinus disease: a review of 85 cases. J Equine Vet Sci 1985;5:268–75.
[14] Lane JG, Longstaffe JA, Gibbs C. Equine paranasal sinus cysts: a report of 15 cases. Equine Vet J 1987;19:537–44.
[15] Cannon JH, Grant BD, Sande RD. Diagnosis and surgical treatment of cystlike lesions of the equine paranasal sinuses. J Am Vet Med Assoc 1976;169:610–3.
[16] Trotter GW. Paranasal sinuses. Vet Clin North Am Equine Pract 1993;9:153–69.
[17] Lane JG. The management of sinus disorders of horses—part 1. Equine Vet Educ 1993;5: 5–9.
[18] Ford TS. Standing surgery and procedures of the head. Vet Clin North Am Equine Pract 1991;7:583–602.
[19] Ruggles AJ, Ross MW, Freeman DE. Endoscopic examination of normal paranasal sinuses in horses. Vet Surg 1991;20:418–23.
[20] Ruggles AJ, Ross MW, Freeman DE. Endoscopic examination and treatment of paranasal sinus disease in 16 horses. Vet Surg 1993;22:508–14.
[21] Worster AA, Hackett RP. Equine sinus endoscopy using a flexible endoscope: diagnosis and treatment of sinus disease in the standing sedated horse. In: Proceedings of the 45th

Annual Convention of the American Association of Equine Practitioners. Lexington (KY): American Association of Equine Practitioners; 1999. p. 128–30.

[22] Solano M. Equine radiography: portable x-ray generators, film-screen technology, and tabletop automatic film processors. Clin Tech Equine Pract 2004;3:328–40.

[23] Behrens E, Schumacher J, Morris E, et al. Equine paranasal sinusography. Vet Radiol 1991; 32:98–104.

[24] Behrens E, Schumacher J, Morris E. Contrast paranasal sinusography for evaluation of disease of the paranasal sinuses of five horses. Vet Radiol 1991;32:105–9.

[25] Archer DC, Blake CL, Singer ER, et al. The normal scintigraphic appearance of the equine head. Equine Vet Educ 2003;15:243–9.

[26] Archer DC, Blake CL, Singer ER, et al. Scintigraphic appearance of selected diseases of the equine head. Equine Vet Educ 2003;15:305–13.

[27] Barakzai SZ, Dixon PM. Effect of sinus trephination on scintigraphy of the equine skull. Vet Rec 2003;152:629–30.

[28] Tucker RL, Farrell E. Computed tomography and magnetic resonance imaging of the equine head. Vet Clin North Am Equine Pract 2001;17:131–44.

[29] Solano M, Brawer RS. CT of the equine head: technical considerations, anatomical guide, and selected diseases. Clin Tech Equine Pract 2004;3:374–88.

[30] Tietje S, Becker M, Bockenhoff G. Computed tomographic evaluation of head diseases in the horse: 15 cases. Equine Vet J 1996;28:98–105.

[31] Henninger W, Frame EM, Willmann M, et al. CT features of alveolitis and sinusitis in horses. Vet Radiol Ultrasound 2003;44:269–76.

[32] Arencibia A, Vazquez JM, Jaber R, et al. Magnetic resonance imaging and cross sectional anatomy of the normal equine sinuses and nasal passages. Vet Radiol Ultrasound 2000;41: 313–9.

[33] Devaiah AK. Adult chronic rhinosinusitis: diagnosis and dilemmas. Otolaryngol Clin North Am 2004;37:243–52.

[34] Lane JG. The management of sinus disorders of horses—part 2. Equine Vet Educ 1993;5: 69–73.

[35] Meginnis PJ. Nasal irrigation in the treatment of nasal catarrh and sinus infections in horses. J Am Vet Med Assoc 1956;128:577–80.

[36] Rabago D, Zgierska A, Mundt M, et al. Efficacy of daily hypertonic saline nasal irrigation among patients with sinusitis: a randomized controlled trial. J Fam Pract 2002;51: 1049–55.

[37] Schumacher J, Crossland LE. Removal of inspissated purulent exudate from the ventral conchal sinus of three standing horses. J Am Vet Med Assoc 1994;205:1312–4.

[38] Schumacher J, Dutton DM, Murphy DJ, et al. Paranasal sinus surgery through a frontonasal flap in sedated, standing horses. Vet Surg 2000;29:173–7.

[39] Selimoglu E. Nitric oxide in health and disease from the point of view of the otorhinolaryngologist. Curr Pharm Des 2005;11:3051–60.

[40] Scrutchfield WL, Schumacher J, Walker M, et al. Removal of an osteoma from the paranasal sinuses of a standing horse. Equine Pract 1994;16:24–8.

[41] Quinn GC, Kidd JA, Lane JG. Modified frontonasal sinus flap surgery in standing horses: surgical findings and outcomes of 60 cases. Equine Vet J 2005;37:138–42.

[42] Wyn-Jones G, Jones RS, Church S. Temporary bilateral carotid artery occlusion as an aid to nasal surgery in the horse. Equine Vet J 1986;18:125–8.

[43] Woodie JB, Ducharme NG, Gleed RD, et al. In horses with guttural pouch mycosis or after stylohyoid bone resection, what arterial ligation(s) could be effective in emergency treatment of a hemorrhagic crisis? Vet Surg 2002;31:498–9.

[44] Mudge MC, MacDonald MH, Owens SD, et al. Comparison of 4 blood storage methods in a protocol for equine pre-operative autologous donation. Vet Surg 2004;33:475–86.

[45] Schumacher J. The present state of equine dentistry. Equine Vet J 2001;33:2–3.

[46] Dixon PM, Tremaine WH, Pickles K, et al. Equine dental disease part 4: a long-term study of 400 cases: apical infections of cheek teeth. Equine Vet J 2000;32:182–94.
[47] Dixon PM, Dacre I. A review of equine dental disorders. Vet J 2005;169:165–87.
[48] Lane JG. A review of dental disorders of the horse, their treatment and possible fresh approaches to management. Equine Vet Educ 1994;6:13–21.
[49] Dacre IT. Equine dental pathology. In: Baker GJ, Easley J, editors. Equine dentistry. 2nd edition. Philadelphia: Elsevier Saunders; 2005. p. 91–109.
[50] Johnson TJ, Porter CM. Periodontal disease and tooth decay in the horse. In: Proceedings of the 50th Annual Convention of the American Association of Equine Practitioners. Lexington (KY): American Association of Equine Practitioners; 2004. p. 19–24.
[51] Dixon PM, Tremaine WH, Pickles K, et al. Equine dental disease part 1: a long-term study of 400 cases: disorders of incisor, canine and first premolar teeth. Equine Vet J 1999;31: 369–77.
[52] Gayle JM, Redding WR, Vacek JR, et al. Diagnosis and surgical treatment of periapical infection of the third mandibular molar in five horses. J Am Vet Med Assoc 1999;215:829–32.
[53] Lowder MQ, Mueller POE. Periradicular dental disease in horses. Compend Contin Educ Pract Vet 1999;21:874–6.
[54] Easley J. Dental and oral examination. In: Baker GJ, Easley J, editors. Equine dentistry. 2nd edition. Philadelphia: Elsevier Saunders; 2005. p. 151–69.
[55] Scrutchfield WL, Easley J, Morton K. Equine dental equipment, supplies and instrumentation. In: Baker GJ, Easley J, editors. Equine dentistry. 2nd edition. Philadelphia: Elsevier Saunders; 2005. p. 205–19.
[56] Gibbs C. Dental imaging. In: Baker GJ, Easley J, editors. Equine dentistry. 2nd edition. Philadelphia: Elsevier Saunders; 2005. p. 171–202.
[57] Dixon PM. Dental extraction in horses: indications and preoperative evaluation. Compend Contin Educ Pract Vet 1997;19:366–75.
[58] Richardson JD, Lane JG. Metaplastic conchal calcification secondary to chronic periapical infection in seven horses. Equine Vet Educ 1993;5:303–7.
[59] Easley J. A new look at dental radiology. In: Proceedings of the 48th Annual Convention of the American Association of Equine Practitioners. Lexington (KY): American Association of Equine Practitioners; 2002. p. 412–20.
[60] Barakzai SZ, Dixon PM. A study of open-mouthed oblique radiographic projections for evaluating lesions of the erupted (clinical) crown. Equine Vet Educ 2003;15:143–8.
[61] Klugh DO. Intraoral radiography of equine premolars and molars. In: Proceedings of the 49th Annual Convention of the American Association of Equine Practitioners. Lexington (KY): American Association of Equine Practitioners; 2003. p. 280–6.
[62] Boswell JC, Schramme MC, Livesey LC, et al. Use of scintigraphy in the diagnosis of dental disease in four horses. Equine Vet Educ 1999;11:294–8.
[63] Ramzan PHL. The head. In: Dyson SJ, Pilsworth RC, Twardock AR, et al, editors. Equine scintigraphy. Newmarket (England): Equine Veterinary Journal Ltd; 2003. p. 225–38.
[64] Semevolos SA, Hackett RP, Scrivani PV. Nuclear scintigraphy as a diagnostic aid in the evaluation of tooth root abscessation. In: Proceedings of the 45th Annual Convention of the American Association of Equine Practitioners. Lexington (KY): American Association of Equine Practitioners; 1999. p. 103–4.
[65] Metcalf MR, Tate LP, Sellett LC. Clinical use of ^{99m}Tc-MDP scintigraphy in the equine mandible and maxilla. Vet Radiol 1989;30:80–7.
[66] Weller R, Livesey L, Maierl J, et al. Comparison of radiography and scintigraphy in the diagnosis of dental disorders in the horse. Equine Vet J 2001;33:49–58.
[67] Boutros CP, Koenig JB. A combined frontal and maxillary sinus approach for repulsion of the third maxillary molar in a horse. Can Vet J 2001;42:286–8.
[68] Dixon PM. Dental extraction and endodontic techniques in horses. Compend Contin Educ Pract Vet 1997;19:628–38.

[69] Prichard MA, Hackett RP, Erb HN. Long-term outcome of tooth repulsion in horses. A retrospective study of 61 cases. Vet Surg 1992;21:145–9.
[70] Tremaine WH, Lane JG. Exodontia. In: Baker GJ, Easley J, editors. Equine dentistry. 2nd edition. Philadelphia: Elsevier Saunders; 2005. p. 267–94.
[71] Evans LH, Tate LP, LaDow CS. Extraction of the equine 4th upper premolar and 1st and 2nd upper molars through a lateral buccotomy. In: Proceedings of the 27th Annual Convention of the American Association of Equine Practitioners. Lexington (KY): American Association of Equine Practitioners; 1981. p. 249–52.
[72] Lowder MQ. Oral extraction of equine teeth. Compend Contin Educ Pract Vet 1999;21: 1150–7.
[73] Dixon PM, Dacre I, Dacre K, et al. Standing oral extraction of cheek teeth in 100 horses (1998–2003). Equine Vet J 2005;37:105–12.
[74] Dacre I, Dixon PM. Oral extraction of cheek teeth in the standing horse: indications and techniques. In: Proceedings of the 50th Annual Convention of the American Association of Equine Practitioners. Lexington (KY): American Association of Equine Practitioners; 2004. p. 25–30.
[75] Tremaine WH. Oral extraction of equine cheek teeth. Equine Vet Educ 2004;16:151–8.
[76] Carmalt JL, Barber SM. Periapical curettage: an alternative surgical approach to infected mandibular cheek teeth in horses. Vet Surg 2004;33:267–71.
[77] Fletcher BW. How to perform effective equine dental nerve blocks. In: Proceedings of the 50th Annual Convention of the American Association of Equine Practitioners. Lexington (KY): American Association of Equine Practitioners; 2004. p. 233–6.
[78] Trostle SS, Juzwiak JS, Santschi EM. How to use antibiotic impregnated plaster of Paris for alveolar packing after tooth removal. In: 46th Annual Convention of the American Association of Equine Practitioners. Lexington (KY): American Association of Equine Practitioners; 2000. p. 180–1.
[79] Schramme MC, Boswell JC, Robinson J, et al. Endodontic therapy for periapical infection of the cheek teeth: a study of 19 horses. In: 46th Annual Convention of the American Association of Equine Practitioners. Lexington (KY): American Association of Equine Practitioners; 2000. p. 113–6.
[80] Baker GJ. Endodontic therapy. In: Baker GJ, Easley J, editors. Equine dentistry. 2nd edition. Philadelphia: Elsevier Saunders; 2005. p. 295–302.
[81] Brannan R. Dental materials in veterinary dentistry. In: Baker GJ, Easley J, editors. Equine dentistry. 2nd edition. Philadelphia: Elsevier Saunders; 2005. p. 303–11.
[82] Baker GJ, Kirkland DK. Endodontic therapy in the horse. In: 38th Annual Convention of the American Association of Equine Practitioners. Lexington (KY): American Association of Equine Practitioners; 1992. p. 329–35.
[83] Kirkland DK, Baker GJ, Manfra Marretta S, et al. Effects of aging on the endodontic system, reserve crown, and roots of equine mandibular cheek teeth. Am J Vet Res 1996;57: 31–8.
[84] Greene SK, Basile TP. Recognition and treatment of equine periodontal disease. In: Proceedings of the 48th Annual Convention of the American Association of Equine Practitioners. Lexington (KY): American Association of Equine Practitioners; 2002. p. 463–6.
[85] Baker GJ. Abnormalities of wear and periodontal disease. In: Baker GJ, Easley J, editors. Equine dentistry. 2nd edition. Philadelphia: Elsevier Saunders; 2005. p. 111–9.
[86] Carmalt JL, Rucker BA, Rach DJ. Treatment of periodontitis associated with diastema formation in the horse—an alternative approach. In: Proceedings of the 50th Annual Convention of the American Association of Equine Practitioners. Lexington (KY): American Association of Equine Practitioners; 2004. p. 37–40.
[87] Perkins GA, Pease A, Crotty E, et al. Diagnosing guttural pouch disorders and managing guttural pouch empyema in adult horses. Compend Contin Educ Pract Vet 2003;25: 966–73.

[88] Lepage OM, Perron MF, Cadore JL. The mystery of fungal infection in the guttural pouches. Vet J 2004;168:60–4.
[89] Cook WR. The auditory tube diverticulum (guttural pouch) in the horse: its radiographic examination. J Am Radiol Soc 1973;14:41–71.
[90] Colles CM, Cook WR. Carotid and cerebral angiography in the horse. Vet Rec 1983;113: 483–9.
[91] Butler JA, Colles CM, Dyson SJ, et al. Miscellaneous techniques. In: Butler JA, Colles CM, Dyson SJ, et al, editors. Clinical radiology of the horse. London: Blackwell Science; 2000. p. 563–84.
[92] Chiesa OA, Lopez C, Domingo M, et al. A percutaneous technique for guttural pouch lavage. Equine Pract 2000;22:8–11.
[93] Chiesa OA, Vidal D, Domingo M, et al. Cytological and bacteriological findings in guttural pouch lavages of clinically normal horses. Vet Rec 1999;144:346–9.
[94] Chiesa OA, Cuenca R, Mayayo E, et al. Cytological and microbiological findings in guttural pouch lavages of clinically normal horses with head restraint. Aust Vet J 2002;80:234–8.
[95] Judy CE, Chaffin MK, Cohen ND. Empyema of the guttural pouch (auditory tube diverticulum) in horses: 91 cases (1977–1997). J Am Vet Med Assoc 1999;215:1666–70.
[96] Verheyen K, Newton JR, Talbot NC, et al. Elimination of guttural pouch infection and inflammation in asymptomatic carriers of Streptococcus equi. Equine Vet J 2000;32:527–32.
[97] Newton JR, Wood JL, Dunn KA, et al. Naturally occurring persistent and asymptomatic infection of the guttural pouches of horses with Streptococcus equi. Vet Rec 1997;140: 84–90.
[98] Ludwig A, Gatineau S, Reynaud MC, et al. Fungal isolation and identification in 21 cases of guttural pouch mycosis in horses (1998–2002). Vet J 2005;169:457–61.
[99] Baptiste KE. The mystery of guttural pouch mycosis: the paradox of advancing knowledge of a rare disease. Vet J 2004;168:1–2.
[100] Guillot J, Sarfati J, Ribot X, et al. Detection of antibodies to Aspergillus fumigatus in serum of horses with mycosis of the auditory tube diverticulum (guttural pouch). Am J Vet Res 1997;58:1364–6.
[101] Gelbmann LM, Vrotsos PD, MacLeay JM, et al. Guttural pouch catheter: production and placement. In: Proceedings of the 43rd Annual Convention of the American Association of Equine Practitioners. Lexington (KY): American Association of Equine Practitioners; 1997. p. 158–9.
[102] White SL, Williamson L. How to make a retention catheter to treat guttural pouch empyema. Veterinary Medicine 1987;82:76–82.
[103] Wilson J. Effects of indwelling catheters and povidone iodine flushes on the guttural pouches of the horse. Equine Vet J 1985;17:242–4.
[104] Bentz BG, Dowd AL, Freeman DE. Treatment of guttural pouch empyema with acetylcysteine irrigation. Equine Pract 1996;18:33–5.
[105] Adams SB, Fessler JF. Modified Whitehouse approach to the guttural pouch. In: Adams SB, Fessler JF, editors. Atlas of equine surgery. Philadelphia: WB Saunders; 2000. p. 171–3.
[106] Hawkins JF, Frank N, Sojka JE, et al. Fistulation of the auditory tube diverticulum (guttural pouch) with a neodymium:yttrium-aluminum-garnet laser for treatment of chronic empyema in two horses. J Am Vet Med Assoc 2001;218:405–7.
[107] Tate LP, Blikslager AT, Little EDE. Transendoscopic laser treatment of guttural pouch tympanites in eight foals. Vet Surg 1995;24:367–72.
[108] Gehlen H, Ohnesorge B. Laser fenestration of the mesial septum for treatment of guttural pouch chondroids in a pony. Vet Surg 2005;34:383–6.
[109] Seahorn TL, Schumacher J. Nonsurgical removal of chondroid masses from the guttural pouches of two horses. J Am Vet Med Assoc 1991;199:368–9.
[110] Adkins AR, Yovich JV, Colbourne CM. Nonsurgical treatment of chondroids of the guttural pouch in a horse. Aust Vet J 1997;75:332–3.

[111] Speirs VC, Harrison IW, van Veenendaal JC, et al. Is specific antifungal therapy necessary for the treatment of guttural pouch mycosis in horses? Equine Vet J 1995;27:151–2.
[112] Lane JG. The management of guttural pouch mycosis. Equine Vet J 1989;21(5):321–4.
[113] Cook WR. The clinical features of guttural pouch mycosis in the horse. Vet Rec 1968;83: 336–45.
[114] Davis EW, Legendre AM. Successful treatment of guttural pouch mycosis with itraconazole and topical enilconazole in a horse. J Vet Intern Med 1994;8:304–5.
[115] Lepage OM, Piccot-Crezollet C. Transarterial coil embolisation in 31 horses (1999–2002) with guttural pouch mycosis: a 2 year follow-up. Equine Vet J 2005;37:430–4.
[116] Caron JP, Fretz PB, Bailey JV, et al. Balloon-tipped catheter arterial occlusion for prevention of hemorrhage caused by guttural pouch mycosis: 13 cases (1982–1985). J Am Vet Med Assoc 1987;191:345–9.
[117] Freeman DE, Ross MW, Donawick WJ, et al. Occlusion of the external carotid and maxillary arteries in the horse to prevent hemorrhage from guttural pouch mycosis. Vet Surg 1989;18:39–47.
[118] Freeman DE, Donawick WJ. Occlusion of internal carotid artery in the horse by means of a balloon-tipped catheter: clinical use of a method to prevent epistaxis caused by guttural pouch mycosis. J Am Vet Med Assoc 1980;176:236–40.
[119] Smith KM, Barber SM. Guttural pouch hemorrhage associated with lesions of the maxillary artery in two horses. Can Vet J 1984;25:239–42.
[120] Adams SB, Fessler JF. Arterial ligation for guttural pouch mycosis. In: Adams SB, Fessler JF, editors. Atlas of equine surgery. Philadelphia: WB Saunders; 2000. p. 181–4.
[121] Church S, Wyn-Jones G, Parks AH, et al. Treatment of guttural pouch mycosis. Equine Vet J 1986;18:362–5.
[122] Greet TR. Outcome of treatment in 35 cases of guttural pouch mycosis. Equine Vet J 1987; 19:483–7.
[123] Freeman DE, Donawick WJ, Klein LV. Effect of ligation on internal carotid artery blood pressure in horses. Vet Surg 1994;23:250–6.
[124] Freeman DE, Donawick WJ. Occlusion of internal carotid artery in the horse by means of a balloon-tipped catheter: evaluation of a method designed to prevent epistaxis caused by guttural pouch mycosis. J Am Vet Med Assoc 1980;176:232–5.
[125] Hardy J, Robertson JT, Wilkie DA. Ischemic optic neuropathy and blindness after arterial occlusion for treatment of guttural pouch mycosis in two horses. J Am Vet Med Assoc 1990; 196:1631–4.
[126] Freeman DE, Ross MW, Donawick WJ. "Steal phenomenon" proposed as the cause of blindness after arterial occlusion for treatment of guttural pouch mycosis in horses. J Am Vet Med Assoc 1990;197:811–2.
[127] Freeman DE, Staller GS, Maxson AD, et al. Unusual internal carotid artery branching that prevented arterial occlusion with a balloon-tipped catheter in a horse. Vet Surg 1993;22: 531–4.
[128] Bacon Miller C, Wilson DA, Martin DD, et al. Complications of balloon catheterization associated with aberrant cerebral arterial anatomy in a horse with guttural pouch mycosis. Vet Surg 1998;27:450–3.
[129] Cheramie HS, Pleasant RS, Dabareiner RM, et al. Detachable latex balloon occlusion of an internal carotid artery with an aberrant branch in a horse with guttural pouch (auditory tube diverticulum) mycosis. J Am Vet Med Assoc 2000;216:888–91.
[130] Leveille R, Hardy J, Robertson JT, et al. Transarterial coil embolization of the internal and external carotid and maxillary arteries for prevention of hemorrhage from guttural pouch mycosis in horses. Vet Surg 2000;29:389–97.
[131] Matsuda Y, Nakanishi Y, Mizuno Y. Occlusion of the internal carotid artery by means of microcoils for preventing epistaxis caused by guttural pouch mycosis in horses. J Vet Med Sci 1999;61:221–5.

[132] Cheramie HS, Pleasant RS, Robertson JL, et al. Evaluation of a technique to occlude the internal carotid artery of horses. Vet Surg 1999;28:83–90.
[133] Kern TJ, Brooks DE, White MM. Equine keratomycosis: current concepts of diagnosis and treatment. Equine Vet J Suppl 1983;2:33–8.
[134] Moore CP, Collins BK, Fales WH, et al. Antimicrobial agents for treatment of infectious keratitis in horses. J Am Vet Med Assoc 1995;207:855–61.
[135] Moore CP, Collins BK, Fales WH. Antibacterial susceptibility patterns for microbial isolates associated with infectious keratitis in horses: 63 cases (1986–1994). J Am Vet Med Assoc 1995;207:928–33.
[136] Edwards A. Equine keratomycosis: a rational approach to therapy. Vet Tech 1989;10: 34–40.
[137] Brooks DE, Andrew SE, Biros DJ, et al. Ulcerative keratitis caused by beta-hemolytic *Streptococcus equi* in 11 horses. Vet Ophthalmol 2000;3:121–5.
[138] Samuelson DA, Andresen TL, Gwin RM. Conjunctival fungal flora in horses, cattle, dogs, and cats. J Am Vet Med Assoc 1984;184:1240–2.
[139] Foster CS. Fungal keratitis. Infect Dis Clin North Am 1992;6:851–7.
[140] Brooks DE. Equine ophthalmology. In: Gelatt KN, editor. Veterinary ophthalmology. 3rd edition. Baltimore (MD): Lippincott, Williams & Wilkins; 1999. p. 1053–116.
[141] Rebhun WC. Corneal stromal abscesses in the horse. J Am Vet Med Assoc 1982;181: 677–9.
[142] Rebhum WC. Corneal stromal infections in horses. Compend Contin Educ Pract Vet 1992; 14:363–71.
[143] Hendrix DVH, Brooks DE, Smith PJ, et al. Corneal stromal abscesses in the horse: a review of 24 cases. Equine Vet J 1995;27:440–7.
[144] Brooks DE, Millichamp NJ, Peterson MG, et al. Nonulcerative keratouveitis in five horses. J Am Vet Med Assoc 1990;196:1985–91.
[145] Gilger BC, Michau TM, Salmon JH. Immune-mediated keratitis in horses: 19 cases (1998–2004). Vet Ophthalmol 2005;8:233–9.
[146] Sauer P, Andrew SE, Lassaline M, et al. Changes in antibiotic resistance in equine bacterial ulcerative keratitis (1991–2000): 65 horses. Vet Ophthalmol 2003;6:309–13.
[147] Brooks DE. Inflammatory stromal keratopathies: medical management of stromal abscesses, eosinophilic keratitis, and band keratopathy in the horse. Vet Clin North Am Equine Pract 2004;20:345–60.
[148] Moore PA, Dietrich UM, Barton MH, et al. The influence of rainfall and temperature on the frequency of equine fungal keratitis [E-abstract 5067]. Invest Ophthalmol Vis Sci 2005; 46:E-abstract 5067.
[149] Thomas PA. Fungal infections of the cornea. Eye 2003;17:852–62.
[150] Belknap EB, Barden CA, Yin C, et al. Real time PCR as a diagnostic tool for equine fungal keratitis: a preliminary study [abstract 7]. In: American College of Veterinary Ophthalmologists 36th Annual Conference Proceedings Notes, Nashville, TN. 2005:7.
[151] Cutler TJ. Corneal epithelial disease. Vet Clin North Am Equine Pract 2004;20:319–43.
[152] Miller TR, Gaskin JM, Whitley RD, et al. Herpetic keratitis in a horse. Equine Vet J Suppl 1990;1:15–7.
[153] Kershaw O, von Oppen T, Glitz F, et al. Detection of equine herpesvirus type 2 (EHV-2) in horses with keratoconjunctivitis. Virus Res 2001;80:93–9.
[154] von Oppen T. Detection of equine herpesvirus type 2 (EHV-2) in horses showing keratitis [doctoral dissertation]. School of Veterinary Medicine, Hanover (Germany); 2000.
[155] von Borstel M. Advanced diagnostic methods for keratitis in horses with particular consideration for the detection of equine herpesvirus type 2 (EHV-2) [doctoral dissertation]. School of Veterinary Medicine, Hanover (Germany); 2003.
[156] Thein P, Böhm D. Ätiologie und Klinik einer virusbedingten Keratokonjuktivitis beim Fohlen. Zentralbl Veterinarmed B 1976;23:507–19.

[157] Hendrix DV, Cox SK. Pharmacokinetics of topically applied ciprofloxacin in equine tears [E-abstract 4897]. Invest Ophthalmol Vis Sci 2005;46:E-abstract 4897.
[158] Hendrix DV, Ward DA, Barnhill MA. Effects of antibiotics on morphologic characteristics and migration of canine corneal epithelial cells in tissue culture. Am J Vet Res 2001;62: 1664–9.
[159] Ball MA, Rebhun WC, Gaarder JE, et al. Evaluation of itraconazole-dimethyl sulfoxide ointment for treatment of keratomycosis in nine horses. J Am Vet Med Assoc 1997;211: 199–203.
[160] Brooks DE, Andrew SE, Dillavou CL, et al. Antimicrobial susceptibility patterns of fungi isolated from horses with ulcerative keratomycosis. Am J Vet Res 1998;59:138–42.
[161] Betbeze CM, Wu CC, Stiles J, et al. *In vitro* fungistatic and fungicidal activity of silver sulfadiazine and natamycin on pathogenic fungi isolated from equine eyes [abstract 26]. In: American College of Veterinary Ophthalmologists 36th Annual Conference Proceedings Notes, Nashville, TN. 2005:26.
[162] Latimer FG, Colitz CM, Campbell NB, et al. Pharmacokinetics of fluconazole following intravenous and oral administration and body fluid concentrations of fluconazole following repeated oral dosing in horses. Am J Vet Res 2001;62:1606–11.
[163] Davis J, Salmon JH, Papich MG. Pharmacokinetics and tissue distribution of itraconazole after oral and intravenous administration to horses. Am J Vet Res 2005;66:1694–701.
[164] Clode AB, Davis JL, Salmon J, et al. Evaluation of concentration of voriconazole in aqueous humor after topical and oral administration in horses. Am J Vet Res 2006;67:296–301.
[165] Stiles J, Townsend WM, Rogers QR, et al. Effect of oral administration of L-lysine on conjunctivitis caused by feline herpesvirus in cats. Am J Vet Res 2002;63:99–103.
[166] Maggs DJ, Naisse MP, Kass PH. Efficacy of oral supplementation with L-lysine infected with feline herpesvirus. Am J Vet Res 2003;64:37–42.
[167] Ollivier FJ. Proteases. In: Gilger BC, editor. Equine ophthalmology. 1st edition. St. Louis (MO): Elsevier; 2005. p. 165–6.
[168] Swank A, Hosgood G. Corneal wound healing and the role of growth factors. Compend Contin Educ Pract Vet 1996;18:1007–16.
[169] Ollivier FJ, Brooks DE, Kallberg ME, et al. Evaluation of various compounds to inhibit activity of matrix metalloproteinases in the tear film of horses with ulcerative keratitis. Am J Vet Res 2003;64:1081–7.
[170] Ollivier FJ, Brooks DE, Van Setten GB, et al. Profiles of matrix metalloproteinase activity in equine tear film during corneal healing in 10 horses with ulcerative keratitis. Vet Ophthalmol 2004;7:397–405.
[171] Strubbe DT, Brooks DE, Schultz GS, et al. Evaluation of tear film proteases in horses with ulcerative keratitis. Vet Ophthalmol 2000;3:111–9.
[172] Slansky HH, Gnadinger MC, Itoi M, et al. Coagenase in corneal ulcerations. Arch Ophthalmol 1969;82:108–11.
[173] O'Brien TP. Bacterial keratitis. In: Krachmer JH, Mannis MJ, Holland EJ, editors. Cornea. St. Louis (MO): Mosby Year Book; 1997. p. 1139–90.
[174] Mastumoto K. Proteases in bacterial keratitis. Cornea 2000;S19(Suppl):160–4.
[175] Gopinathan U, Ramakrishna T, Willcox M, et al. Enzymatic, clinical and histological evaluation of corneal tissues in experimental fungal keratitis in rabbits. Exp Eye Res 2001;72: 433–42.
[176] Brooks DE, Ollivier F, Lassaline ME, et al. MMP production by microbial isolates from equine corneal ulcers. In: American College of Veterinary Ophthalmologists 34th Annual Conference Proceedings Notes, Coeur D'Alene, ID. 2003:71.
[177] Schultz G, Chegini N, Grant M, et al. Effects of growth factors on corneal wound healing. Acta Ophthalmol Suppl 1992;202:60–6.
[178] Burling KB, Seguin MS, Marsh P, et al. Effect of topical administration of epidermal growth factor on healing of corneal epithelial defects in horses. Am J Vet Res 2000;61: 1150–5.

[179] Gilger BC. Bacterial ulcer. In: Gilger B, editor. Equine ophthalmology. 1st edition. St. Louis (MO): Elsevier; 2005. p. 175–92.
[180] Gelatt KN, Gelatt JP. Handbook of small animal ophthalmic surgery, vol. 1. Extraocular procedures. New York: Pergamon; 1994. p. 165–88.
[181] Denis HM. Equine corneal surgery and transplantation. Vet Clin North Am Equine Pract 2004;20:361–80.
[182] Whitaker CJG, Smith PJ, Brooks DE, et al. Therapeutic penetrating keratoplasty for deep corneal stromal abscesses in eight horses. Vet Comp Ophthalmol 1997;7:19–28.
[183] Andrew SE. Corneal stromal abscess in a horse. Vet Ophthalmol 1999;2(4):207–11.
[184] Andrew SE, Brooks DE, Biros DJ, et al. Posterior lamellar keratoplasty for treatment of deep stromal abscesses in nine horses. Vet Ophthalmol 2000;3:99–103.
[185] Brooks DE, Lassaline ME, Kallberg ME, et al. Deep lamellar endothelial keratoplasty (DLEK) in six horses. In: American College of Veterinary Ophthalmologists 34th Annual Conference Proceedings Notes, Coeur D'Alene, ID. 2003:70.
[186] Bussieres M, Krohne SG, Stiles J, et al. The use of porcine small intestinal submucosa for the repair of full-thickness corneal defects in dogs, cats and horses. Vet Ophthalmol 2004;7: 352–9.
[187] Lassaline ME, Brooks DE, Ollivier FJ, et al. Equine amniotic membrane transplantation for corneal ulceration and keratomalacia in three horses. Vet Ophthalmol 2005;8: 311–7.
[188] Heiligenhaus A, Li HF, Yang Y, et al. Transplantation of amniotic membrane in murine herpes stromal keratitis modulates matrix metalloproteinases in the cornea. Invest Ophthalmol Vis Sci 2005;46:4079–85.
[189] Hick S, Demers PE, Brunette I, et al. Amniotic membrane transplantation and fibrin glue in the management of corneal ulcers and perforations: a review of 33 cases. Cornea 2005;24: 369–77.
[190] Bentley E, Murphy CJ, Li F, et al. Biosynthetic corneal substitute implantation in dogs [abstract 57]. In: American College of Veterinary Ophthalmologists 36th Annual Conference Proceedings Notes, Nashville, TN. 2005:57.
[191] Bruining MJ, Pijpers PA, Kingshott P, et al. Studies on new polymeric biomaterials with tunable hydrophilicity, and their possible utility in corneal repair surgery. Biomaterials 2002;23:1213–9.
[192] Rebhun WC. Diagnosis and treatment of equine uveitis. J Am Vet Med Assoc 1979;175: 803–8.
[193] Schwink KL. Equine uveitis. Vet Clin North Am Equine Pract 1992;8:557–74.
[194] Abrams K, Brooks DE. Equine recurrent uveitis: current concepts in diagnosis and treatment. Equine Pract 1990;12:27–35.
[195] Davidson MG. Anterior uveitis. In: Robinson N, editor. Current therapy in equine medicine. 4th edition. Philadelphia: WB Saunders; 1992. p. 592–3.
[196] Dwyer A, Gilger BC. Equine recurrent uveitis. In: Gilger BC, editor. Equine ophthalmology. 1st edition. St. Louis (MO): Elsevier; 2005. p. 285–322.
[197] Deeg CA, Kaspers B, Gerhards H, et al. Immune responses to retinal autoantigens and peptides in equine recurrent uveitis. Invest Ophthalmol Vis Sci 2001;42:393–8.
[198] Deeg CA, Ehrenhoffer M, Thurau SR, et al. Immunopathology of recurrent uveitis in spontaneously diseased horses. Exp Eye Res 2002;75:127–33.
[199] Deeg CA, Thurau SR, Gerhards H, et al. Uveitis in horses induced by photoreceptor retinoid-binding protein is similar to the spontaneous disease. Eur J Immunol 2002;32: 2598–606.
[200] Deeg CA, Marti E, Gaillard C, et al. Equine recurrent uveitis is strongly associated with the MHC class I haplotype ELA-A9. Equine Vet J 2004;36:73–5.
[201] Kaese HJ, Flickinger G, Valberg SJ, et al. Microsatellite association with uveitis in the Appaloosa horse [abstract 29]. In: American College of Veterinary Ophthalmologists 36th Annual Conference Proceedings Notes, Nashville, TN. 2005:29.

[202] Faber NA, Crawford M, LeFebvre RB, et al. Detection of *Leptospira* spp. in the aqueous humor of horses with naturally acquired recurrent uveitis. J Clin Microbiol 2000;38:2731–3.
[203] Parma AE, Santisteban CG, Villalba JS, et al. Experimental demonstration of an antigenic relationship between Leptospira and equine cornea. Vet Immunol Immunopathol 1985;10: 215–24.
[204] Tizard I. Veterinary immunology: an introduction. Philadelphia: WB Saunders; 1992. p. 445–6.
[205] Lucchesi PM, Parma AE, Arroyo GH. Serovar distribution of a DNA sequence involved in the antigenic relationship between *Leptospira* and equine cornea. BMC Microbiol 2002;2:3.
[206] Dwyer AE, Crockett RS, Kalsow CM. Association of leptospiral seroreactivity and breed with uveitis and blindness in horses: 372 cases (1986–1993). J Am Vet Med Assoc 1995;207: 1327–31.
[207] Dwyer AE. Equine recurrent uveitis and leptospirosis. In: Gilger B, editor. Equine ophthalmology. 1st edition. St. Louis (MO): Elsevier; 2005. p. 303–7.
[208] Roberts SR, York C, Robinson J. An outbreak of leptospirosis in horses on a small farm. J Am Vet Med Assoc 1952;121:237–42.
[209] Roberts SJ. Sequela of leptospirosis in horses on a small farm. J Am Vet Med Assod 1958; 133:189–94.
[210] Morter RL, Williams RD, Bolte H, et al. Equine leptospirosis. J Am Vet Med Assoc 1969; 155:436–42.
[211] Williams RD, Morter RL, Freeman MJ, et al. Experimental chronic uveitis. Ophthalmic signs following equine leptospirosis. Invest Ophthalmol 1971;10:948–54.
[212] Swart KS, Calvert K, Meney C. The prevalence of antibodies to serovars of *Leptospira interrogans* in horses. Aust Vet J 1982;59:25–7.
[213] Schwink KL. Equine uveitis. Vet Clin North Am Equine Pract 1992;8:557–74.
[214] Wollanke B, Rohrbach BW, Gerhards H. Serum and vitreous humor antibody titers in and isolation of Leptospira interrogans from horses with recurrent uveitis. J Am Vet Med Assoc 2001;219:795–800.
[215] Gerhards H, Wollanke B. Antibody titers against Borrelia in horses in serum and in eyes and occurrence of equine recurrent uveitis. Berl Munch Tierarztl Wochenschr 1996;109: 273–8.
[216] Rohrback BW, Ward DA, Hendrix DVH, et al. Effect of vaccination against leptospirosis on the frequency, days to recurrence and progression of disease in horses with equine recurrent uveitis. Vet Ophthalmol 2005;8:171–9.
[217] Chang YF, Ku YW, Chang CF, et al. Antibiotic treatment of experimentally *Borrelia burgdorferi* infected ponies. Vet Microbiol 2005;107:285–94.
[218] Frühauf B, Ohnesorge B, Deegen E, et al. Surgical management of equine recurrent uveitis with single port pars planta vitrectomy. Vet Ophthalmol 1998;1:137–51.
[219] Diamond JG, Kaplan HJ. Lensectomy and vitrectomy for complicated cataract secondary to uveitis. Arch Ophthalmol 1978;96:1798–804.
[220] Diamond JG, Kaplan HJ. Uveitis: effect of vitrectomy combined with lensectomy. Ophthalmology 1979;86:1320–9.
[221] Verbraeken H. Therapeutic pars plana vitrectomy for chronic uveitis: a retrospective study of long term results. Graefes Arch Clin Exp Ophthalmol 1996;234:288–93.
[222] Wollanke B. Die equine rezidivierende Uveitis (ERU) als intraokulare Leptospirose, Tieraerztliche Fakultaet. Munich (Germany): Ludwig-Maximilians-Universitaet; 2002.
[223] Brooks DE, Cutler TJ, Andrew SE, et al. Outcome of pars plana vitrectomy in 24 eyes of 18 horses with equine recurrent uveitis. In: American College of Veterinary Ophthalmologists 32nd Annual Conference Proceeding Notes, Sarasota, FL. 2001:38.
[224] Pinard CL, Piétrement E, Macieira S, et al. Intravitreal injections of gentamicin for the treatment of *Leptospira*-associated equine recurrent uveitis [abstract 74]. In: American College of Veterinary Ophthalmologists 36th Annual Conference Proceedings Notes, Nashville, TN. 2005:74.

[225] Gilger BC, Malok E, Stewart T, et al. Effect of an intravitreal cyclosporine implant on experimental uveitis in horses. Vet Immunol Immunopathol 2000;76:239–55.
[226] Benezre D, Maftzir G. Ocular penetration of cyclosporin A: the rabbit eye. Invest Ophthalmol Vis Sci 1990;31:1362–6.
[227] Benezre D, Maftzir G, DeCourten D, et al. Ocular penetration of cyclosporin A. III: the human eye. Br J Ophthalmol 1990;74:350–2.
[228] Gilger BC, Malok E, Stewart T, et al. Long-term effect on the equine eye of an intravitreal device used for sustained release of cyclosporine A. Vet Ophthalmol 2000;3:105–10.
[229] Gilger BC, Salmon JH, Wilkie DA, et al. A novel bioerodible deep scleral lamellar cyclosporine implant for uveitis. Invest Ophthalmol Vis Sci 2006;47:2596–605.
[230] Colitz CMH, Davis JL. Ocular manifestations of systemic disease. In: Gilger BC, editor. Equine ophthalmology. 1st edition. St. Louis (MO): Elsevier; 2005. p. 421–47.
[231] MacKay RJ. Equine protozoal myelitis. In: Robinson NE, editor. Current therapy in equine medicine. 5th edition. Philadelphia: WB Saunders; 2000. p. 69–74.
[232] Fontaine-Rodgerson G. Viral encephalitides. In: Robinson NE, editor. Current therapy in equine medicine. 5th edition. Philadelphia: WB Saunders; 2000. p. 47–50.
[233] Schlipf J. Alphavirus and flavivirus encephalitis of horses. In: Smith BP, editor. Large animal internal medicine. 3rd edition. St. Louis (MO): Mosby; 2002. p. 888–90.
[234] Porter MB, Long MT, Getman LM, et al. West Nile virus encephalomyelitis in horses: 46 cases (2001). J Am Vet Med Assoc 2003;222:1241–7.
[235] Solomon T, Fisher AF, Beasley DW, et al. Natural and nosocomial infection in a patient with West Nile encephalitis and extrapyramidal movement disorders. Clin Infect Dis 2003;36:140–5.

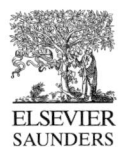

Advanced Techniques in the Diagnosis and Management of Infectious Pulmonary Diseases in Horses

Valerie A. Brown, DVM*, Pamela A. Wilkins, DVM, MS, PhD

New Bolton Center, University of Pennsylvania School of Veterinary Medicine, 382 West Street Road, Kennett Square, PA 19348, USA

Novel diagnostic and management techniques for infectious equine pulmonary disease continue to be developed. The rapidity with which infectious pulmonary diseases can spread necessitates rapid accurate diagnosis and appropriate management. Measures can then be taken to devise therapeutic and prophylactic protocols for the management of the pulmonary disease. Although culture and subsequent identification of the infectious organisms still remains an approach of great diagnostic value, new diagnostic modalities based on the detection of antibodies and antigens using immunologic assays as well as on the detection of nucleic acid using nucleic acid probes and amplification techniques have been developed. These diagnostic capabilities provide a distinct advantage in the rapidity with which results can be made available. Although parenteral administration of pharmacotherapeutic agents still forms the basis of treatment for infectious pneumonic disease of bacterial etiology, alternative delivery routes of the pharmacotherapeutic agents may serve as a useful adjunct to treatment. Prevention of pulmonary disease through increasing host resistance to infection is essential. Novel strategies for immunization have been developed and include nucleic acid plasmid vaccines. The use of novel diagnostic, therapeutic, and prophylactic techniques may assist in the control of infectious pulmonary disease.

---

* Corresponding author.
  E-mail address: brown@vet.penn.edu (V.A. Brown).

Diagnostic techniques

Infectious pulmonary disease represents a diagnostic challenge for the equine practitioner. A presumptive diagnosis can often be made based on the history, physical examination, clinical impression, complete blood cell count, radiography, and endoscopy. Definitive identification of the etiologic agent(s) is necessary to ensure that the appropriate therapeutic and prophylactic protocols are instituted.

The "gold standard" diagnostic technique for the detection of infectious pulmonary pathogens is culture. Culture of infectious pathogens is an indispensable diagnostic technique and should be attempted in all cases of pulmonary disease. By recovering the infectious pathogen, it can be characterized, undergo pharmacologic testing, and be used in the development of novel diagnostic test vaccines for its identification and prophylaxis, respectively. The ability to cultivate infectious pulmonary pathogens from clinical specimens is time-consuming, however, and may require from days to months before an organism is identified [1]. Consequently, delays in the most appropriate management regimens may ensue if the causative pathogen is not rapidly and correctly identified. The ability to cultivate infectious pathogens is also influenced by transport conditions of the clinical specimen. For example, to maximize sensitivity in the isolation of equine influenza virus, Dacron nasopharyngeal swabs that have been chilled in virus transport medium and inoculated in allantoic fluid of embryonated hens' eggs within 24 hours of collection should be used [2]. Molecular recognition systems that can be used for rapid identification can improve response time and reduce the number of susceptible animals exposed to the infectious pathogen.

Several technologic innovations have improved the rapidity and sensitivity with which microorganisms are identified [1]. Immunologic assays and nucleic acid–based methods for the identification of bacterial, viral, and fungal pathogens have found clinical application in the diagnosis of equine pulmonary disease.

Immunologic techniques

Immunologic techniques for the detection of bacterial, viral, and fungal pulmonary pathogens have been developed. Immunoassays rely on interaction between the bacterial, viral, and fungal antigens and enzyme- or fluorescent-labeled antibody. The antibody is the major factor determining the sensitivity and specificity of an assay [3]. Polyclonal antibodies, antibodies produced by immunizing animals with the target antigen and harvesting the antisera, can be produced for use in immunoassays. The use of polyclonal antibodies tends to increase the sensitivity of the assay, because the preparation may contain antibodies to multiple epitopes on the target antigen, thus increasing the chance of antigen detection [4]. Polyclonal antibody preparations tend to decrease assay specificity because of their heterogenous nature, which consists of a variety of different antibodies with varying affinities for different epitopes on the target immunogen [3]. As a consequence, there is a greater chance of cross-reactivity between epitopes on target and nontarget proteins [5]. Test specificity can be improved by the use of monoclonal antibodies, however, because these antibodies interact with only a single well-defined epitope or similar epitopes [6]. Briefly, monoclonal antibodies are produced by immunizing mice with purified antigen, harvesting B lymphocytes from the spleen after an immune response has been elicited, fusing the harvested B lymphocytes with myeloma cells to produce immortal cell lines (hybridomas), and selecting the hybridoma that produces the desired antibody specific for a single epitope [6]. Therefore, if monoclonal antibodies are used in diagnostic assays, the target epitope to which monoclonal antibodies are produced must be chosen carefully so as to avoid target epitopes that are frequent sites of mutation. In this situation, the antibodies may no longer be capable of binding to the target epitope [6,7].

Immunohistochemistry is rapidly becoming a standard diagnostic tool for the identification of viral, bacterial, and protozoal pathogens in tissue sections [8]. Immunohistochemistry depends on polyclonal or monoclonal antibodies binding to a target antigen and the demonstration of this interaction by colored histochemical reactions visible by light microscopy or by emittance of fluorescence detectable after ultraviolet light illumination [4]. Immunohistochemistry is highly versatile, and assays have been developed to detect a variety of equine pulmonary pathogens in tissue sections, including but not limited to equine herpesviruses [9,10], equine viral arteritis virus [11], Hendra virus [12], *Rhodococcus equi* [13], and *Pneumocystis carinii* [14]. Recent advancements in methodology have increased the ability to detect antigens in formalin-fixed tissues. Antigen retrieval techniques using proteases [15] and heat [16] have been developed and result in reversion of some of the conformational changes of proteins and their epitopes that occurred during the fixation process.

The antigen-capture ELISA is the most widely used immunologic assay [17]. The ELISA can be used to detect antigen of pulmonary pathogens directly from an animal before or during clinical disease. The ELISA commonly follows a sandwich assay format and uses capture and detecting antibodies. Briefly, antigen of the test sample is captured by an antibody that has been bound to a solid-phase support, and this interaction is detected by a second fluoro- or enzyme-labeled antibody [7]. One such ELISA, the Directigen FLU-A (Becton Dickinson Microbiology Systems, Cockeysville, Maryland) was developed for use in human medicine to detect influenza A virus. The assay uses monoclonal antibodies that detect influenza A viral nucleoprotein [18,19]. The assay could be adopted for use in veterinary medicine, because the amino acid sequences and antigens of influenza A viral nucleoprotein are similar and relatively conserved among different species [18]. The Directigen FLU-A was evaluated for the diagnosis of equine influenza, with good results [18,20,21]. The Directigen FLU-A did not react with other viruses and bacteria commonly found in the equine respiratory tract [20]. Results of the Directigen FLU-A are available in 15 minutes [18–21]. The ability to detect antigen is highly dependent on the timing of nasopharyngeal swab specimen collection; antigen detection tests for equine influenza are able to identify infectious horses at the peak of infection but are not sensitive enough to reliably detect low levels of viral shedding [18].

Nucleic acid–based techniques

Nucleic acid–based techniques for the diagnosis of equine pulmonary disease are becoming widely accepted because of the sensitivity, specificity, and speed with which results can be obtained [17]. These assays can detect nucleic acid of live and dead pathogens at low concentrations, often less than 100 copies per microliter [22]. Bacterial, viral, and fungal pulmonary pathogens can be discriminated based on nucleic acid sequences unique to that particular organism [1]. Once a sequence is identified that may serve as a useful target able to discriminate between the particular pathogen in question and other microorganisms, the sequence can be compared with all other possible homologous sequences in a current nucleic acid database (GenBank; National Institute of Health, Bethesda, Maryland) using a nucleic acid alignment program (BLAST; National Center for Biotechnology Information, National Library of Medicine, Bethesda, Maryland) [23]. Refinement of methodologies has compressed the time frame for analysis of nucleic acid–based techniques from several hours to several minutes [22].

The polymerase chain reaction (PCR) is the most widely used molecular diagnostic technique in research and clinical laboratories [24]. The PCR assay involves the enzymatic replication of a target region of DNA as defined by a set of oligonucleotide primers [1]. DNA polymerase synthesizes each complimentary strand of the target region in the $5'$ to $3'$ direction, and the amount of DNA that is synthesized increases exponentially [25]. For viruses whose genome is composed of RNA, an initial reverse transcriptase step is required to generate a complimentary strand of nucleic acid, because the DNA polymerase requires a double-stranded template to amplify the target sequence [1]. PCR techniques have been described for the detection of equine influenza virus [26–28], equine herpesviruses [29–32], Hendra virus [33], *P carinii* [34], *R equi* [35,36], and fungal pneumonic pathogens [37].

Conventional methods for the detection of PCR products involve the use of gel electrophoresis and radioactive or fluorogenic markers. Accurate quantification of the amount of the template present initially is not possible using conventional methods [25]. A real-time PCR assay combines PCR amplification with detection of the amplified products, allowing quantification of PCR products [25]. In a real-time PCR assay, the PCR reaction is performed in a reaction tube to which an optical device is attached to read the fluorescent signal generated during each cycle of PCR reaction.

Increases in the reporter fluorescence are proportional to the increase in PCR product. By monitoring the changes in degree of fluorescence, the time in which a transition from exponential to log phase amplification occurs can be determined and compared with that of a standard control to determine the initial template concentration [25].

Nonspecific and specific techniques have been described to detect nucleic acid amplification products in real time. One approach uses a double-stranded DNA (dsDNA) fluorescent dye that becomes intercalated in dsDNA and emits fluorescence when bound to dsDNA [25]. When used in an assay to detect equine influenza virus in nasopharyngeal swabs, the quantitative PCR assay was more sensitive compared with an ELISA and with virus isolation [38]. Specific means of detecting and quantifying nucleic acids rely on nucleic acid primer or probe constructs and include hydrolysis probes [39,40], black hole quenchers [41], molecular beacons [42], and lux primers [43]. Each method has a slightly different method of generating fluorescence during the amplification process [25]. Hydrolysis probes, such as TaqMan (Applied Biosystems, Foster City, California), are commercially available and can be tailored for use as a diagnostic test to detect specific pathogens. This technology has been used to develop an assay for the diagnosis of Hendra virus in tissue homogenates [44]. In the TaqMan assay, a probe is labeled with fluorescence and binds to a nucleic acid sequence within the target region. During amplification, the *Thermus aquaticus* (Taq) polymerase hydrolyses the probe that separates the fluorescein from a quenching dye and allows the emission of fluorescence [25]. The amount of fluorescence emitted is proportional to the accumulation of specific PCR product [44]. TaqMan assays reduce the risk of contamination, because there is less sample handling compared with traditional PCR techniques, and the results are produced rapidly [44].

With the increased use of the PCR assay as a diagnostic test, there is increased demand for standardized techniques and internal control measures [45]. The PCR assay is a highly sensitive test and may produce false-positive results, which are commonly attributed to contamination [46]. False-negative results may occur as a result of the presence of enzyme inhibitors in the sample that suppress DNA amplification [47]. Chemical, enzymatic, and thermal techniques used to extract nucleic acid from the microorganism may damage the nucleic acid and result in false-negative results [47,48]. A standardized method was developed for the detection of equine herpesvirus-1 to minimize false-negative results [29]. A control plasmid containing a DNA sequence that would be amplified at the same time as the target DNA but was sufficiently mutated so that it could be distinguished from the target DNA sequence after the PCR assay was used [29]. In this way, the presence of inhibitory molecules in the PCR reaction that prevented amplification of viral DNA could be identified, because the target and control are affected equally by variation in amplification efficiency [49]. In a similar manner, a 16S ribosomal RNA (rRNA) universal bacterial primer was incorporated into an assay for the detection of *R equi* [50]. The 16S rRNA gene is a conserved DNA sequence of the bacterial genome, and its use in a multiplex PCR assay for the detection of virulent *R equi* allowed direct detection of DNA extraction efficiency as well as confirmation of template presence so as to prevent erroneous interpretation of false-negative results [50].

Treatment

Regardless of the etiologic agent causing pulmonary disease, stall rest and supportive care are essential in the treatment of pulmonary disease. An adequate duration of stall rest is necessary for complete recovery of the respiratory tract [51]. Exercise during clinical disease may exacerbate the clinical signs of disease [52]. A guideline for viral pulmonary diseases states that horses should be stall rested for as many weeks as the number of days they had a fever [51,53]. For bacterial pulmonary diseases, horses should be rested for at least 3 weeks after clinical and clinicopathologic resolution [54]. During the convalescent period, the animal should be stabled in a well-ventilated area that is free of drafts and marked changes in temperature [54,55]. Good-quality hay and clean water should be provided at all times [55].

Specific antiviral treatment is possible for a limited number of viral pulmonary diseases. Antiviral agents have been used for the prevention and treatment of influenza. The M2 inhibitors, such as amantadine and rimantadine, are antiviral agents that inhibit the M2 protein of influenza viruses. The M2 protein is a membrane protein required for efficient nucleocapsid release after viral fusion with the endosomal membrane [56]. Inhibition of the M2 protein therefore prevents influenza viral replication [56]. The efficacy of amantadine and rimantadine has been demonstrated in human patients with influenza [56,57]. In horses, the administration of rimantadine starting 12 hours before challenge exposure to equine influenza virus and continuing for 7 days ameliorated clinical signs of influenza infection [58]. Resistance to amantadine and rimantadine is rare among wild-type viral strains but emerges rapidly within 2 to 4 days after the start of therapy in up to 30% of human patients [59]. The development of resistance to an M2 inhibitor confers cross-resistance to all M2 inhibitors but not to neuraminidase inhibitors or ribavirin [56]. Neuraminidase inhibitors, such as zanamivir and oseltamivir, prevent the influenza virus from effectively passing through respiratory secretions and decrease viral spread [60]. Clinical trials in human influenza have supported the use of neuraminidase inhibitors in influenza viral infection [61–66]. Ribavirin, a guanosine analogue, exhibits antiviral activity by depleting guanine pools, inhibiting influenza virus RNA polymerase activity, and inhibiting guanosine triphosphate–dependent 5′-capping of viral mRNA [56]. Clinical benefit has been shown after the administration of ribavirin in human patients [67–79]. Although antiviral drugs are often cost-prohibitive for use in equine patients with influenza, they may be beneficial for the protection of valuable horses during influenza outbreaks [53].

Treatment of bacterial infectious pulmonary diseases has traditionally relied on parenteral or oral administration of antimicrobials. The outcome of therapy depends on the concentration of antimicrobials in the airways rather than in the serum [70,71]. Many parenterally administered antimicrobials exhibit low bioavailability in the lungs and distal airways of the respiratory tract [72–75]. Furthermore, bronchial secretions may inactivate aminoglycosides and β-lactam antimicrobials, necessitating larger concentrations to achieve bactericidal effects [76]. To overcome effects of low bioavailability and inactivation in the pulmonary tree, antimicrobials must be administered in high doses so as to achieve adequate drug concentrations in the airways for antibacterial activity, which increases the risk of systemic toxicity [77,78].

The direct delivery of antimicrobials to the lower airways through aerosolization has been investigated with great interest because it presents the potential to maximize drug concentrations at the site of infection while minimizing systemic exposure. The efficient delivery of antimicrobial aerosols to the lower airways is influenced by the characteristics of the nebulizer, the patient, and the aerosol. An aerosol is defined as a gas containing finely dispersed solid- or liquid-suspended particles [79]. It is believed that the size of the aerosol particles is of importance in determining the proportion of drug that reaches and distributes within the lungs. Aerosol particle sizes between 1 and 5 μm are thought to be ideal; particles less than 1 μm have insufficient mass for effective drug delivery and are exhaled, whereas particles greater than 5 μm are usually deposited in the oropharynx and subsequently cleared by swallowing [80]. The efficiency with which a nebulizer aerosolizes a solution and produces particles of ideal size varies with its design. Ultrasonic and jet nebulizers are capable of delivering aerosol to the peripheral regions of the lungs [81]. Improvements in nebulizer design, for example, breath-actuated jet nebulizers, which only produce medication during inspiration, and breath-enhanced nebulizers, which improve aerosolization of the solution, increase the efficiency with which solutions are aerosolized [82–85]. Although nebulizer performance plays an important role, variation in antimicrobial delivery to the lower airways seems to be more a result of patient-specific variables than of particle size or other nebulizer variables [86]. The route of breathing, respiratory rate, and respiratory pattern are all factors that can significantly reduce the efficiency of aerosol delivery [87]. Nasal breathing alone reduces lung deposition of nebulized drugs by approximately 50% in human adults [88]. For most nebulizer systems, it has been estimated that approximately 10% of the initial drug mass nebulized reaches the lungs and the remaining 90% is deposited in the delivery system and nasopharynx or is exhaled into the surrounding atmosphere [89,90]. As airway disease worsens, the distribution of aerosols to the distal airways decreases; excessive mucus secretions and bronchospasm favor the deposition of aerosols in the central airways [91–94]. The ideal respiratory pattern is that of a deep slow inhalation accompanied by breath holding [95]. During larger breaths, aerosol is likely to penetrate further into the lung, increasing peripheral deposition, whereas during higher flows of deep and fast breathing, turbulence is more likely to occur and deposition in the upper airways and major bronchi increases [96]. Because respiration cannot be controlled in conscious horses, the alteration of respiratory pattern cannot be used to optimize lung deposition of aerosols. Characteristics of the therapeutic nebulized solution can have a major impact on the characteristics of the aerosol produced and on the patient's response to aerosol administration [97]. Increases in the concentration of solute, surface tension, or viscosity of the solution can independently decrease aerosol output and increase particle size [98–100]. Solutions that are hypertonic, hypotonic, or acidic may induce coughing, bronchoconstriction, or both [101–103]. Furthermore, antimicrobial solutions marketed for intravenous use may induce coughing and bronchoconstriction because of the presence of preservatives in the solution, such as sodium metabisulfite, benzalkonium chloride, or EDTA [98,99,104]. To avoid bronchoconstriction and the unwanted effects from additives, a preservative-free tobramycin solution, Tobramycin for Inhalation (TOBI; Chiroh Corporation, Emeryville, California), has been developed and marketed for nebulization therapy.

Regardless of technical limitations compromising maximal efficiency, aerosolization of antimicrobials can achieve high concentrations in the pulmonary epithelial lining fluid and mucosa of the respiratory tract [105–107] and decrease the severity or duration of respiratory tract bacterial infection [108–110]. Approximately 80% of human adolescent and adult patients with cystic fibrosis develop chronic *Pseudomonas aeruginosa* pulmonary infection [111,112], which, when established, is associated with progressive deterioration of lung function [113]. Nebulization of these patients with tobramycin was found to decrease *P aeruginosa* bacterial density in sputum, improve pulmonary function, and decrease the number of hospitalizations attributable to acute pulmonary exacerbations [110,113,114]. When compared with placebo, treatment with inhaled tobramycin did not significantly increase the isolation of intrinsically tobramycin-resistant gram-negative isolates, such as *Burkholderia cepacia*, *Stenotrophomonas maltophilia*, and *Alcaligenes xylosoxidans* [115,116]. Long-term administration of preservative-free tobramycin in rodent models showed a high degree of safety with no irreversible toxic effects on the respiratory tract epithelium if less than 12 times the intended human dose is used for aerosolization [80]. After once- or twice-daily aerosolization for consecutive days, no apparent accumulation of tobramycin was detected in the pulmonary tree [75,89]. Ototoxicity, nephrotoxicity, and pneumotoxicity have not been reported in short- and long-term studies of tobramycin aerosols in human patients [117–120]. Although clinical trials have not yet been published using horses, nebulization of antimicrobials remains promising. McKenzie and Murray

[75] showed that nebulization of gentamicin in healthy adult horses achieved bronchoalveolar fluid concentrations 12 times greater than serum concentrations. There was low systemic absorption of gentamicin at all times. Thus, the aerosolization of antimicrobials offers the advantage of direct delivery of the antimicrobial in high concentrations directly to the site of infection while minimizing systemic side effects.

The pharmacokinetics of the chemotherapeutic drug after nebulization should have a great impact on therapeutic efficacy. Although aminoglycosides, semisynthetic penicillins, and polymyxins have demonstrated variable clinical benefit, adequately powered trials have not been performed, with the exception of studies using preservative-free tobramycin [80]. Aminoglycosides are the most commonly reported aerosolized antimicrobial agents because they remain bioactive when aerosolized, are poorly absorbed across epithelial surfaces, and thus remain within the pulmonary tree, where they exert their concentration-dependent effect [80]. Another therapeutic approach that has been investigated produces high antimicrobial drug concentrations in the pulmonary tree to liposome-encapsulated antimicrobials. Liposomes are spherically shaped vesicles consisting of one or more natural or synthetic lipid bilayers surrounding an aqueous space [120]. Aqueous soluble drugs, such as aminoglycosides, can be encapsulated in the internal aqueous compartment, whereas lipid-soluble drugs may bind or are incorporated in the lipid bilayer [120]. Experimental trials using aerosolized liposome-encapsulated antimicrobial drugs have demonstrated their potential use [121–124]. The nebulization of liposomal amphotericin B has been shown to be effective in the prevention of pulmonary aspergillosis in rodent models [121,122]. Treatment of severely immunocompromised rats with invasive pulmonary aspergillosis using aerosolized liposomal amphotericin B significantly prolonged survival when compared with placebo-treated animals [123]. In another study, mice were infected with *Francisella tularensis*, and only those treated with liposome-encapsulated ciprofloxacin survived the pulmonary infection [124]. Conventional liposomes are naturally taken up by pulmonary macrophages [125]. It has been speculated that the intracellular delivery of antimicrobials may partly account for the effective eradication of intracellular bacteria from the lungs [124]. Experimental studies using intracellularly infected phagocytic cells have shown that the phagocytosis of aminoglycoside-encapsulated liposomes yielded therapeutic intracellular drug concentrations and enhanced killing of intracellular microorganisms [120]. Because liposome-encapsulated antimicrobials are retained in the lower respiratory tract, systemic toxicity after aerosol administration is minimized [121,126]. After the aerosol administration of liposome-encapsulated amphotericin B, little or no drug was deposited in organs other than the lungs [121,126]. No detrimental effect of liposome-encapsulated amphotericin B on surfactant function was found in vitro [127]. To the authors' knowledge, there are no published reports involving the use of liposome-encapsulated antimicrobials in equids. Aerosol delivery of liposome-encapsulated antimicrobials may provide an approach to the treatment of infectious pulmonary diseases in the future, however.

Prevention

Vaccination has become a major tool in the management of infectious pulmonary disease. Although currently available, parenterally administered, inactivated equine influenza virus and equine herpesvirus vaccines elicit a systemic immune response, protection from clinical disease is incomplete and short-lived [127,128]. To provide protective immunity against pulmonary pathogens, the immune system must be primed at the respiratory mucosal surfaces. Novel vaccination strategies, including the use of live-attenuated virus strains and plasmid DNA, have been developed with the goal of stimulating local humoral and cell-mediated immune responses similar to those occurring with natural infection. In this way, infection may be prevented by neutralizing the pathogen at the portal of entry.

Live-attenuated virus vaccines

Live-attenuated virus vaccines have the potential to produce an immune response similar to that of natural pulmonary infection. When delivered intranasally, the virus vaccine strain mimics that of natural infection, and thus, theoretically, stimulates a similar protective immune response. A cold-adapted, temperature-sensitive, live-attenuated virus equine influenza vaccine (FluAvert IN Vaccine; Heska Corporation, Fort Collins, Colorado) has been developed and licensed for use in the United States. After vaccination, a systemic immune response similar to the response that occurs after natural influenza infection was elicited, generated IgGa and IgGb antibodies, and induced protection from clinical disease for 3 months [129]. The intranasal administration of the vaccine did not result in detectable nasal IgA, however, which is the response required for protective immunity. Consequently, the vaccine did not produce sterile immunity [129–133].

Nucleic acid–based vaccines

Since the first reports of genetic immunization were published [132–134], there has been a tremendous interest in developing this technology further. Genetic immunization, or DNA immunization, is based on inoculation of plasmid DNA containing open reading frames with appropriate eukaryotic transcription and translation control signals that result in the synthesis of a protein by cells of the host. The endogenously produced proteins have conformation and posttranslational modifications identical to those produced during natural infection [135]. The protein is expressed in association with major histocompatability complex classes I and II and elicits a T-lymphocyte helper 1 (Th1) and T-lymphocyte helper 2 (Th2) immune response [136,137]. Genetic immunization can induce immune responses in neonates, even in the presence of maternal antibodies [137–140]. Investigations have shown that genetic immunization may be capable of inducing an immune response in the fetus [141]. This may provide individuals with immunity to pathogens to which they may be exposed early in life [135].

The efficacy of genetic immunization depends on the identification of antigens that elicit a protective immune response. Prime candidates include those antigens involved in the infection process, including those proteins involved in virus adsorption, penetration, and cell-to-cell spread. Hemagglutinin (HA) glycoproteins of equine influenza virus [142] and glycoproteins (gI, gD gI, gL), of equine herpesviruses 1 and 4 [142–145] have been investigated as potential protective antigens because of their central role in the initial viral infection.

The efficiency of genetic immunization depends on the efficiency of gene expression after transfection of host cells. Galvin and colleagues [146] proposed that the level of humoral and cell-mediated immunity induced by a DNA vaccine is directly correlated with the eukaryotic promoter strength. Several different promoters have been used in studies on genetic immunization; however, the human cytomegalovirus immediate early promoter has induced superior immune responses in comparison to other promoters [146,147]. The incorporation of costimulatory molecules, such as CD80, CD86, intracellular adhesion molecule 1 (ICAM 1), and CD40L, has been shown to enhance the cytotoxic T-lymphocyte response [148–150]. Furthermore, gene-encoded cytokines, including interleukin (IL)-6, IL-12, and granulocyte-monocyte colony-stimulating factor [151–153], have been used to modulate and enhance humoral and cell-mediated immune responses.

Numerous delivery systems have been proposed to enhance plasmid uptake by host cells; however, "gene gun" delivery, a high-energy microparticle bombardment method that fires DNA-coated gold beads into target tissues, is the most efficient [154,155]. Gene gun delivery seems to be efficient for transfecting Langerhans cells or dendritic cells [156]. These cells then migrate to lymph nodes and generate an immune response [157,158]. Lunn and coworkers [159] used a gene gun delivery system to vaccinate ponies using HA DNA of influenza A virus. Ponies were vaccinated at skin locations and mucosal sites. IgGa and IgGb mucosal antibodies were produced and significantly reduced clinical signs in ponies when challenged with influenza virus 30 days after the final vaccination [142]. In a similar experiment, Soboll and colleagues [160] compared gene gun–delivered HA DNA with a gene gun–delivered combination of IL-6 DNA and HA DNA (IL-6/HA DNA). Those ponies vaccinated with IL-6/HA DNA produced significantly higher levels of serum IgG(T) compared with the ponies vaccinated with HA DNA [159]. This IgG(T) response suggests that a shift toward a Th2-like response in the systemic compartment may have occurred [160]. Although neither experiment resulted in the production of nasal mucosal IgA, both resulted in increased concentrations of IgGa and IgGb, which exerted a protective effect against clinical disease.

Summary

Techniques for novel approaches to the diagnosis and management of equine pulmonary disease continue to be developed and used in clinical practice. Diagnostic techniques involving immunoassays and nucleic acid–based tests not only decrease the time in which results become available but increase the sensitivity and specificity of test results. These assays do not substitute for careful clinical evaluation but can shorten the time to a confirmed accurate diagnosis, and thus permit early initiation of therapeutic strategies and prevention protocols. With further understanding of the molecular biology and immunology of equine pulmonary disease, diagnostic and management techniques should become further refined.

References

[1] Iqbal SS, Mayo MW, Bruno JG, et al. A review of molecular recognition technologies for detection of biological threat agents. Biosens Bioelectron 2000;15:549–78.
[2] Mumford EL, Traub-Dargatz JL, Salman MD, et al. Monitoring and detection of acute viral respiratory tract disease in horses. J Am Vet Med Assoc 1998;213:385–90.
[3] Ronald A, Stimson WH. The evolution of immunoassay technology. Parasitology 1998;117(Suppl):S13–27.
[4] Ramos-Vara JA. Technical aspects of immunohistochemistry. Vet Pathol 2005;42:405–26.
[5] Mighell AJ, Hume WJ, Robinson PA. An overview of the complexities and subtleties of immunohistochemistry. Oral Dis 1998;4:217–23.
[6] Berry JD. Rational monoclonal antibody development to emerging pathogens, biothreat agents and agents of foreign animal disease: the antigen scale. Vet J 2005;170:193–211.
[7] Andreotti PE, Ludwig GV, Peruski AH, et al. Immunoassay of infectious agents. Biotechniques 2003;35:850–9.
[8] Procop GW, Wilson M. Infectious disease pathology. Clin Infect Dis 2001;32:1589–601.
[9] Kydd JH, Smith KC, Hannant D, et al. Distribution of equid herpesvirus-1 (EHV-1) in the respiratory tract of ponies: implications for vaccination strategies. Equine Vet J 1994;26:466–9.
[10] Kydd JH, Smith KC, Hannant D, et al. Distribution of equid herpesvirus-1 (EHV-1) in respiratory tract associated lymphoid tissue: implications for cellular immunity. Equine Vet J 1994;26:470–3.
[11] Del Piero F. Equine virus arteritis. Vet Pathol 2000;37:287–96.
[12] Murray PK, Hooper PT, Hyatt AD, et al. A morbillivirus that caused fatal disease in horses and humans. Science 1995;268:94–7.
[13] Szeredi L, Makrai L, Dénes B. Rapid immunohistochemical detection of *Rhodococcus equi* in impression smears from affected foals on postmortem examination. J Vet Med B Infect Dis Vet Public Health 2001;48:751–8.
[14] Jensen TK, Boye M, Bille-Hansen V. Application of fluorescent in situ hybridization for specific diagnosis of *Pneumocystis carinii* pneumonia in foals and pigs. Vet Pathol 2001;38:269–74.
[15] Huang SN, Minassian H, More JD. Application of immunofluorescent staining on paraffin sections improved by trypsin digestion. Lab Invest 1976;35:383–90.
[16] Shi SR, Key ME, Kalra KL. Antigen retrieval in formalin-fixed, paraffin-embedded tissue: an enhancement method for immunohistochemical staining based on microwave oven heating of tissue sections. J Histochem Cytochem 1991;39:741–8.

[17] Peruski LF Jr, Peruski AH. Rapid diagnostic assays in the genomic biology era: detection and identification of infectious disease and biologic weapon agents. Biotechniques 2003;35: 840–6.
[18] Chambers TM, Shortridge KF, Li PH, et al. Rapid diagnosis of equine influenza by the Directigen FLU-A enzyme immunoassay. Vet Rec 1994;135:275–9.
[19] Johnston SL, Bloy H. Evaluation of a rapid enzyme immunoassay for detection of influenza A virus. J Clin Microbiol 1993;31:142–3.
[20] Morley PS, Bogdan JR, Townsend HG, et al. Evaluation of Directigen Flu A assay for detection of influenza antigen in nasal secretions of horses. Equine Vet J 1995;27:131–4.
[21] Van Maanen C, Van Essen GJ, Minke J, et al. Diagnostic methods applied to analysis of an outbreak of equine influenza in a riding school in which vaccine failure occurred. Vet Microbiol 2003;93:291–306.
[22] Ivnitski D, O'Neil DJ, Gattuso A, et al. Nucleic acid approaches for detection and identification of biological warfare and infectious disease agents. Biotechnology 2003;35:862–9.
[23] Benson DA, Karsch-Mizrachi I, Lipman DJ, et al. GenBank. Nucleic Acids Res 2005;33: D34–8.
[24] Pfaller MA. Molecular approaches to diagnosing and managing infectious diseases: practicality and costs. Emerg Infect Dis 2001;7:312–8.
[25] Cai HY, Archambault M, Gyles CL, et al. Molecular genetic methods in the veterinary clinical bacteriology laboratory: current usage and future applications. An Health Res Rev 2003;4:73–93.
[26] Donofrio JC, Coonrod JD, Chambers TM. Diagnosis of equine influenza by the polymerase chain reaction. J Vet Diagn Invest 1994;24:20–5.
[27] Fouchier RA, Bestebroer TM, Van Der Kemp L, et al. Detection of influenza A viruses from different species by PCR amplification of conserved sequences in the matrix gene. J Clin Microbiol 2000;38:4096–104.
[28] Oxburgh L, Hagstrom AA. PCR based method for the identification of equine influenza virus from clinical samples. Vet Microbiol 1999;67:161–74.
[29] Daly P, Doyle S. The development of a competitive PCR-ELISA for the detection of equine herpesvirus-1. J Virol Methods 2003;107:237–44.
[30] Kirisawa R, Endo A, Iwai H, et al. Detection and identification of equine herpesvirus-1 and -4 by polymerase chain reaction. Vet Microbiol 1993;36:57–67.
[31] Sharma PC, Cullinane AA, Onions DE, et al. Diagnosis of equid herpesviruses-1 and -4 by polymerase chain reaction. Equine Vet J 1992;24:20–5.
[32] Varrasso A, Dynon K, Ficorilli N, et al. Identification of equine herpesvirus 1 and 4 by polymerase chain reaction. Aust Vet J 2001;79:563–9.
[33] Hooper PT, Gould AR, Hyatt AD, et al. Identification and molecular characterization of Hendra virus in a horse in Queensland. Aust Vet J 2000;78:281–2.
[34] Ribes JA, Limper AH, Espy MJ, et al. PCR detection of *Pneumocystis carinii* in bronchoalveolar lavage specimens: analysis of sensitivity and specificity. J Clin Microbiol 1997;35: 830–5.
[35] Sellon DC, Walker K, Suyemoto M, et al. Nucleic acid amplification for rapid detection of *Rhodococcus equi* in equine blood and tracheal wash fluids. Am J Vet Res 1997;58: 1232–7.
[36] Takai S, Vigo G, Ikushima H, et al. Detection of virulent *Rhodococcus equi* in tracheal aspirate samples by polymerase chain reaction for rapid diagnosis of *Rhodococcus equi* pneumonia in foals. Vet Microbiol 1998;61:59–69.
[37] Skladny H, Bucheidt D, Baust C, et al. Specific detection of *Aspergillus* species in blood and bronchoalveolar lavage samples of immunocompromised patients by two-step PCR. J Clin Microbiol 1999;37:3865–71.
[38] Quinlivan M, Dempsey E, Ryan F, et al. Real-time reverse transcription PCR for detection and quantitative analysis of equine influenza virus. J Clin Microbiol 2005;43: 5055–7.

[39] Holland P, Abramson R, Watson R, et al. Detection of specific polymerase chain reaction product by utilizing the 5′ to 3′ exonuclease activity of *Thermus aquaticus* DNA polymerase. Proc Natl Acad Sci USA 1991;88:7276–80.
[40] Livak KJ, Flood SJ, Marmaro J, et al. Oligonucleotides with fluorescent dyes at opposite ends provide a quenched probe system useful for detecting PCR product and nucleic acid hybridization. PCR Methods Appl 1995;4:357–62.
[41] Johansson MK, Cook RM. Intramolecular dimmers: a new design strategy for fluorescence-quenched probes. Chemistry (Easton) 2003;9:3466–71.
[42] Tyagi S, Kramer FR. Molecular beacons: probes that fluoresce upon hybridization. Nat Biotechnol 1996;14:303–8.
[43] Nazarenko I, Lowe B, Darfler M, et al. Multiplex quantitative PCR using self-quenched primers labeled with a single fluorophore. Nucleic Acids Res 2002;30:e37.
[44] Smith IL, Halpin K, Warrilow D, et al. Development of a fluorogenic RT-PCR assay (TaqMan) for the detection of Hendra virus. J Virol Methods 2001;98:33–40.
[45] Hoorfar J, Cook N, Malorny B, et al. Diagnostic PCR: making internal amplification control mandatory. J Appl Microbiol 2004;96:221–2.
[46] Borst A, Box AT, Fluit AC. False-positive results and contamination in nucleic acid amplification assays: suggestions for a prevent and destroy strategy. Eur J Clin Microbiol Infect Dis 2004;23:289–99.
[47] Burkardt HJ. Standardization and quality control of PCR analyses. Clin Chem Lab 2000;38:87–91.
[48] Ivnitski D, O'Neil DJ, Gattuso A, et al. Nucleic acid approaches for detection and identification of biologic warfare and infectious disease agents. Biotechniques 2003;35:862–9.
[49] Drews K, Bashir T, Dorries K. Quantification of human polyomavirus JC in brain tissue and cerebrospinal fluid of patients with progressive multifocal leukoencephalopathy by competitive PCR. J Virol Methods 2000;84:23–36.
[50] Halbert ND, Reitzel RA, Martens RJ, et al. Evaluation of a multiplex polymerase chain reaction assay for simultaneous detection of Rhodococcus equi and the vapA gene. Am J Vet Res 2005;66:1380–5.
[51] Wilson WD. Equine influenza. Vet Clin North Am Equine Pract 1993;9:257–81.
[52] Gross DK, Hinchcliff KW, French PS, et al. Effect of moderate exercise on the severity of clinical signs associated with influenza virus infection in horses. Equine Vet J 1998;30:489–97.
[53] Chambers TM, Holland RE Jr, Lai AC. Equine influenza—current veterinary perspectives, part 2. Equine Pract 1995;17:26–30.
[54] Traub-Dargatz JL. Bacterial pneumonia. Vet Clin North Am Equine Pract 1991;7:53–61.
[55] Van Maanen C, Cullinane A. Equine influenza virus infections: an update. Vet Q 2002;24:79–94.
[56] Ison MG, Hayden FG. Therapeutic options for the management of influenza. Curr Opin Pharmacol 2001;1:482–90.
[57] Rees WA, Chambers TM, Fenger CK, et al. Pharmacokinetics and bioavailability of amantadine in the horse: a preliminary report. In: Proceedings of the American Association of Equine Practitioners. Lexington (KY); 1995. p. 270–1.
[58] Rees WA, Harkins JD, Woods WE, et al. Amantadine and equine influenza: pharmacology, pharmacokinetics, and neurological effects in the horse. Equine Vet J 1997;29:104–10.
[59] Rees WA, Harkins JD, et al. Pharmacokinetics and therapeutic efficacy of rimantadine in horses experimentally infected with influenza virus A2. Am J Vet Res 1999;60:888–94.
[60] Hayden FG. Amantadine and rimantadine: clinical aspects. In: Richman DD, editor. Antiviral drug resistance. New York: J Wiley and Sons; 1996. p. 78–92.
[61] Colman PM. Influenza virus neuraminidase: structure, antibodies, and inhibitors. Protein Sci 1994;3:1687–96.

[62] Hayden FG, Osterhaus AD, Treanor JJ, et al. Efficacy and safety of the neuraminidase inhibitor zanamivir in the treatment of influenzavirus infections. GG167 Influenza Study Group. N Engl J Med 1997;337:874–80.
[63] Monto AS, Fleming DM, Henry D, et al. Efficacy and safety of the neuraminidase inhibitor zanamivir in the treatment of influenza A and B virus infections. J Infect Dis 1999;180: 254–61.
[64] Makela MJ, Pauksens K, Rostila T, et al. Clinical efficacy and safety of the orally inhaled neuraminidase inhibitor zanamivir in the treatment of influenza: a randomized, double-blind, placebo-controlled European study. J Infect 2000;40:42–8.
[65] McClellan K, Perry CM. Oseltamivir: a review of its use in influenza. Drugs 2001;61: 263–83.
[66] Treanor JJ, Hayden FG, Vrooman PS, et al. Efficacy and safety of the oral neuraminidase inhibitor oseltamivir in treating acute influenza: a randomized controlled trial. US Oral Neuraminidase Study Group. JAMA 2000;283:1016–24.
[67] Whitley RJ, Haydan FG, Reisinger KS, et al. Oral oseltamivir treatment of influenza in children. Pediatr Infect Dis J 2001;20:127–33.
[68] Bernstein DI, Reuman PD, Sherwood JR, et al. Ribavirin small-particle-aerosol treatment of influenza B virus infection. Antimicrob Agents Chemother 1988;32:761–4.
[69] Stein DS, Creticos CM, Jackson GG, et al. Oral ribavirin treatment of influenza A and B. Antimicrob Agents Chemother 1987;31:1285–7.
[70] Valcke Y, Pauwels R, Van Der Straeten M. The penetration of aminoglycosides into the alveolar lining fluid of rats. The effect of airway inflammation. Am Rev Respir Dis 1990; 142:1099–103.
[71] Goldstein I, Wallet F, Nicolas-Robin A, et al. Lung deposition and efficacy of nebulized Amikacin during *Escherichia coli* pneumonia in ventilated pigs. Am J Respir Crit Care Med 2002;166:1375–81.
[72] Wong GA, Pierce TH, Golstein E, et al. Penetration of antimicrobial agents into bronchial secretions. Am J Med 1975;59:219–23.
[73] Valcke Y, Pauwels R, Van Der Straeten M. Pharmacokinetics of antibiotics in the lungs. Eur Respir J 1990;3:715–22.
[74] Godber LM, Walker RD, Stein GE, et al. Pharmacokinetics, nephrotoxicosis, and in vitro antibacterial activity associated with single versus multiple (three times) daily gentamicin treatments in horses. Am J Vet Res 1995;56:613–8.
[75] Mckenzie HC, Murray MJ. Concentrations of gentamicin in serum and bronchial lavage fluid after intervenous and aerosol administration of gentamicin to horses. Am J Vet Res 2000;61:1185–90.
[76] Thys JP, Aoun M, Klastersky J. Local antibiotic therapy for bronchopulmonary infections. In: Pennington JE, editor. Respiratory infections: diagnosis and management. 3rd edition. New York: Raven Press; 1994. p. 741–66.
[77] Cheer SM, Waugh J, Noble S. Inhaled tobramycin (TOBI®): a review of its use in the management of *Pseudomonas aeruginosa* infections in patients with cystic fibrosis. Drugs 2003; 63:2501–20.
[78] Geller DE, Rosenfeld M, Waltz DA, et al. AeroDose TOBI Study Group. Efficiency of pulmonary administration of tobramycin solution for inhalation in cystic fibrosis using an improved drug delivery system. Chest 2003;123:28–36.
[79] Duvivier DH, Votion D, Vandenput S, et al. Aerosol therapy in the equine species. Vet J 1997;154:189–202.
[80] Campbell PW, Saiman L. Use of aerosolized antibiotics in patients with cystic fibrosis. Chest 1999;116:775–88.
[81] Votion D, Ghafir Y, Munsters K, et al. Aerosol deposition in equine lungs following ultrasonic nebulization versus jet aerosol delivery system. Equine Vet J 1997;29:388–93.
[82] Lueng K, Louca E, Coates AL. Comparison of breath-enhanced to breath-actuated nebulizers for rate, consistency, and efficiency. Chest 2004;126:1619–27.

[83] Coates AL, MacNeish CF, Lands LC, et al. A comparison of the availability of tobramycin for inhalation from vented versus unvented nebulizers. Chest 1998;113:951–6.
[84] Katz SL, Ho SL, Coates AL. Nebulizer choice for treatment of cystic fibrosis patients with inhaled colistin. Chest 2001;119:250–5.
[85] Wilson D, Burnstein M, Moya E, et al. Improvement of nebulised antibiotic delivery in cystic fibrosis. Arch Dis Child 1990;80:348–52.
[86] Weber A, Smith A, Williams-Warren J, Ramsey B, et al. Nebulizer delivery of tobramycin to the lower respiratory tract. Pediatr Pulmonol 1994;17:331–9.
[87] Barry PW, O'Callaghan C. Nebuliser therapy in childhood. Thorax 1997;52(Suppl): S78–88.
[88] Everard ML, Hardy JG, Milner AD. Comparison of nebulized aerosol disposition in the lungs of healthy adults following oral and nasal inhalation. Thorax 1993;48:1045–6.
[89] Geller DE, Pitlick WH, Nardella PA, et al. Pharmacokinetics and bioavailability of aerosolized tobramycin in cystic fibrosis. Chest 2002;122:219–26.
[90] Touw DJ, Brimicombe RW, Hodson ME, et al. Inhalation of antibiotics in cystic fibrosis. Eur Respir J 1995;8:1594–604.
[91] Chung KF, Jeyasingh K, Snashall PD. Influence of airway caliber on the intrapulmonary dose and distribution of inhaled aerosol in normal and asthmatic subjects. Eur Respir J 1988;1:890–5.
[92] Ilowite JS, Gorvoy JD, Smaldone GC. Quantitative deposition of aerosolized gentamicin in cystic fibrosis. Am Rev Respir Dis 1987;136:1445–9.
[93] Diot P, Palmer LB, Smaldone A, et al. RhDNase I aerosol deposition and related factors in cystic fibrosis. Am J Respir Crit Care Med 1997;156:1662–8.
[94] Mukhopadhyay S, Staddon GE, Eastman C, et al. The quantitative distribution of nebulized antibiotic in the lung in cystic fibrosis. Respir Med 1994;88:203–11.
[95] Pavia D, Thomson ML, Clarke SW, et al. Effect of lung function and mode of inhalation on penetration of aerosol into the human lung. Thorax 1977;32:194–7.
[96] Ryan G, Dolovich MB, Obminski G, et al. Standardization of inhalation provocation tests: influence of nebulizer output, particle size, and method of inhalation. J Allergy Clin Immunol 1981;67:156–61.
[97] Moren F. Aerosol dosage forms and formulations. In: Moren F, Dolovich MB, Newhouse MT, et al, editors. Aerosols in medicine: principles, diagnosis and therapy. Amsterdam: Elsevier; 1993. p. 321–49.
[98] Weber A, Morlin G, Cohen M, et al. Effect of nebulizer type and antibiotic concentration on device performance. Pediatr Pulmonol 1997;23:249–60.
[99] O'Callaghan C, Barry PW. The science of nebulized drug delivery. Thorax 1997;52(Suppl): S31–44.
[100] McKenzie HC. Characterization of antimicrobial aerosols for administration to horses. Vet Ther 2003;4:110–9.
[101] Chua HL, Collis GG, Le Souef PN. Bronchial response to nebulized antibiotics in children with cystic fibrosis. Eur Respir J 1990;3:1114–6.
[102] Dally MB, Kurrle S, Breslin AB. Ventilatory effects of aerosol gentamicin. Thorax 1978;33: 54–6.
[103] Dickie KJ, De Groot WJ. Ventilatory effects of aerosolized kanamycin and polymyxin. Chest 1973;63:694–7.
[104] Beasley CR, Rafferty R, Holgate ST. Bronchoconstrictor properties of preservative in ipratropium bromide (Atrovent) nebulizer solution. BMJ 1987;294:1197–8.
[105] Montgomery AB, Debs RJ, Luce JM, et al. Selective delivery of pentamidine to the lung by aerosol. Am Rev Respir Dis 1988;137:477–8.
[106] Vermeersch H, Vandenbossche G, Remon JP, et al. Pharmacokinetics of nebulized sodium ceftiofur in calves. J Vet Pharmacol Ther 1996;19:152–4.
[107] Baran D, De Vuyst P, Ooms HA. Concentration of tobramycin given by aerosol in the fluid obtained by bronchoalveolar lavage. Respir Med 1990;84:203–4.

[108] Orcutt TA, Godwin CR, Pizzo PA, et al. Aerosolized pentamidine: a well-tolerated mode of prophylaxis against *Pneumocystis carinii* in older children with human immunodeficiency virus infection. Pediatr Infect Dis J 1992;11:290–4.
[109] Sustronck B, Deprez P, Muylle E, et al. Evaluation of the nebulization of sodium ceftiofur in the treatment of experimental *Pasteurella haemolytica* bronchopneumonia in calves. Res Vet Sci 1995;59:267–71.
[110] Ramsey BW, Dorkin HL, Eisenberg JD, et al. Efficacy of aerosolized tobramycin in patients with cystic fibrosis. N Engl J Med 1993;328:1740–6.
[111] FitzSimmons SC. The changing epidemiology of cystic fibrosis. J Pediatr 1993;122:1–9.
[112] Gibson RL, Emerson J, McNamara S, et al. Significant microbiological effect of inhaled tobramycin in young children with cystic fibrosis. Am J Respir Crit Care Med 2003;167: 841–9.
[113] Ramsey BW, Pepe MS, Quan JM, et al. Intermittent administration of inhaled tobramycin in patients with cystic fibrosis. N Engl J Med 1999;340:23–30.
[114] Moss RB. Long-term benefits of inhaled tobramycin in adolescent patients with cystic fibrosis. Chest 2002;121:55–63.
[115] Burns JL, Van Dalfsen JM, Shawar RM, et al. Effect of chronic intermittent administration of inhaled tobramycin on respiratory microbial flora in patients with cystic fibrosis. J Infect Dis 1999;179:1190–6.
[116] Moss RB. Administration of aerosolized antibiotics in cystic fibrosis patients. Chest 2001; 120(Suppl):S107–13.
[117] MacLusky IB, Gold R, Corey M, et al. Long-term effects of inhaled tobramycin in patients with cystic fibrosis colonized with *Pseudomonas aeruginosa*. Pediatr Pulmonol 1989;7:42–8.
[118] Stephens D, Garey N, Isles A, et al. Efficiency of inhaled tobramycin in the treatment of pulmonary exacerbations in children with cystic fibrosis. Pediatr Infect Dis 1983;2:209–11.
[119] Steinkamp G, Tummler B, Gappa M, et al. Long-term tobramycin aerosol therapy in cystic fibrosis. Pediatr Pulmonol 1989;6:91–8.
[120] Schiffelers RM, Storm G, Bakker-Woudenberg IA. Liposome-encapsulated aminoglycoside in pre-clinical and clinical studies. J Antimicrob Chemother 2001;48:333–44.
[121] Allen SD, Sorensen KN, Nejdl MJ, et al. Prophylactic efficacy of aerosolized liposomal (AmBiosome) and non-liposomal (Fungizone) amphotericin B in murine pulmonary aspergillosis. J Antimicrob Chemother 1994;34:1001–13.
[122] Cicogna CE, White MH, Bernard EM, et al. Efficacy of prophylactic aerosol amphotericin B lipid complex in a rat model of pulmonary aspergillosis. Antimicrob Agents Chemother 1997;41:259–61.
[123] Ruijgrok EJ, Vulto AG, Van Etten EW. Efficacy of aerosolized amphotericin B desoxycholate and liposomal amphotericin B in the treatment of invasive pulmonary aspergillosis in severely immunocompromised rats. J Antimicrob Chemother 2001;48:89–95.
[124] Conley J, Yang H, Wilson T, et al. Aerosol delivery of liposome-encapsulated ciprofloxacin: aerosol characterization and efficacy against *Francisella tularensis* infection in mice. Antimicrob Agents Chemother 1997;41:1288–92.
[125] Gonzalez-Rothi RJ, Straub L, Cacace J, et al. Liposomes and pulmonary alveolar macrophages: function and morphological interactions. Exp Lung Res 1991;17:687–705.
[126] Lambros MP, Bourne DW, Abbas SA, et al. Disposition of aerosolized liposomal amphotericin B. J Pharm Sci 1997;86:1066–9.
[127] Cullinane A, Weld J, Osborne M, et al. Field studies on equine influenza vaccination regimes in Thoroughbred foals and yearlings. Vet J 2001;161:174–85.
[128] Heldens JG, Hannant D, Cullinane AA, et al. Clinical and virological evaluation of the efficacy of an inactivated EHV1 and EHV4 whole virus vaccine (Duvaxyn EHV1, 4). Vaccination/challenge experiments in foals and pregnant mares. Vaccine 2001;19:4307–17.
[129] Lunn D, Hussey S, Sebring R, et al. Safety, efficacy, and immunogenicity of a modified-live equine influenza virus vaccine in ponies after induction of exercised-induced immunosuppression. J Am Vet Med Assoc 2001;218:900–6.

[130] Chambers TM, Holland RE, Tudor LR, et al. A new modified live equine influenza virus vaccine: phenotypic stability, restricted spread and efficacy against heterologous virus challenge. Equine Vet J 2001;33:630–6.

[131] Townsend HG, Penner SJ, Watts TC, et al. Efficacy of a cold-adapted, intranasal equine influenza vaccine: challenge trials. Equine Vet J 2001;33:637–43.

[132] Tang DC, DeVit M, Johnston SA. Genetic immunization is a simple method for eliciting an immune response. Nature 1992;356:152–4.

[133] Cox GJ, Zamb TJ, Babiuk LA. Bovine herpesvirus-1: immune responses in mice and cattle infected with plasmid DNA. J Virol 1993;67:5664–7.

[134] Ulmer JB, Donnelly JJ, Parker SE, et al. Heterologous protection against influenza by injection of DNA encoding a viral protein. Science 1993;259:1745–9.

[135] Babiuk LA, Pontarallo R, Babiuk S, et al. Induction of immune responses by DNA vaccines in large animals. Vaccine 2003;21:649–58.

[136] Ulmer JB, Fu TM, Deck RR, et al. Protective CD4+ and CD8+ T cells against influenza virus induced by vaccination and nucleoprotein DNA. J Virol 1993;72:5648–53.

[137] Robinson HL. DNA vaccines: basic mechanism and immune responses. Int J Mol Med 1999;4:549–55.

[138] Lewis PJ, Van Drunen Little-Van Den Hurk S, Babiuk LA. Induction of immune responses to bovine herpesvirus type 1 gD in passively immune mice after immunization with a DNA-based vaccine. J Gen Virol 1999;80:2829–37.

[139] Van Drunen Little-Van Den Hurk S, Braun RP, Lewis PJ, et al. Immunization of neonates with DNA encoding a bovine herpesvirus glycoprotein is effective in the presence of maternal antibody. Viral Immunol 1999;12:67–77.

[140] Fischer J, Barzu S, Andreoni C, et al. DNA vaccination of neonate piglets in the face of maternal immunity induces humoral memory and protection against a virulent pseudorabies virus challenge. Vaccine 2003;21:1732–41.

[141] Gerdts V, Babiuk LA, Van Drunen Little-Van Den Hurk S, et al. Fetal immunization by a DNA vaccine delivered orally into the amniotic fluid. Nat Med 2000;6:929–32.

[142] Ruitenberg KM, Walker C, Wellington JE, et al. DNA-mediated immunization with glycoprotein D of equine herpesvirus 1 (EHV-1) in a murine model of EHV-1 respiratory infection. Vaccine 1999;17:237–44.

[143] Ruitenberg KM, Love DN, Gilkerson JR, et al. Equine herpesvirus 1 (EHV-1) glycoprotein D DNA inoculation in horses with pre-existing EHV-1/EHV-4 antibody. Vet Microbiol 2000;76:117–27.

[144] Soboll G, Whalley JM, Koen MT, et al. Identification of equine herpesvirus-1 antigens recognized by cytotoxic T lymphocytes. J Gen Virol 2003;84:2625–34.

[145] Zhang Y, Smith PM, Tarbet EB, et al. Protective immunity against equine herpesvirus type-1 (EHV-1) infection in mice induced by recombinant EHV-1 gD. Virus Res 1998;56: 11–24.

[146] Galvin TA, Muller J, Khan AS. Effect of different promoters on immune responses elicited by HIV-1 gag/env multigenic DNA vaccine in *Macaca mulatta* and *Macaca nemestrina*. Vaccine 2000;18:2566–83.

[147] Lee AH, Suh YS, Sung JH, et al. Comparison of various expression plasmids for the induction of immune response by DNA immunization. Mol Cells 1997;7:495–501.

[148] Santra S, Barouch DH, Jackson SS, et al. Functional equivalency of B7-1 and B7-2 for co-stimulating plasmid DNA vaccine-elicited CTL responses. J Immunol 2000;165: 6791–5.

[149] Kim LL, Tsai A, Nottingham LK, et al. Intracellular adhesion molecule-1 modulates beta-chemokines and directly co-stimulates T cells in vivo. J Clin Invest 1999;103:869–77.

[150] Sin JI, Kim JJ, Zhang D, et al. Modulation of cellular responses by plasmid CD40L: CD40L plasmid vectors enhance antigen-specific helper T cell type 1 CD4+ T cell-mediated protective immunity against herpes simplex virus type 2 in vivo. Hum Gene Ther 2001;12: 1091–102.

[151] Larsen DL, Dybdahl-Sissoko N, McGregor MW, et al. Coadministration of DNA encoding interleukin-6 and hemagglutinin confers protection from influenza virus challenge in mice. J Virol 1998;72:1704–8.
[152] Iwasaki A, Stiernholm BJ, Chan AK, et al. Enhanced CTL responses mediated by plasmid DNA immunogens encoding co-stimulatory molecules and cytokines. J Immunol 1997;158: 4591–601.
[153] Okada E, Sasaki S, Ishii N, et al. Intranasal immunization of a DNA vaccine with IL-12 and granulocyte-macrophage colony-stimulating factor (GM-CSF)-expressing plasmids in liposomes induces strong mucosal and cell-mediated immune responses against HIV-1 antigens. J Immunol 1997;159:3638–47.
[154] Pertmer TM, Eisenbraun MD, McCabe D, et al. Gene gun-based nucleic acid immunization: elicitation of humoral and cytotoxic T-lymphocyte responses following epidermal delivery of nanogram quantities of DNA. Vaccine 1995;13:1427–30.
[155] Fynan EF, Webster RG, Fuller DH, et al. DNA vaccines: protective immunizations by parenteral, mucosal, and gene-gun inoculations. Proc Natl Acad Sci USA 1993;90:11478–82.
[156] Roz E, Carson DA, Parker SE, et al. Intradermal gene immunization: the possible role of DNA uptake in the induction of cellular immunity to viruses. Proc Natl Acad Sci USA 1994;91:9519–23.
[157] Falo LD Jr. Targeting the skin for genetic immunization. Proc Assoc Am Physicians 1999; 111:211–9.
[158] Tuting T, Storkus WJ, Falo LD Jr. DNA immunization targeting the skin: molecular control of adaptive immunity. J Invest Dermatol 1998;111:183–8.
[159] Lunn DP, Soboll G, Schram BR, et al. Antibody responses to DNA vaccination of horses using the influenza hemagglutinin gene. Vaccine 1999;17:2245–58.
[160] Soboll G, Horohov DW, Aldridge BM, et al. Regional antibody and cellular immune responses to equine influenza virus infection, and particle mediated DNA vaccination. Vet Immunol Immunopathol 2003;94:47–62.

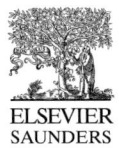

Index

Note: Page numbers of article titles are in **boldface** type.

A

Abdomen
　infections in
　　in horses, **419–436.** See also specific infection.

Abdominal abscess
　in horses, 428–432
　　complications of, 431–432
　　diagnosis of, 429–431
　　pathophysiology of, 428–429
　　prognosis of, 431–432
　　treatment of, 431

Abortion
　in horses, 530–531

Abscess(es)
　abdominal
　　in horses, 428–432. See also *Abdominal abscess, in horses.*
　perirectal
　　in horses, 419–424. See also *Perirectal abscess, in horses.*

Acyclovir
　for equine herpesvirus myeloencephalitis, 571–573

Adsorbent(s)
　in enterocolitis treatment, 467–468

AIPMMA implants. See *Antimicrobial-impregnated polymethylmethacrylate (AIPMMA) implants.*

Amikacin
　for infections of nonpregnant uterus, 532–533

Aminoglycoside(s)
　for infections of nonpregnant uterus, 532
　for septic synovitis, 371

Ampicillin
　indications for, 298

Antibacterial agents
　for infections of nonpregnant uterus, 531–534

Antibiotic(s). See *Antimicrobial agents.*

Antifungal agents
　for infections of nonpregnant uterus, 534–535
　in infectious corneal disease management, 612–613

Antigen(s)
　detection of
　　in equine herpesvirus myeloencephalitis diagnosis, 569–570

Anti-inflammatory agents
　for equine herpesvirus myeloencephalitis, 571
　in meningitis management in horses, 561–562

Anti-inflammatory drugs
　nonsteroidal (NSAIDs)
　　for septic synovitis, 372–374
　　in enterocolitis treatment, 469

Antimicrobial agents
　biodegradable antimicrobial-impregnated implants, 303–306
　collagen, 303–305
　constant rate infusion of, 306–307
　delivery methods
　　local *vs.* systemic, 284
　diarrhea due to, 291–292
　direct intra-articular injection of, 308
　for postoperative fever, 287–288
　for septic synovitis, 369–372
　　intrasynovial agents, 376–377
　　repositol agents, 378–380
　hyaluronan, 306
　hydroxyapatite, 305
　in critically ill surgical patients, 285
　in infectious corneal disease management, 611–612
　in meningitis management in horses, 557–561

Antimicrobial (continued)
    in UTI management in horses, 506–509
    indications for, 286–288, 297–299
    indwelling systems for, 306–307
    new agents, **297–322**
    nonbiodegradable antimicrobial-impregnated implants, 301–303
    perioperative use of
        duration of, 282–284
        specific agents, 284–285
    pharmacodynamics of, 300–301
    pharmacokinetics of, 300–301
    PMMA, 301–303
    polyanhydrides, 305–306
    polylactide-polyglycolide, 306
    POP, 305
    prophylactic use of, **279–296**
        indications for, 281–282
    regional perfusion of, 308–317
        clinical use of, 313–314
        described, 308–311
        distribution of perfusate after, 316
        dose considerations in, 314–315
        number of perfusions, 317
        procedure selection for, 317
        selection criteria for, 311–313
        volume of perfusate solution for, 315–316
    selection of, 297–299
    systemic
        for osteomyelitis in horses, 397–398
        in POIs prevention in horses, 328–329

Antimicrobial drug resistance, 288–291

Antimicrobial-impregnated implants
    biodegradable, 303–306
    nonbiodegradable, 301–303

Antimicrobial-impregnated polymethylmethacrylate (AIPMMA) implants
    for osteomyelitis in horses, 399–407

Antiviral agents
    in infectious corneal disease management, 613–614

Arterial blood pressure
    in enterocolitis diagnosis, 461–462

B

Bacterial nephritis
    hematogenous
        UTIs in horses and, 511–512

Biodegradable antimicrobial-impregnated implants, 303–306

Biopsy
    in female reproductive tract infection diagnosis, 525–526
    in male reproductive tract infection diagnosis, 541

Blood culture
    in meningitis diagnosis in horses, 555

Blood pressure
    arterial
        in enterocolitis diagnosis, 461–462

Bone graft
    for osteomyelitis in horses, 399

C

Cardiovascular infections
    septicemia and
        in horses, **481–495**

Catheterization
    urinary
        in UTI management in horses, 511–512

Cefepime
    in UTI management in horses, 508

Ceftiofur
    in UTI management in horses, 507–508
    indications for, 298

Cellulitis
    in horses, 352–354

CEM. See *Contagious equine metritis (CEM)*.

Central venous pressure
    in enterocolitis diagnosis, 462

Cephalosporin(s)
    for infections of nonpregnant uterus, 532
    in UTI management in horses, 507

Cerebrospinal fluid (CSF) analysis
    in equine herpesvirus myeloencephalitis diagnosis, 568
    in meningitis diagnosis in horses, 555–557

Chronic degenerative endometritis
    in horses, 529

Chronic infectious endometritis
    in horses, 529

Clostridial enterocolitis, **444–452**

diagnosis of, 444–449
treatment of, 449–452

Clostridium difficile infection
diagnosis of, 445–447
treatment of, 449–451

Clostridium perfringens infection
diagnosis of, 447–449
treatment of, 451–452

Colitis
in horses, **437–479**

Collagen, 303–305

Colloid(s)
in enterocolitis treatment, 468–469

Colloid osmotic pressure
in enterocolitis diagnosis, 462–463

Constant rate infusion
of antimicrobial agents, 306–307

Contagious equine metritis (CEM)
in females, 528–529
in males, 541–542

Corneal diseases
infectious, 608–616. See also *Infectious corneal diseases*.

Counterirritant therapy
for infections of nonpregnant uterus, 536–537

Cranberry products
in UTI management in horses, 510

CSF analysis. See *Cerebrospinal fluid (CSF) analysis*.

Curettage
for osteomyelitis in horses, 398

Cytology
in female reproductive tract infection diagnosis, 523–525
in male reproductive tract infection diagnosis, 539–540

D

Dexamethasone
in meningitis management in horses, 561–562

Diarrhea
antimicrobial-induced, 291–292

DIC. See *Disseminated intravascular coagulopathy (DIC)*.

Diffuse peritonitis
in horses, 432–433

Dimethyl sulfoxide (DMSO)
for septic synovitis, 373–374

Direct intra-articular injection
of antimicrobial agents, 308

Disseminated intravascular coagulopathy (DIC)
heparin and, 469–471

Di-tri-octahedral (DTO)–smectite
in enterocolitis treatment, 464–465

DMSO. See *Dimethyl sulfoxide (DMSO)*.

DPJ. See *Duodenitis–proximal jejunitis (DPJ)*.

Drug(s)
for septic synovitis, 382–383

Drug resistance
antimicrobial, 288–291

DTO–smectite. See *Di-tri-octahedral (DTO)–smectite*.

Duodenitis–proximal jejunitis (DPJ), 457–459

E

EDTA. See *Ethylenediaminetetraacetic acid (EDTA)*.

Electrolyte(s)
in enterocolitis diagnosis, 460–461

Empyema
guttural pouch
in horses, 603–605

Encephalitis
West Nile virus, **575–581**. See also *West Nile virus encephalitis*.

Endocarditis, 481–483

Endometritis
chronic degenerative
in horses, 529
chronic infectious
in horses, 529
in horses, 528–529
persistent breeding-induced
in horses, 529

Endoscopy
in female reproductive tract infection diagnosis, 526–527
in male reproductive tract infection diagnosis, 540–541

Enrofloxacin
for infections of nonpregnant uterus, 533

Enrofloxacin (*continued*)
　　for septic synovitis, 371–372
　　in UTI management in horses, 509
　　indications for, 299
Enteritis
　　in horses, **437–479**
　　parasitic, 455–457
Enterocolitis
　　clostridial, 444–452. See also *Clostridial enterocolitis*.
　　diagnosis of, 460–464
　　　　arterial blood pressure in, 461–462
　　　　central venous pressure in, 462
　　　　clinical assessment in, 460
　　　　colloid osmotic pressure in, 462–463
　　　　electrolytes in, 460–461
　　　　lactate in, 463–464
　　monitoring of
　　　　advances in, 459–469
　　treatment of, 464–469
　　　　adsorbents in, 467–468
　　　　colloids in, 468–469
　　　　DTO–smectite in, 464–465
　　　　immune products in, 467–468
　　　　NSAIDs in, 469
　　　　probiotics in, 465–467
Enteropathy
　　equine proliferative, 452–455. See also *Equine proliferative enteropathy (Lawsonia intracellularis)*.
Environment(s)
　　wound
　　　　in POIs in horses, 325–328
Equine herpesvirus myeloencephalitis, **567–575**
　　clinical signs of, 568
　　control of, 573–574
　　described, 567
　　diagnosis of, 568–571
　　　　antigen detection in, 569–570
　　　　CSF analysis in, 568
　　　　patient history in, 568
　　　　postmortem, 570–571
　　　　serology in, 568–569
　　management of, 571–573
　　prevention of, 573–574
　　vaccines for
　　　　research trends in, 574–575
Equine proliferative enteropathy (*Lawsonia intracellularis*), 452–455
　　diagnosis of, 452–455
　　treatment of, 455

Equine protozoal myeloencephalitis, **563–565**
Equine recurrent uveitis
　　causes of, 616–618
　　diagnosis of, 616–618
　　in horses, 616–620
　　treatment of, 618–620
Equine viral arteritis, 542
Ethylenediaminetetraacetic acid (EDTA)
　　for infections of nonpregnant uterus, 534
　　in infectious corneal disease management, 614

F

Female reproductive tract
　　infections of
　　　　in horses, **519–539**
　　　　　　abortion, 530–531
　　　　　　anatomic barriers to, 519–520
　　　　　　CEM, 528–529
　　　　　　chronic degenerative endometritis, 529
　　　　　　chronic infectious endometritis, 529
　　　　　　diagnosis of, 523–528
　　　　　　　　biopsy in, 525–526
　　　　　　　　culture in, 523
　　　　　　　　cytology in, 523–525
　　　　　　　　endoscopy in, 526–527
　　　　　　　　hormonal and peptide markers in, 527–528
　　　　　　　　ultrasonography in, 526
　　　　　　endometritis, 528
　　　　　　immunologic mechanisms in, 520–522
　　　　　　metritis, 530
　　　　　　nonpregnant uterus
　　　　　　　　treatment of, 531–537
　　　　　　persistent breeding-induced endometritis, 529
　　　　　　physical uterine clearance in, 519–520
　　　　　　placentitis, 530–531
　　　　　　pregnant uterus
　　　　　　　　treatment of, 537–539
　　　　　　STDs, 528–529
Fever
　　postoperative
　　　　antimicrobial agents for, 287–288
Fluoroquinolone(s)
　　indications for, 299

G

Gentamicin
    for infections of nonpregnant uterus, 532–533
    indications for, 298–299

Guttural pouch empyema
    in horses, 603–605
        described, 603
        diagnosis of, 603–604
        management of, 604–605

H

Head
    infections of
        in horses, **591–631**. See also specific infections.

Hematogenous bacterial nephritis
    UTIs in horses and, 511–512

Hematology
    in meningitis diagnosis in horses, 555

Heparin
    DIC and, 469–471

Herpesvirus myeloencephalitis
    equine, **567–575**. See also Equine herpesvirus myeloencephalitis.

Hoof structures
    infections of, 383–385

Hormonal and peptide markers
    in female reproductive tract infection diagnosis, 527–528

Hyaluronan, 306

Hydroxyapatite, 305

I

Idoxuridine
    in infectious corneal disease management, 613–614

Imipenem-cilastin
    for septic synovitis, 372

Immune products
    in enterocolitis treatment, 467–468

Immune system
    POIs in horses and, 324–325

Immunomodulation
    for infections of nonpregnant uterus, 536

Implant(s)
    AIPMMA
        for osteomyelitis in horses, 399–407

Implant removal
    for osteomyelitis in horses, 398

Indwelling systems
    for antimicrobial agents, 306–307

Infection(s). See also specific sites and types.
    of head
        in horses, **591–631**
    of hoof structures, 383–385
    of ocular structures
        in horses, **591–631**
    of teeth and supporting structures
        in horses, 597–603
    postoperative
        in horses
            prevention of, **323–334**. See also Postoperative infections (POIs), in horses, prevention of.

Infectious corneal diseases
    in horses, 608–616
        causes of, 608–610
        described, 608
        diagnosis of, 608–610
        treatment of, 611–616
            antifungal agents in, 612–613
            antimicrobial agents in, 611–612
            antiviral agents in, 613–614
            EDTA in, 614
            medical therapy in, 611
            MMPs in, 614
            surgical, 614–616

Infectious pulmonary diseases
    in horses
        diagnosis of
            advanced techniques in, **633–638**
            nucleic acid–based techniques in, 636–638
        prevention of, 642–643
            live-attenuated virus vaccines in, 642
            nucleic acid–based vaccines in, 642–643
        treatment of
            advanced techniques in, **638–642**

Inflammatory mediators
    in male reproductive tract infection assessment of, 541

Intracranial pressure (ICP)
    increased
        in meningitis in horses
            management of, 563

Intraosseous perfusion
    for septic synovitis, 376
Intraosseous regional perfusion
    for osteomyelitis in horses, 407–413
Intrauterine ceftiofur sodium
    for infections of nonpregnant uterus, 532
Intravenous regional perfusion
    for osteomyelitis in horses, 407–413
Itraconazole
    in infectious corneal disease management, 612–613

K

Klebsiella pneumoniae
    in horses, 542–543

L

ß-Lactam(s)
    for infections of nonpregnant uterus, 531–532
Lactate
    in enterocolitis diagnosis, 463–464
Lactobacillus spp.–containing suppositories
    in UTI management in horses, 509
Lavage
    for septic synovitis, 380–381
Lawsonia intracellularis, 452–455. See also *Equine proliferative enteropathy (Lawsonia intracellularis)*.
Live-attenuated virus vaccines
    in prevention of infectious pulmonary diseases in horses, 642–643

M

Macrolide(s)
    indications for, 298
Male reproductive tract
    in horses
        defense mechanisms of, 539
        infections of
            in horses, **539–543**
                CEM, 541–542
                diagnosis of, 539–541
                    biopsy in, 541
                    culture in, 539–540
                    cytology in, 539–540
                    endoscopy in, 540–541
                    inflammatory mediators assessment in, 541
                    ultrasonography in, 540
                equine viral arteritis, 542
                Klebsiella pneumoniae, 542–543
                Pseudomonas aeruginosa, 542–543
                treatment of, 543
Matrix metalloproteinases (MMPs)
    in infectious corneal disease management, 614
Mechanical curettage
    for infections of nonpregnant uterus, 537
Meningitis
    in horses, **553–563**
        causes of, 553–554
        diagnosis of, 554–557
            CSF analysis in, 555–557
            hematology and blood culture in, 555
            patient history in, 554–555
            physical examination in, 554–555
        increased ICP in
            management of, 563
        management of, 557–563
            anti-inflammatory agents in, 561–562
            antimicrobial agents in, 557–561
            dexamethasone in, 561–562
Metritis
    in horses, 530
MMPs. See *Matrix metalloproteinases (MMPs)*.
Mycosis
    in horses
        management of, 606–608
Myeloencephalitis
    equine herpesvirus, **567–575**. See also *Equine herpesvirus myeloencephalitis*.
    equine protozoal, 563–565
Myocarditis, 483–484
Myositis
    in horses, 354–357

N

National Research Council Operative Wound Classification, 336

Neorickettsia risticii, 441–444. See also
    Potomac horse fever (Neorickettsia risticii).
Nephritis
    bacterial
        hematogenous
            UTIs in horses and, 511–512
Nonbiodegradable antimicrobial-impregnated implants, 301–303
NSAIDs. See *Anti-inflammatory drugs, nonsteroidal (NSAIDs)*.
Nucleic acid–based techniques
    in infectious pulmonary diseases in horses, 636–638
Nucleic acid–based vaccines
    in prevention of infectious pulmonary diseases in horses, 642–643

O

Ocular structures
    in horses
        infectious corneal diseases, 608–616. See also *Infectious corneal diseases, in horses*.
    infections of
        in horses, **591–631**. See also specific infections.
Osteomyelitis
    defined, 389–390
    in horses, **389–417**
        clinical findings in, 393–397
        described, 389–390
        diagnosis of, 393–397
        organisms associated with, 391–392
        treatment of, 397–413
            AIPMMA implants in, 399–407
            bone graft in, 399
            curettage in, 398
            implant removal in, 398
            innovative treatments, 399–407
            intravenous and intraosseous regional limb perfusion in, 407–413
            PMMA in, 400–407
            POP in, 405–406
            systemic antimicrobial agents in, 397–398
            traditional treatments, 397–399
        pathophysiology of, 390–391

P

Paranasal sinusitis
    in horses, **592–597**
        described, 592
        diagnosis of, 592–595
        management of, 595–597
Parasitic enteritis, 455–457
Pelvis
    infections in
        in horses, **419–436**. See also specific infection.
Penicillin(s)
    in UTI management in horses, 507
    indications for, 298
Peptide markers
    in female reproductive tract infection diagnosis, 527–528
Perfusion
    intraosseous
        for septic synovitis, 376
    regional
        for septic synovitis, 374–376
Pericarditis, 484–486
Perirectal abscess
    in horses, **419–436**
        complications of, 423–424
        described, 419
        diagnosis of, 420–421
        pathophysiology of, 419–420
        prognosis of, 423–424
        treatment of, 422–423
Peritonitis
    diffuse
        in horses, 432–433
    in horses, 428
Persistent breeding-induced endometritis
    in horses, 529
Physical therapy
    for septic synovitis, 382
Placentitis
    in horses, 530–531
Plaster of Paris (POP), 305
    for osteomyelitis in horses, 405–406
PMMA. See *Polymethylmethacrylate (PMMA)*.
POIs. See *Postoperative infections (POIs)*.
Polyanhydride(s), 305–306
Polyene(s)
    in infectious corneal disease management, 612

Polymethylmethacrylate (PMMA), 301–303
  for osteomyelitis in horses, 400–407
POP. See *Plaster of Paris (POP)*.
Postoperative fever
  antimicrobial agents for, 287–288
Postoperative infections (POIs)
  described, 323
  in horses
    immune system of host and, 324–325
    patient factors in, 324–325
    prevention of, **323–334**
      surgical procedure in, 329–332
      systemic antimicrobial agents in, 328–329
      wound environment and, 325–328
Potomac horse fever *(Neorickettsia risticii)*, 441–444
  diagnosis of, 441–443
  treatment of, 443–444
Probiotic(s)
  in enterocolitis treatment, 465–467
Pseudomonas aeruginosa
  in horses, 542–543

R

Regional perfusion
  for septic synovitis, 374–376
  intravenous and intraosseous
    for osteomyelitis in horses, 407–413
  of antimicrobial agents, 308–317. See also *Antimicrobial agents, regional perfusion of*.
Rehabilitation
  for septic synovitis, 382–383
Repositol antimicrobial agents
  for septic synovitis, 378–380
Reproductive tract infections
  in horses, **519–552**
    female-related, **519–539**. See also *Female reproductive tract, infections of, in horses*.
    male-related, **539–543**. See also *Male reproductive tract, infections of, in horses*.

S

Salmonellosis, 438–441
  diagnosis of, 438–440
  treatment of, 440–441

Septacin, 305–306
Septic synovitis, **363–388**
  diagnosis of, 364–369
  pathogenesis of, 363–364
  treatment of, 369–381
    aminoglycosides in, 371
    antimicrobial agents in, 369–372
      intrasynovial, 376–377
    DMSO in, 373–374
    enrofloxacin in, 371–372
    imipenem-cilastin in, 372
    intraosseous perfusion in, 376
    lavage in, 380–381
    NSAIDs in, 372–374
    pharmaceutical, 382–383
    physical therapy in, 382
    regional perfusion in, 374–376
    rehabilitation in, 382–383
Septicemia, 489–491
Serology
  in equine herpesvirus myeloencephalitis diagnosis, 568–569
Sexually transmitted diseases (STDs)
  in horses, 528–529
Sinusitis
  paranasal
    in horses, 592–597. See also *Paranasal sinusitis, in horses*.
STDs. See *Sexually transmitted diseases (STDs)*.
Sulfonamide(s)
  for infections of nonpregnant uterus, 534
Suppositories
  Lactobacillus spp.–containing
    in UTI management in horses, 509
Surgical wound infections
  in horses, **335–361**
    diagnosis of, 339–340
    pathophysiology of, 336–339
    treatment of, 339–340
Synovitis
  septic, **363–388**. See also *Septic synovitis*.
Systemic antimicrobial agents
  for osteomyelitis in horses, 397–398
Systemic diseases
  ocular manifestations of
    in horses, 620

T

Teeth
  infection of
    in horses, 597–603
      described, 597
      diagnosis of, 597–601
      management of, 601–603

Tenosynovitis, **363–388**

Tetracycline(s)
  for infections of nonpregnant uterus, 534

Traumatic wound infection
  in horses, 340

Trifluridine
  in infectious corneal disease management, 613–614

Trimethoprim-sulfonamides
  in UTI management in horses, 507

U

Ultrasonography
  in female reproductive tract infection diagnosis, 526
  in male reproductive tract infection diagnosis, 540

Umbilical remnant infections
  described, 424
  in horses, 424–428
    complications of, 428
    diagnosis of, 426–427
    pathophysiology of, 424–425
    prognosis of, 428
    treatment of, 427–428

Urinary catheterization
  in UTI management in horses, 511–512

Urinary tract infections (UTIs)
  in horses, **497–517**
    causes of, 502–503
    described, 497–498
    diagnosis of, 503–506
    hematogenous bacterial nephritis and, 511–512
    host-agent interactions in, 498–502
    management of, 506–510
      antimicrobial agents in, 506–509
      cranberry products in, 510
      Lactobacillus spp.-containing suppositories in, 509
      special considerations in, 510–512
    urinary catheterization in, 511–512
    vaccinations in, 510
    populations for, 506

Uterotonic(s)
  for infections of nonpregnant uterus, 535–536

Uterus
  nonpregnant
    infections of
      treatment of
        antibacterial agents in, 531–534
        antifungal agents in, 534–535
        counterirritant therapy in, 536–537
        immunomodulation in, 536
        mechanical curettage in, 537
        uterotonics in, 535–536
  pregnant
    infections of
      treatment of, 537–539

UTIs. See *Urinary tract infections (UTIs)*.

Uveitis
  equine recurrent, 616–620. See also *Equine recurrent uveitis*.

V

Vaccination(s)
  in UTI management in horses, 510

Vaccine(s)
  for equine herpesvirus myeloencephalitis
    research trends in, 574–575
  in prevention of infectious pulmonary diseases in horses, 642–643

Vasculitis, 486–489

W

West Nile virus encephalitis, **575–581**
  described, 575–576
  diagnosis of, 576–577
  prevention of, 579–581
  treatment of, 578–579

Wound environment
  in POIs in horses, 325–328

Wound evaluation
  in horses, 343–351

Wound healing
 in horses, 341–343

Wound infections
 in horses, **335–361**
  cellulitis, 352–354
  evaluation of, 343–351
  healing of, 341–343
  myositis, 354–357
 surgical
  in horses, **335–361.** See also
   *Surgical wound infections, in
   horses.*
 traumatic
  in horses, 340

Moving?

Make sure your subscription moves with you!

To notify us of your new address, find your **Clinics Account Number** (located on your mailing label above your name), and contact customer service at:

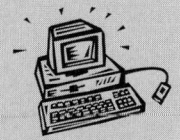

E-mail: elspcs@elsevier.com

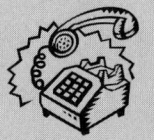

800-654-2452 (subscribers in the U.S. & Canada)
407-345-4000 (subscribers outside of the U.S. & Canada)

Fax number: 407-363-9661

Elsevier Periodicals Customer Service
6277 Sea Harbor Drive
Orlando, FL 32887-4800

*To ensure uninterrupted delivery of your subscription, please notify us at least 4 weeks in advance of move.

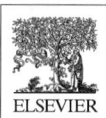